Precision in CT Imaging for Personalized Implants and Surgical Planning

Soobia Saeed
Taylor's University, Malaysia

Mohsin Qadeer
National Medical Center, Pakistan

IGI Global Scientific Publishing
Publishing Tomorrow's Research Today

Vice President of Editorial	Melissa Wagner
Director of Acquisitions	Mikaela Felty
Director of Book Development	Jocelynn Hessler
Production Manager	Mike Brehm
Cover Design	Jose Rosado

Published in the United States of America by
IGI Global Scientific Publishing
701 East Chocolate Avenue
Hershey, PA, 17033, USA
Tel: 717-533-8845
Fax: 717-533-7115
Website: https://www.igi-global.com E-mail: cust@igi-global.com

Library of Congress Cataloging-in-Publication Data

Names: Saeed, Soobia, 1987- editor | Qadeer, Mohsin, 1981- editor
Title: Precision in CT imaging for personalized implants and surgical planning / edited by Soobia Saeed, Mohsin Qadeer.
Description: Hershey, PA : IGI Global Scientific Publishing, [2026] | Includes bibliographical references and index. | Summary: "This book plans to general framework for implementing imaging protocols into effective personalized healthcare solutions"-- Provided by publisher.
Identifiers: LCCN 2025018920 (print) | LCCN 2025018921 (ebook) | ISBN 9798337328072 h/c | ISBN 9798337328089 s/c | ISBN 9798337328096 ebook
Subjects: LCSH: Tomography | Surgery--Planning | Implants, Artificial | Precision medicine | Artificial intelligence--Medical applications
Classification: LCC RC78.7.T6 P74 2026 (print) | LCC RC78.7.T6 (ebook)
LC record available at https://lccn.loc.gov/2025018920
LC ebook record available at https://lccn.loc.gov/2025018921

British Cataloguing in Publication Data
A Cataloguing in Publication record for this book is available from the British Library.

Editors dedicated this book to their respective Families and colleagues

Editorial Advisory Board

Table of Contents

Detailed Table of Contents

The use of autologous platelet-rich plasma (PRP) and adipose-derived stem cells (ADSC) has shown therapeutic effectiveness in various conditions such as diabetic ulcers, ocular infections, cataract surgery, and dermatological disorders. This case report presents a novel approach to the treatment of cervical spinal cord injury by combining artificial intelligence (AI) with PRP and ADSC therapy. In total, the patient received two treatment sessions of PRP and ADSC therapy lasting 15 days each, while an AI – based gait, posture and deep tendon reflexes assessments were conducted before and after treatment. At baseline, hyperreflexia was noted, the patient could not stand unaided or hold himself upright; the first therapy session did not elicit any changes.

Intracranial aneurysms are a significant neurosurgical issue in low- to middle-income countries. This study evaluates a CT-based anatomical mapping system for enhancing surgical accuracy in cerebral aneurysm treatment. In a retrospective analysis of 82 patients operated in Karachi, Pakistan, at a tertiary care center. The female predominance of(65.9%) and high prevalence of hypertension (82.9%) were identified as major risk factors. All patients had acute hemorrhage and headache. CT scan enabled precise localization of aneurysms and showed statistically significant correlations between Glasgow Coma Scale (GCS) scores and locations of aneurysms ($p = 0.029$), and between seizure types and locations of aneurysms ($p = 0.003$).

Cerebral infarction was also strongly correlated with the need for decompressive surgery (p < 0.001).

Managing intracranial aneurysms is a tightrope balancing act for any neurosurgeon, especially in low- and middle- income countries where lack of resources threatens an optimal care. A retrospective study was carried out to observe how a CT-based anatomical mapping system influenced the diagnostic accuracy and surgical precision in managing cerebral aneurysms at a tertiary care center in Karachi, Pakistan. Analyzing data from 82 patients showed a female preponderance (65.9%) and a high incidence of hypertension in relation to risk factors (82.9%). All patients presented with acute hemorrhage and headache. CT localized the aneurysms with precision and yielded statistically significant correlations between GCS and aneurysm sites (p = 0.029) and between types of seizures and aneurysm locations (p = 0.003). Cerebral infarction highly correlated with decompressive surgery (p < 0.001). These findings further elaborate how the state-of-the-art CT-based anatomical mapping allows for early diagnosis, risk stratification, and targeted surgical intervention.

Traumatic Brain Injury (TBI) is a significant morbidity and mortality cause worldwide, and post-traumatic seizures (PTS) are a common and severe complication. TBI can be followed by early (within seven days of injury) or late-onset (beyond seven days) seizures, both of which are linked to neurological deterioration and poor patient prognosis. The Brain Trauma Foundation recommends anticonvulsants for the prophylaxis of early seizures. Its high bioavailability and low drug interactions were responsible for increased tolerability and long-term efficacy. Brivaracetam is a desirable choice for early seizure prophylaxis in TBI patients with greater efficacy and fewer adverse effects compared to traditional anticonvulsants. More large-scale randomized controlled trials are necessary to validate these findings and establish Brivaracetam as a standard of care in post-traumatic seizure management.

Aneurysmal subarachnoid hemorrhage (aSAH) outcomes depend on demographic, clinical, and imaging features, as demonstrated through examination of an 82-patient series. Demographically, the series' mean age was 49.7 years (range: 30–70) with a female predominance (65.8%). Clinically, there were lower Glasgow Coma Scale (GCS) scores (mean: 13.3) and increased Hunt and Hess grades (mean: 1.87, range: 1–3), while hydrocephalus requiring intervention was encountered in 6.1% of cases. Imaging predictors were an overall CT-confirmed subarachnoid hemorrhage, 18.3% of which developed cerebral infarction and 6.2% required ventricular-peritoneal shunting. Large interventions such as surgical clipping (100% of patients) and external ventricular drainage (8.5% use) were associated with management outcomes. Despite limited by the fineness of outcome information, this assessment delineates the prognostically significant contribution of acute clinical state (GCS, Hunt and Hess grade) and secondary complication (infarction, hydrocephalus) in a SAH.

The quality of life of every patient suffering from Parkinson's disease is significantly hindered by tremors, muscle rigidity, and other symptoms of general backed-up stages of the disorder. Early detection in some instances has improved treatment, leading to higher quality of living. This study aims to devise a predictive model utilizing biomedical voice data to allow for early diagnosis of Parkinson's disease. By studying voice signals and extracting crucial features from them, the model will seek to discover factors that can be traced to the disease. Findings from this study would aid in initiating early and necessary interventions towards furthering treatment and provide insights into the role of voice-based biomarkers for the diagnosis of other neurological diseases.

The integration of intraoperative CT and AR exemplifies major leaps toward ever-increasing surgical precision and safety in the neurosurgical setting. This systematic literature review synthesized results from articles published between 2015 and 2025 concerning the clinical and educational implications of AR combined with iCT in neurosurgical operations. Data have been extracted from 25 articles selected according to strict inclusion criteria pointing toward PRISMA guidelines. Results show that AR-iCT systems considerably promote surgical accuracy, reduce operative time by a median of 19%, lower intraoperative complication percentages, and provide better visualization with real-time 3D overlays. On the other hand, it fosters neurosurgical education by improving spatial cognition and procedural planning. Despite these promising results, the system's high latency, registration errors, costs, and lack of a cross-platform standard remain problematic.

Traumatic Brain Injury, commonly referred to as TBI, is an important issue that concerns worldwide health; it generates permanent disabilities or death, depending on its severity and treatment delay. In any case, early diagnosis and accurate diagnosis are vital for an intervention outcome. This research project, BrainView AI, is an ML-based solution to classify TBI from brain CT scans as an adjunct to fast-tracking clinical decision-making. The Mixed ML approach utilized Support Vector Machines, K-means Clustering, as well as Convolutional Neural Networks to ensure flexible and performant classification methods. The TBI research project is that the researchers also develop UI and user acceptance testing of their web-based prototype with complete stack operating in full functional mode covering backend logic, user-friendly front-end interface, and orderly manage data system.

Computed tomography (CT) imaging has become a vital instrument in personalized medicine, allowing accurate diagnosis, customized treatment planning, and enhanced patient outcomes. New developments in AI, radiomics, and 3D imaging have further maximized its use in different medical fields, ranging from oncology and cardiology to neurology and orthopedics. With advancing technology, the integration of CT imaging with personalized medicine will become more sophisticated, enhancing clinical decision-making and healthcare delivery. With the resolution of current challenges and exploration of future innovations, CT imaging will remain a cornerstone of modern personalized healthcare. Raw patient data employed in this research was sourced from Jinnah Medical and Dental College and approved by the Sohail Trust Hospital Ethical Review Board. The dataset is made up of de-identified patient data that includes CT imaging to enable comprehensive insight into the use of CT imaging in personalized medicine, including oncology, cardiology, neurology, and orthopedic diseases.

Intracranial hemorrhage (ICH) is a critical condition requiring timely and accurate diagnosis, especially in craniocerebral trauma. This chapter presents two deep learning-based models for classifying ICH in CT images. The first employs a convolutional neural network (CNN) for spatial feature extraction and classification via SoftMax or Sigmoid layers. The second proposes a hybrid approach, combining an autoencoder for unsupervised feature extraction with a gradient boosting machine (GBM) for classification. The autoencoder compresses image data to extract essential features, which are classified by GBM through ensemble learning. This chapter outlines the models' design, data preprocessing, training strategies, and evaluation metrics. The aim is to enhance classification accuracy through CNN-based spatial-temporal modeling and efficient feature extraction via autoencoder-GBM. The chapter also explores the hybrid model's potential to outperform traditional CNNs and its feasibility in clinical use.

The combination of high-end Computed Tomography (CT) imaging and Artificial Intelligence (AI) is revolutionizing surgical accuracy and individualized treatment planning. This chapter discusses how such technological innovations improve diagnostic confidence, refine surgical planning, and maximize patient outcomes. The development of CT imaging, from initial uses through high-definition and dual-energy imaging, has led to extremely refined anatomical renderings. Paired with AI-driven analysis and predictive modeling, these innovations enable real-time decision-making, individualized surgical intervention, and improved post-operative rehabilitation planning. Further, the application of augmented reality (AR) and virtual reality (VR) for surgical planning introduces new dimensions of preoperative visualization and intraoperative navigation. Despite these advances, constraints related to radiation exposure, economic feasibility, regulatory limitations, and the need for specialized training persist.

Traumatic Brain Injury (TBI) significantly increases the risk of post-traumatic seizures (PTS), and their long-term implications on neurological health and quality of life. While global evidence shows a seizure incidence of 10–25% following moderate to severe TBI, regional evidence from Pakistan, particularly from tertiary care institutions, is sparse. In order to determine the incidence and patterns of seizures in head-injured patients presented to a tertiary care facility in Pakistan, with implications for their early diagnosis and management. A descriptive cross-sectional study was conducted at the Neurosurgical Ward of Abbasi Shaheed Hospital and Karachi Medical and Dental College, Karachi, Pakistan, for a duration of six months. A sample of 140 patients aged 1–60 years with established head injuries was assessed for the occurrence of seizures, type of seizure, and timing (immediate, early, or late). Clinical assessment was supplemented with radiological investigations (CT, MRI) and follow-up of patients.

The merger of 3D printing and additive manufacturing with surgical practice has almost revolutionized personalized medicine. This review searches how these new technologies allow surgical procedures to be executed with greater precision with patient-specific anatomical models, implants, and bioprinted tissues generated by these technologies. The process of translating medical imaging into physical models allows realizing more accurate preoperative planning, intraoperative guidance, and patient outcomes in disciplines including neurosurgery, orthopedics, and maxillofacial surgery. The combination of AI and point of care manufacturing with 3D printing is also facilitating real-time design and rapid prototyping in hospital environments. That said, clinical adoption is still hindered by expense, regulatory bottlenecks, material and standardization concerns. Emerging applications for bioprinting and smart implants are also forthrightly discussed, hinting at a future where surgical interventions will be tailored but also anticipatory and responsive.

Foreword

With the resurgence of precision and customization in patientcare, CT imaging remains one of the most transformative options to transition from a diagnostic tool to that of a personalized surgical plan and implant design. This book has come at a moment of revolution when AI, 3-D printing, and personalized treatment protocols are setting new standards for surgical outcomes. By covering the optimization of CT parameters such as voxel size, slice thickness, matrix resolution, and reconstruction algorithms, it helps the clinician, biomedical engineer, and the researcher-some three key players in manipulation-based interventions-to break all limitations so far in the field of accuracy.

What makes this book particularly impactful is its emphasis on real-world clinical applications, including neurosurgery and orthopedics. The thoughtful combination of foundational knowledge, advanced image processing techniques, and case-based insights offers a holistic guide for both seasoned professionals and emerging scholars. Moreover, its exploration of AI-driven analysis and additive manufacturing underscores the interdisciplinary synergy that is shaping the future of personalized medicine.

I would like to congratulate Dr. Mohsin Qadeer and Dr. Soobia Saeed on their vision, determination, and willingness to work hard to assemble contributors from around the world for this important work.

The work of the editors guarantees that this book will be a thorough academic resource as well as a pragmatic guide to foster precision in clinical practice. As the field of medicine shifts towards more individualized, data-driven care, readers of this volume will find the contributions valuable for their purposes aimed towards innovation and precision in the hopes of better patient outcomes.

Zeelaf Shahid
Jinnah Medical and Dental College (JMDC), Pakistan

Preface

The field of medical imaging has experienced rapid advancements over the past decade, with computed tomography (CT) emerging as a cornerstone in both diagnostic and interventional medicine. As the demand for personalized and patient-centered care increases, the precision of CT imaging plays an increasingly vital role in improving surgical outcomes, enabling the development of customized implants, and advancing clinical decision-making.

Precision in CT Imaging: A Guide to Optimizing Scans for Personalized Implants and Surgical Planning was conceived to address the growing need for a comprehensive resource that bridges technical innovations with practical clinical applications. This book presents an in-depth exploration of CT imaging optimization, highlighting critical parameters such as matrix size, voxel resolution, slice thickness, and reconstruction algorithms that directly influence diagnostic accuracy and preoperative planning.

This volume also brings together interdisciplinary knowledge in image processing, artificial intelligence, and additive manufacturing, showcasing how these technologies are revolutionizing surgical planning and patient-specific treatments. Real-world clinical applications, including neurosurgery and orthopedics, are featured to demonstrate the practical value of optimized CT imaging protocols in enhancing patient outcomes.

Through this collaborative effort, we aim to provide a valuable reference for radiologists, surgeons, biomedical engineers, and researchers alike. The book is intended to serve not only as an academic resource but also as a practical guide to inform imaging protocols, surgical workflows, and the future integration of AI-driven technologies in medical imaging.

We extend our sincere gratitude to the contributors who shared their expertise and to the global research community for its continued pursuit of excellence in medical imaging.

THE ORGANIZATION OF THE BOOK

Chapter 1: Advancements in CT Imaging for Personalized Implants and Surgical Planning: A Stem Cell Therapy Perspective

Rubina Ghani

The use of autologous platelet-rich plasma (PRP) and adipose-derived stem cells (ADSC) has shown therapeutic effectiveness in various conditions such as diabetic ulcers, ocular infections, cataract surgery, and dermatological disorders. This case report presents a novel approach to the treatment of cervical spinal cord injury by combining artificial intelligence (AI) with PRP and ADSC therapy. In total, the patient received two treatment sessions of PRP and ADSC therapy lasting 15 days each, while an AI – based gait, posture and deep tendon reflexes assessments were conducted before and after treatment. At baseline, hyperreflexia was noted, the patient could not stand unaided or hold himself upright; the first therapy session did not elicit any changes. Still, at reassessment after the second session, the patient demonstrated remarkable improvement in lower limb control and was able to sustain an upright position without any help. The patient's inability to walk progressively improved, to the point where she was able to ambulate independently. The results provide support for the use of PRP and ADSC therapy in spinal cord injuries, thus justifying the conduction of randomized clinical trials to evaluate the treatment modality and the application of AI in treatment response assessing.

Chapter 2: Anatomical Mapping of Intracranial Aneurysms: A CT-Based Framework for Precision Neurosurgery

Amanullah Khan, Mohsin Qadeer, Salman Shareef

Intracranial aneurysms are a significant neurosurgical issue in low- to middle-income countries. This study evaluates the use of a CT-based anatomical mapping system for enhancing surgical accuracy in cerebral aneurysm treatment. In a retrospective analysis of 82 patients operated on at a Karachi, Pakistan, tertiary care center, female predominance (65.9%) and high prevalence of hypertension (82.9%) were identified as major risk factors. All patients had acute hemorrhage and headache. CT scan enabled precise localization of aneurysms and showed statistically significant correlations between Glasgow Coma Scale (GCS) scores and locations of aneurysms ($p = 0.029$), and between seizure types and locations of aneurysms ($p = 0.003$). Cerebral infarction was also strongly correlated with the need for decompressive surgery ($p < 0.001$). These findings show the value of CT-based anatomic mapping in facilitating early diagnosis, risk stratification, and targeted surgical intervention—an evidence-based approach to improving neurosurgical outcomes in resource-constrained settings.

Chapter 3: Clinical Management of Intracranial Aneurysms: Enhancing Diagnostic Accuracy and Surgical Precision

Amanullah Khan, Salman Shareef, Mehak Hafiz

Managing intracranial aneurysms is a tightrope balancing act for any neurosurgeon, especially in low- and middle- income countries where lack of resources threatens an optimal care. A retrospective study was carried out to observe how a CT-based anatomical mapping system influenced the diagnostic accuracy and surgical precision in managing cerebral aneurysms at a tertiary care center in Karachi, Pakistan. Analyzing data from 82 patients showed a female preponderance (65.9%) and a high incidence of hypertension in relation to risk factors (82.9%). All patients presented with acute hemorrhage and headache. CT localized the aneurysms with precision and yielded statistically significant correlations between GCS and aneurysm sites ($p = 0.029$) and between types of seizures and aneurysm locations ($p = 0.003$). Cerebral infarction highly correlated with decompressive surgery ($p < 0.001$). These findings further elaborate how the state-of-the-art CT-based anatomical mapping allows for early diagnosis, risk stratification, and targeted surgical intervention. The incorporation of contemporary imaging modalities, multidisciplinary care, and established protocols is certainly an avenue of hope for better neurosurgical outcomes in resource-deficient areas.

Chapter 4: CT Imaging in Neurosurgical Interventions: Optimizing Seizure Management and Surgical Planning for Traumatic Brain Injury

Soobia Saeed, Mohsin Qadeer

Traumatic Brain Injury (TBI) is a significant morbidity and mortality cause worldwide, and post-traumatic seizures (PTS) are a common and severe complication. TBI can be followed by early (within seven days of injury) or late-onset (beyond seven days) seizures, both of which are linked to neurological deterioration and poor patient prognosis. The Brain Trauma Foundation recommends anticonvulsants for the prophylaxis of early seizures; however, traditional medications such as phenytoin and carbamazepine have limitations, including narrow therapeutic windows and adverse effects. Brivaracetam (BRV), a novel antiepileptic, has demonstrated efficacy and safety in a variety of seizure types. The study contrasts the efficacy of Brivaracetam in the prophylaxis of post-traumatic seizures in TBI patients with the effectiveness of traditional anticonvulsants such as phenytoin and levetiracetam. A cohort study was conducted at Medicare Cardiac and General Hospital, Karachi, between September 2023 and December 2024. Patients who met Brain Trauma Foundation criteria for seizure prophylaxis were administered IV phenytoin as a loading dose, then enteral Brivaracetam (100 mg/kg/dose, three times daily). A comparison was made with a historical cohort that had been administered levetiracetam. Seizure occurrence, Glasgow Coma Scale (GCS) scores, neurobehavioral symptom inventory (NSI), and EEG reports were compared at 7, 14, and 30 days. Statistical analysis included Mann-Whitney U tests and correlation regression analysis, and p-values <0.05 were considered significant. Brivaracetam had a statistically significant decrease in the incidence of early post-traumatic seizures when compared to levetiracetam and phenytoin (p=0.02). Seizure control was found to be improved, with less loss of consciousness and better functional outcomes in patients treated with Brivaracetam. Its high bioavailability and low drug interactions were responsible for increased tolerability and long-term efficacy. Brivaracetam is a desirable choice for early seizure prophylaxis in TBI patients with greater efficacy and fewer adverse effects compared to traditional anticonvulsants. More large-scale randomized controlled trials are necessary to validate these findings and establish Brivaracetam as a standard of care in post-traumatic seizure management.

Chapter 5: Demographic, Clinical, and Imaging Predictors of Outcome in Aneurysmal Subarachnoid Hemorrhage

Amanullah Khan, Salman Shareef

Aneurysmal subarachnoid hemorrhage (aSAH) outcomes depend on demographic, clinical, and imaging features, as demonstrated through examination of an 82-patient series. Demographically, the series' mean age was 49.7 years (range: 30–70) with a female predominance (65.8%). Clinically, there were lower Glasgow Coma Scale (GCS) scores (mean: 13.3) and increased Hunt and Hess grades (mean: 1.87, range: 1–3), while hydrocephalus requiring intervention was encountered in 6.1% of cases. Imaging predictors were an overall CT-confirmed subarachnoid hemorrhage, 18.3% of which developed cerebral infarction and 6.2% required ventricular-peritoneal shunting. Large interventions such as surgical clipping (100% of patients) and external ventricular drainage (8.5% use) were associated with management outcomes. Despite limited by the fineness of outcome information, this assessment delineates the prognostically significant contribution of acute clinical state (GCS, Hunt and Hess grade) and secondary complication (infarction, hydrocephalus) in a SAH. Such findings are concordant with traditional outcome predictive schemes but point to the critical role of prompt imaging and early clinical stratification.

Chapter 6: Early Detection of Parkinson's Disease for Developing a Predictive Model Using Biomedical Voice Data: Developing a Predictive Model Using Biomedical Voice Data

Muhammad Zubair, Bushra Khalid

The quality of life of every patient suffering from Parkinson's disease is significantly hindered by tremors, muscle rigidity, and other symptoms of general backed-up stages of the disorder. Early detection in some instances has improved treatment, leading to higher quality of living. This study aims to devise a predictive model utilizing biomedical voice data to allow for early diagnosis of Parkinson's disease. By studying voice signals and extracting crucial features from them, the model will seek to discover factors that can be traced to the disease. Findings from this study would aid in initiating early and necessary interventions towards furthering treatment and provide insights into the role of voice-based biomarkers for the diagnosis of other neurological diseases.

Chapter 7: Enhancing Neurosurgical Precision Integration of Intraoperative CT and Augmented Reality Systematic Literature Review

Bilal Ashraf

The integration of intraoperative CT and AR exemplifies major leaps toward ever-increasing surgical precision and safety in the neurosurgical setting. This systematic literature review synthesized results from articles published between 2015 and 2025 concerning the clinical and educational implications of AR combined with iCT in neurosurgical operations. Data has been extracted from 25 articles selected according to strict inclusion criteria pointing toward PRISMA guidelines. Results show that AR-iCT systems considerably promote surgical accuracy, reduce operative time by a median of 19%, lower intraoperative complication percentages, and provide better visualization with real-time 3D overlays. On the other hand, it fosters neurosurgical education by improving spatial cognition and procedural planning. Despite these promising results, the system's high latency, registration errors, costs, and lack of a cross-platform standard remain problematic. This review underpins the strong potential of an AR-iCT fusion to revolutionize neurosurgical workflows while emphasizing the greatest needs for multidimensional clinical validation and improved technical interoperability. As this technology matures, integration with AI could offer even more precision and personalization to future neurosurgical interventions.

Chapter 8: Hybrid Machine Learning Model for Classifying Traumatic Brain Injury (TBI): CT Scan Analysis

Sabrina Tang, Ashley Teong Ling Kuan, Lee Yee Jeen, Tia'a Faang Der, Harrel Xu Hao Yang

Traumatic Brain Injury, commonly referred to as TBI, is an important issue that concerns worldwide health; it generates permanent disabilities or death, depending on its severity and treatment delay. In any case, early diagnosis and accurate diagnosis are vital for an intervention outcome. This research project, BrainView AI, is an ML-based solution to classify TBI from brain CT scans as an adjunct to fast-tracking clinical decision-making. The Mixed ML approach utilized Support Vector Machines, K-means Clustering, as well as Convolutional Neural Networks to ensure flexible and performant classification methods. The TBI research project is that the researchers also develop UI and user acceptance testing of their web-based prototype with complete stack operating in full functional mode covering backend logic, user-friendly front-end interface, and orderly manage data system. This web platform is implemented with essential security means to ensure sensitive medical records' privacy. BrainView AI should hence act as a proof of concept for real-world diagnostic purpose gear supporting the medical personnel in making timely and trustworthy diagnostics that will help them in making critical decisions. Thus, this interdisciplinary research project emphasizes that artificial intelligence and software development translate into healthcare, where such scalable, flexible, and cost-friendly technologies will improve patient outcomes in emergency medical settings.

Chapter 9: Introduction to CT Imaging for Personalized Medicine and Its Impact on Patients'

Zeelaf Shahid, Rubina Ghani

Computed tomography (CT) imaging has become a vital instrument in personalized medicine, allowing accurate diagnosis, customized treatment planning, and enhanced patient outcomes. New developments in AI, radiomics, and 3D imaging have further maximized its use in different medical fields, ranging from oncology and cardiology to neurology and orthopedics. With advancing technology, the integration of CT imaging with personalized medicine will become more sophisticated, enhancing clinical decision-making and healthcare delivery. With the resolution of current challenges and exploration of future innovations, CT imaging will remain a cornerstone of modern personalized healthcare. Raw patient data employed in this research was sourced from Jinnah Medical and Dental College and approved by the Sohail Trust Hospital Ethical Review Board. The dataset is made up of de-identified patient data that includes CT imaging scans, clinical history, and treatment outcomes gathered meticulously to enable comprehensive insight into the use of CT imaging in personalized medicine, which includes a wide variety of conditions, including oncology, cardiology, neurology, and orthopedic diseases.

Chapter 10: Optimized Feature Extraction and Spatial-Temporal Analysis for Accurate Intracranial Hemorrhage Classification

Yanxu, Soobia Saeed

Intracranial hemorrhage (Intracranial Hemorrhage, ICH) is a 1 critical medical condition, especially in cases of craniocerebral trauma, and timely and accurate diagnosis is essential to improve patient outcomes. This paper presents two deep learning-based models for the classification of intracranial hemorrhage from CT images. The first model uses a traditional convolutional neural network (CNN) architecture with multiple convolutional layers, pooling layers, and fully connected layers, focusing on spatial feature extraction and final classification by SoftMax or Sigmoid layers to determine whether there is bleeding. The second method introduces a hybrid model based on an autoencoder (Autoencoder) for unsupervised feature extraction, combined with a gradient hoist (GBM) for classification. The autoencoder compresses the high-dimensional CT image into a low-dimensional potential space to capture important image features, which are then input into the GBM, and through an iterative ensemble learning process, the image is classified into bleeding or non-bleeding categories. This paper introduces the design and implementation of these two models in detail, including data preprocessing, model architecture, training and testing strategies and their evaluation indicators. The purpose of this study is to develop a hybrid model combining CNN for spatial and time series modeling, as well as an efficient feature extraction model based on autoencoder, aiming to improve the accuracy of intracranial hemorrhage classification. The study also explores the potential for improved classification efficiency by combining autoencoder and GBM over traditional CNN methods. Future work will verify the performance of these two models in classification performance through experiments and further evaluate their feasibility in practical clinical applications.

Chapter 11: Radiological Assessment of Bilateral Occipital Lesions with Vasogenic Edema: A Meta Analysis

Waqas Mughis Rajpoot, Muhammad Adil Khatri

This meta-analysis combines radiological and clinical information from 200 cases of seizure and unconsciousness patients, all of whom presented with bilateral occipital lesions with vasogenic edema on neuroimaging. The aim was to identify consistent diagnostic features indicative of metastatic brain disease and assess the role of multimodal imaging and multidisciplinary management in diagnosis and treatment. Data were derived from non-contrast CT, which consistently demonstrated ill-defined hyperdense lesions in the bilateral occipital lobes with extensive vasogenic edema extending to the frontoparietal, temporal, and occipital regions. Contrast-enhanced MRI imaging, DWI, and perfusion imaging were then performed to further delineate lesion vascularity and cellularity. Systemic diagnostic evaluation entailed PET-CT and histopathological correlation on CSF examination and stereotactic biopsy. 63% of lesions proved to be hypervascular on perfusion MRI, 91% exhibited correlation between DWI and histopathology, and PET-CT identified primary malignancies in 82% of cases—the majority being lung cancer (56%). The right cerebral hemisphere was affected more frequently with common occurrences like mass effect, midline shift, and lateral ventricle compression. Neither acute hemorrhage nor fracture occurred in any case. The aggregate data highlights the prognostic significance of high-field neuroimaging and confirms the working hypothesis that bilateral occipital lesions with vasogenic edema are consistent predictors of metastatic intracranial disease. Early recognition by CT and MRI, augmented by complete systemic evaluation and multidisciplinary input, is mandatory to early diagnosis and individualized treatment planning. These findings underpin the contribution of a formalized, image-based approach in the management of difficult neuro-oncological cases.

Chapter 12: Revolutionizing Neurosurgery and Orthopedics: Case Studies at the Intersection of Robotics and Personalized Medicine

Zeelaf Shahid

The convergence of robotics and personalized medicine is revolutionizing orthopedic and neurosurgical practice with unmatched precision, improved patient outcomes, and personalized treatment plans. This chapter presents a case study-based review exploring daily applications of robotic-assisted surgery and 3D-printed patient-specific implants. Robotic systems demonstrate enhanced spine and cranial procedure accuracy, resulting in a noteworthy reduction in intraoperative complications and postoperative recovery time by enhancing image-guided navigation and intraoperative precision. Concurrently, patient-specific medicine in the form of 3D-printed implants from patient anatomy showed profound improvement in implant fit, biomechanics, and long-term surgical outcome, with reductions in revision rates and operative time being noted. Research data were derived from peer-reviewed literature, surgeon interviews, and clinical case data from Sohail Trust Hospital in Karachi, Pakistan. While the findings underscore the disruptive potential of such technologies, the research also flags the big challenges, including astronomical implementation costs, extensive training needs, and ethical concerns around AI-driven decision-making and patient consent. Despite such challenges, clinical adoption is growing, provided there are sufficient regulatory frameworks, training facilities, and patient education systems in place. This review finds that robotic-assisted surgery and customized implants represent a significant advance in modern surgical intervention. In order to become fully established and accessed fairly, health systems must invest in policy formation and technological infrastructure. The continued evolution of these technologies through interdisciplinary research and clinical expertise has the potential to redefine standards of care in surgery in the future.

Chapter 13: Revolutionizing Surgical Precision: The Intersection of Advanced CT Imaging, AI Integration, and Personalized Approaches

Zeelaf Shahid, Syed Imran Mehmood

The combination of high-end Computed Tomography (CT) imaging and Artificial Intelligence (AI) is revolutionizing surgical accuracy and individualized treatment planning. This chapter discusses how such technological innovations improve diagnostic confidence, refine surgical planning, and maximize patient outcomes. The development of CT imaging, from initial uses through high-definition and dual-energy imaging, has led to extremely refined anatomical renderings. Paired with AI-driven analysis and predictive modeling, these innovations enable real-time decision-making, individualized surgical intervention, and improved post-operative rehabilitation planning. Further, the application of augmented reality (AR) and virtual reality (VR) for surgical planning introduces new dimensions of preoperative visualization and intraoperative navigation. Despite these advances, constraints related to radiation exposure, economic feasibility, regulatory limitations, and the need for specialized training persist. This chapter provides a detailed review of the current trends, newer technologies, and real-time applications in oncology, neurosurgery, and orthopedics, among others, while commenting on the future of AI-aided surgeries. By reviewing case studies and clinical applications, it reflects on the impact of personalized surgical methods and how they are revolutionizing patient care globally.

Chapter 14: Seizures in Head Injury Patients: A Cross-Sectional Study

Rubina Ghani, Waqas Mughis Rajpoot, Amanullah Khan

Traumatic Brain Injury (TBI) significantly increases the risk of post-traumatic seizures (PTS), and their long-term implications on neurological health and quality of life. While global evidence shows a seizure incidence of 10–25% following moderate to severe TBI, regional evidence from Pakistan, particularly from tertiary care institutions, is sparse. In order to determine the incidence and patterns of seizures in head-injured patients presented to a tertiary care facility in Pakistan, with implications for their early diagnosis and management. A descriptive cross-sectional study was conducted at the Neurosurgical Ward of Abbasi Shaheed Hospital and Karachi Medical and Dental College, Karachi, Pakistan, for a duration of six months. A sample of 140 patients aged 1–60 years with established head injuries was assessed for the occurrence of seizures, type of seizure, and timing (immediate, early, or late). Clinical assessment was supplemented with radiological investigations (CT, MRI) and follow-up of patients. Initial results indicate a rate of seizure attacks in agreement with world patterns, with generalized seizures being most prevalent. Numerous patients who developed intracranial hemorrhage and skull fracture developed seizures; the majority of first attacks within a week after trauma. Early identification of high-risk TBI patients is able to guide prophylactic antiepileptic treatment in order to reduce morbidity. The importance of national surveillance and standardized protocols for seizure management in head trauma is underscored by this study.

Chapter 15: Transforming Surgical Precision, The Role of 3D Printing and Additive Manufacturing in Personalized Medicine

Bilal Ashraf

The merger of 3D printing and additive manufacturing with surgical practice has almost revolutionized personalized medicine. This review searches how these new technologies allow surgical procedures to be executed with greater precision with patient-specific anatomical models, implants, and bioprinted tissues generated by these technologies. The process of translating medical imaging into physical models allows realizing more accurate preoperative planning, intraoperative guidance, and patient outcomes in disciplines including neurosurgery, orthopedics, and maxillofacial surgery. The combination of AI and point of care manufacturing with 3D printing is also facilitating real-time design and rapid prototyping in hospital environments. That said, clinical adoption is still hindered by expense, regulatory bottlenecks, material and standardization concerns. Emerging applications for bioprinting and smart implants are also forthrightly discussed, hinting at a future where surgical interventions will be tailored but also anticipatory and responsive. With the continual growth of interdisciplinary collaboration, 3D printing is becoming a founding principle of precision-guided, patient-specific surgical care.

Soobia Saeed
Taylor's University, Malaysia

Mohsin Qadeer
National Medical Center, Pakistan

Acknowledgment

We would like to extend our heartfelt appreciation to all those who contributed to the successful completion of this project. This endeavor would not have been possible without the collective support and collaboration of many individuals.

First and foremost, we owe sincere thanks to all authors who shared their knowledge, insights, and experience in their chapter contributions. They were ardent supporters of this project and so observed the time limits for the various stages with great discipline, without which this book could never have reached completion.

We are also eternally grateful for the reviewers' excellent work. Their thoughtful and constructive comments greatly improved the chapters' quality, clarity, and coherence. Many of the authors were also reviewers, to whom we extend especial thanks for their commitment and time.

Of course, a last but not least, profound thanks are due to our families and friends for their endless support, love, prayers, and understanding. Their encouragement and sacrifices were paramount for our timely completion of this project.

Soobia Saeed
Taylor's University, Malaysia

Mohsin Qadeer
National Medical Center, Pakistan

Chapter 1
Advancements in CT Imaging for Personalized Implants and Surgical Planning: A Stem Cell Therapy Perspective

Rubina Ghani
https://orcid.org/0000-0003-1923-7924
Sohail University, Pakistan

ABSTRACT

The use of autologous platelet-rich plasma (PRP) and adipose-derived stem cells (ADSC) has shown therapeutic effectiveness in various conditions such as diabetic ulcers, ocular infections, cataract surgery, and dermatological disorders. This case report presents a novel approach to the treatment of cervical spinal cord injury by combining artificial intelligence (AI) with PRP and ADSC therapy. In total, the patient received two treatment sessions of PRP and ADSC therapy lasting 15 days each, while an AI – based gait, posture and deep tendon reflexes assessments were conducted before and after treatment. At baseline, hyperreflexia was noted, the patient could not stand unaided or hold himself upright; the first therapy session did not elicit any changes.

1. INTRODUCTION

Application of regenerative medicine has significantly enhanced the process of tissue repair and quickened response to injury. One of the most studied elements of

DOI: 10.4018/979-8-3373-2807-2.ch001

regenerative medicine is Platelet-Rich Plasma (PRP), and it has been discovered to have immense potential for enhancing tissue regeneration. PRP is a bio-product that is extracted through plasma centrifugation and contains autologous platelets that are involved in the stimulation of cell growth, tissue repair, and healing. The regenerative potential of PRP has been widely researched, and it has been reported to induce mitosis and angiogenesis, which are critical for the repair and healing of damaged tissues. This makes PRP a potential therapeutic agent, particularly in the treatment of injuries such as spinal cord injury (Hussen et al., 2024).

Spinal cord injury, potentially leading to disastrous results, are responsible for causing feelings of loss, pain, spasm, paralysis, and urinary incontinence. Spinal cord injuries pose a large clinical challenge because the spinal cord has no spontaneous capacity for regeneration. The latest advances in regenerative medicine have focused on the use of stem cells, particularly mesenchymal stem cells (MSCs), which have been shown to promote progenitor cell proliferation and inhibit apoptosis. The past 15 years have witnessed extensive research aimed at an understanding of the regenerative potential of MSCs, especially spinal cord injury (Yu et al., 2019; Panni et al., 2019).

Among the various sources of MSCs, adipose-derived stem cells (ADSCs) are of special interest due to their superior regenerative potential, particularly in cartilage regeneration. ADSCs are derived from fat, which is relatively easy to harvest and plentiful in supply and hence are highly desired for therapeutic applications in regenerative medicine. Their ease of handling and capacity to differentiate into numerous cell types make ADSCs eligible for the repair of various injuries, such as spinal injuries (Gupta et al., 2024).

In combination with PRP, ADSCs have also delivered promising results for the repair of spinal injuries. PRP's regenerative capabilities, such as facilitating angiogenesis and cell proliferation, match the reparative capabilities of ADSCs. Together, these agents would facilitate repair of damaged spinal cord and restoration of function. Spinal cord injury treatment by autologous ADSCs and administration of PRP is a new promising approach to potential significant improvement in patient outcome and as a new platform for clinical application in regenerative medicine (Abusalah et al., 2024; Abouchenari et al., 2024).

2. LITERATURE REVIEW

Computed Tomography (CT) imaging technology has largely been responsible for precision medicine, particularly in terms of personalized implants and surgical planning. The blending of artificial intelligence (AI), 3D modeling, and high-resolution imaging technologies in CT imaging enable real-time, high-definition information needed to optimize patient-specific interventions. This article addresses the application of CT imaging in individualized surgical planning, particularly in the context of its application in stem cell therapy for regenerative medicine. CT imaging has emerged as a useful tool for clinicians involved in preoperative assessment and treatment planning (Pathak et al., 2023; Saeed et al., 2018). Technology allows for the reconstruction of three-dimensional anatomical structures, thus enabling patient-specific implant design. Evidence has demonstrated that AI-aided CT imaging improves structural abnormality detection, facilitating precision-guided interventions. Furthermore, the ability to integrate biomechanical modeling with CT imaging makes it possible for surgeons to virtually simulate surgery, thereby reducing intraoperative risks and improving patient outcomes (Saeed et al., 2017).

Stem cell therapy is also a possible pathway for tissue regeneration and repair, particularly in orthopedic and neurosurgical procedures. CT imaging also plays a critical role in the monitoring of stem cell location, viewing tissue reaction, and therapeutic response assessment. Multidetector CT technology, dual-energy CT, and spectral imaging offer better contrast for stem cell differentiation and incorporation into host tissues detection. In addition, contrast agents based on nanoparticle have also been explored for the purpose of visualizing distribution of stem cells post-transplantation, supporting improved monitoring of treatment (Farias et al., 2019; Jain, 2025). Additionally, application of AI algorithms has further enabled the expansion of CT application in personalized medicine. Deep learning algorithms have also been set to perform automated segmentation, anomaly identification, and quantification analysis from CT scans with improved accuracy diagnoses (Liu et al., 2020; Saeed et al., 2022). AI predictive modeling also facilitates the assessment of patient-specific biomechanical response to implants, their ideal design, and reduced failure rates. Studies have also shown that diagnostic performance is well maintained while employing AI-assisted CT scanning with significant reduction in radiation exposure (Saeed et al., 2021; He et al., 2021).

While it has come a long way, CT imaging in individualized surgery planning and stem cell therapy is faced with several challenges. These include radiation exposure, cost constraints, and the need for standardized imaging protocols (Bhandari et al., 2023; Jayawickrama et al., 2024; Zoabi et al., 2022). Future research should target the development of low-dose imaging techniques, hybrid imaging technologies, and AI-based automation to enhance accuracy and minimize patient risks. In addition, further clinical trials are needed to validate the long-term efficacy of CT-guided stem cell treatments in regenerative medicine. CT imaging has revolutionized personalized implants and surgical planning, offering unprecedented accuracy and diagnostic performance (Jehanzeb, 2024; Mohammadi et al., 2024; Saeed et al., 2023). Its integration with AI and state-of-the-art imaging technologies continues to refine preoperative planning, with enhanced patient outcomes. In regenerative medicine, CT-guided stem cell treatment holds enormous potential for advancing therapeutic interventions. Conquering today's challenges by technological progress and clinical validation will be crucial to defining the future of precision medicine (Saeed et al., 2024; Saeed et al., 2024).

3. PROPOSED METHODOLOGY

This study will employ a methodical approach to review the evolution in CT imaging towards individualized implants and surgical planning for stem cell therapy use. The process starts with a comprehensive literature review of peer-reviewed studies on CT imaging technology, AI-driven developments, and their uses in surgical planning and regenerative medicine. This will comprise analysis of peer-reviewed journal articles, summaries of clinical trials, and developments in imaging technologies. Second, data will be obtained on the basis of clinical imaging datasets, focusing on patient cases with stem cell treatment and individualized implants being utilized. The selected datasets will be preprocessed through noise removal, contrast enhancement, and segmentation using AI-based optimization algorithms for optimal visualization.

The third process is the design and deployment of deep learning models for computer-aided analysis of CT images. AI algorithms like convolutional neural networks (CNNs) and machine learning techniques will be utilized to perform feature extraction, anomaly detection, and generate patient-specific surgical planning. The models will be validated with ground truth datasets to ensure accuracy and reliability. The fourth step will be biomechanical modeling and simulation, wherein patient-specific CT imaging data will be combined with finite element analysis to assess the mechanical performance of tailored implants. This will provide insight into the optimization of implant design and increased surgical accuracy.

Following model validation, the methodology will proceed with experimental testing through retrospective and prospective case studies. Retrospective analysis will involve a comparison of existing CT scans and surgical outcomes, while prospective case studies will consist of real-time utilization of AI-enhanced CT imaging for planning surgeries and observing stem cell therapy. Finally, statistical analysis and performance comparison of the proposed methods will conclude the study with the use of AI-based CT imaging in comparison with conventional imaging techniques. The outcomes will be assessed for efficacy, accuracy, and clinical significance to determine the impact of CT imaging innovation upon personal medicine and regenerative therapies.

Figure 1. Flowchart of Proposed Methodology

```
             Start
               |
               v
Comprehensive Literature Review
   - Analyze existing research on CT imaging technologies, AI-driven enhancements, anc
   - Examine peer-reviewed journal articles, clinical trial reports, and technological
               |
               v
      Data Collection
   - Gather clinical imaging datasets focusing on patient cases involving stem cell tr
   - Perform preprocessing: noise reduction, contrast enhancement, segmentation using
               |
               v
Development & Implementation of AI Models
   - Utilize deep learning techniques (CNNs, machine learning algorithms) for feature
   - Develop AI models for patient-specific surgical planning
   - Validate models against ground truth datasets
               |
               v
Biomechanical Modeling & Simulation
   - Integrate patient-specific CT imaging data with finite element analysis
   - Assess mechanical behavior of personalized implants
   - Optimize implant design and improve surgical precision
               |
               v
Experimental Evaluation
   - Conduct retrospective analysis using pre-existing CT scans and surgical outcomes
   - Perform prospective case studies applying AI-enhanced CT imaging in real-time sur
               |
               v
Statistical Analysis & Performance Evaluation
   - Compare AI-driven CT imaging with conventional imaging techniques
   - Assess findings based on accuracy, efficiency, and clinical applicability
   - Determine impact on personalized medicine and regenerative therapies
               |
               v
             End
```

Figure 2. Flowchart of Proposed Methodology

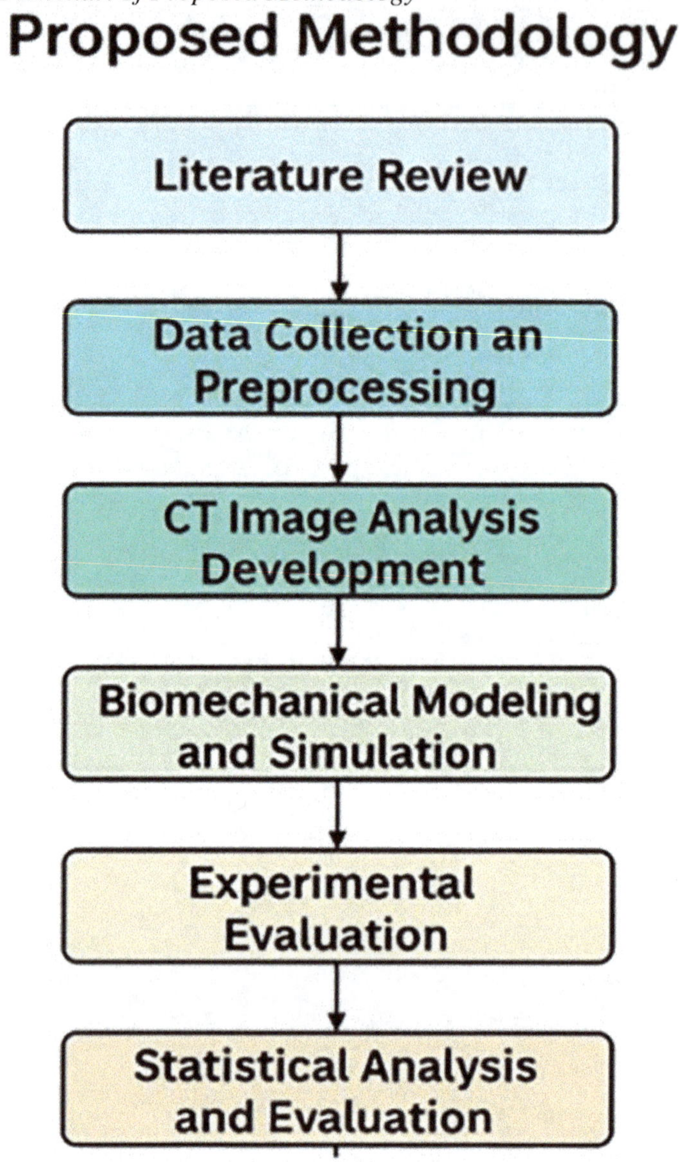

3.1 Case Report

A 35-year-old man with no history of illness had been involved in a road traffic accident in 2006 that resulted in cervical spine injuries. Magnetic resonance imaging showed loss of disc space between C6 and C7 vertebrae consistent with the cervical spine injury, accompanied by motor injury and hemiparesis where the left side was involved. In between it all, physiotherapy achieved success in allowing sensations and motor control of his limbs. However, unfortunately, deterioration occurred, and he needed to be assisted to maintain the erect position and to walk. Signs were that of upper motor neuron lesions presenting as spastic paralysis and associated presentations of clonus, more pronounced on the left side. The subject was free from any compounding comorbidities. His first visit to the Musavvir Stem Cell Clinic, Karachi, Pakistan, took place in March 2017. MRI was done. Detailed explanation of the procedure and the possible side effects of treatment were told to the patient. After obtaining his written consent, treatment was initiated. This was the first case from the region that showed the possibilities of ADSCs and Stromal Vascular Fraction in spinal cord injury patients.

The study was approved by the ethical committee of Musavvir Stem Cell Clinic and were conducted according to all principles of Helsinki Declaration. SVF was harvested by liposuction. Some small incisions were made on the patient thigh, and a hypothetical 100 g of fat was extracted. The lipoaspirate was washed with 0.9% normal saline. The matrix of the adipose tissue was centrifuged in the next process to separate out the stem cells and the SVF was taken to be the pellet formed at the bottom of the centrifuge. Blood was drawn and transferred to the PRP kit from the patient, delivered in a volume of 20 cc. The blood sample was spun for 5 minutes at 2500 rpm to separate. The blood PRP tube should be locked and spun for 8 minutes at 3000 rpm. The PRP was then collected with the hollow needle into a sterile falcon tube. To this PRP was added the already extracted SVF. The final assay was then placed on AdiLight-2 for a period of 20 minutes. AdiLight-2 (AdiLight-2; AdiStem Ltd, Hong Kong) is a Plasma/cell Activation Device, which applies selected monochromatic frequencies within the colored spectrum of light. Cells were photo-activated for 20 minutes using 3 laser-diode transmitting 3 frequencies each in red, green, and yellow. Multiple IV and intrathecal infusion of stem cells took place. No improvement was noted after the first panel. After two weeks, the patient was called for phase two treatment. However, after two days of the second sequence of treatment, the patient reported that he was able to stand for 2 minutes and 30 seconds. That gradually, a remarkable control of the lower limbs and upright standing without any support was achieved. Following that, he could walk for 3 minutes and 30 seconds without support, as shown in a supporting patient video. After five panels of treatment, an MRI was done; it showed hyper intense signals within the spinal cord at the C5 and C6 level, signifying post-intervention changes. These findings have been compared with the previously done MRI.

3.2 Role of Artificial Intelligence in Case Patient

There are many attributions that could be allotted to AI in the present case study, especially with the augmentation of diagnostics, treatment planning, and outcome assessment.

1. Imaging analysis and diagnosis support: Various AI-based imaging-analysis tools, most prominently convolutional neural networks (CNNs), could be used to analyze MRI scans taken pre- and post-treatment. They can recognize subtle changes in disc height, spinal cord signal intensities, and surrounding tissue condition that may be undetectable by the human eye. It could yield a quantitative evaluation of their spinal cord architecture and precise assessment of therapy effect.
2. Progress monitoring and motor recovery: AI algorithms in, specifically speaking, computer vision could analyze video footage of the patient's gait, balance, and posture. It can break movement patterns phone-by-phone to make an objective measurement of improvements in motor control, stability, and muscle coordination over time. Such algorithms can also track involuntary jerk and spasticity, giving clinicians a roadmap for quantifying the adjustments they need to make in therapy sessions.
3. Predictive Modeling for Outcomes-Guided Patient Treatment: Drawing on patient data, AI models may be constructed that allow treatment predictions as to effectiveness-response possibility for such therapies as stem cell and PRP. Such models will be fed with such variables as injury type and initial treatment response, along with physiotherapy history. These predictive models would greatly assist in forming personalized treatment schedules and expected recovery timelines for future patients sustaining similar injuries.
4. Integration of Data for Comparative Analysis: AI could aggregate this one treated case with similar cases in regional or global databases from which insights on treatment efficacy, adverse effects, and recovery timelines could be drawn. Such comparative approaches should confirm findings in rare cases as well as lend support to future clinical recommendations.
5. Natural Language Processing for Documentation and Consent: NLP by AI offers a way to record case histories in detail by generating progress notes and automatic updates. NLP models may allow the generation of consent documents customized by accessing the relevant information from similar case studies in order to convey patient individuality.

There exists a backdrop for AI implementation in improving diagnostic precision, enhancing assessment and monitoring recovery metrics, and ensuring individualization in treatment to lead to improved outcomes for spinal cord injury patients.

Figure 3. Role of AI in health care

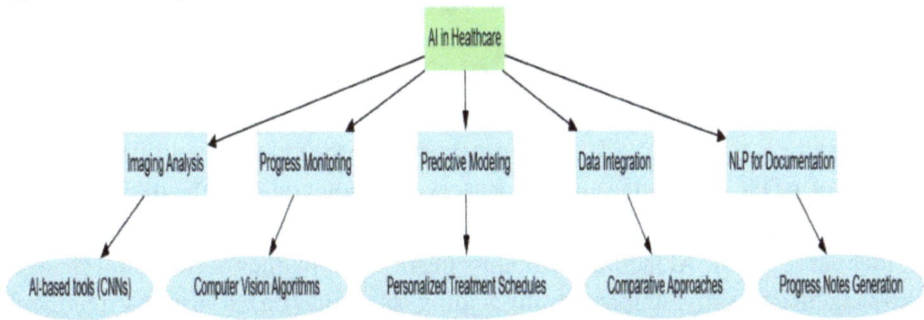

5. RESULT AND DISCUSSION

One of the notable contributions from artifice Intelligence (AI) in the management of SCI is analysis of massive datasets from medical imaging and biomarker analyses to provide a holistic overview of tissue regeneration and nerve repair. For example, AI-based tools capture evidence of subtle gait, postural, and reflex changes, offering an extension of high-resolution tracking of progress that conventional evaluations may miss. In this circumstance, AI's analytical capacities detailed specified improvements in hyperreflexia, chorea ballism, and the influence on his postural control, revealing a refined view of the recovery journey [7,8].

The vast literature supports this conclusion, raising doubts about the credibility of many challenges to be surmounted in developing the best SCI management practices. For instance, AI-powered tools quantify subtle changes in gait, posture, and reflexes, giving high-resolution progress tracking that traditional assessments might miss. In this case, AI's analytical power highlighted detailed improvements in hyperreflexia, chorea ballism, and outpouring on his postural control, revealing an enjoined view of the patient preparedness[9,10].

In addition to pharmacological treatments, AI-based tools complement the evaluation of PRP efficacy by quantifying the concentration of growth factors-such as fibroblast growth factor (FGF), platelet-derived growth factor (PDGF), and insulin-like growth factor (IGF)-and their effect on cell proliferation, angiogenesis, and inflammation modulation. By assessing several cellular outcomes, AI can arrange its applications to best suit the needs of the patient for tissue repair and therefore provide customized modes of treatment to harden regeneration. In the same breath, such technology also provides the basis for forecasting the long-term effects of PRP in nerves and tissue regeneration, which will, in the long haul, bolster clinical decision-making and personalized care initiatives.

The use of AI in this respect stands to include tracking migration and proliferation of stem cells, monitoring implantation into damaged tissues. The complex processes by which ADSCs generate stimulation for neurogenic stem cell activation and cytokine production to inhibit inflammation, become more complete with a deeper insight of AI analytical tools. Provide some prospect for proliferation and differentiation potential of ADSCs, which in another act served as potential therapeutic application by isolating ADSCs as the best nerve regenerative candidate in spinal cord injury. Besides nerve repair, AI facilitates monitoring of the dynamics of structural changes following PRP therapy, supplementing findings of studies on nerve injury treatment. Algorithms have demonstrated progression of axonal regeneration, use of muscle atrophy recovery, and scarring measured decreases as indicated by studies on PRP therapy in Pudendal neuralgia and Carpal tunnel syndrome. Such observations backed by AI imply the role of PRP towards tissue regeneration-characterized by tissue repair and functional recovery. In conclusion, AI enhances the application of PRP and ADSCs in spinal cord injuries by enabling precise, data-driven insights into nerve regeneration, healing, and functional improvement. As demonstrated in this case, AI's advanced analytical capabilities ensure a targeted and effective approach to treatment, showing potential for wider implementation in SCI and related neurological therapies. Future research may explore the further integration of AI with regenerative medicine, with the aim of optimizing therapeutic outcomes for SCI patients and advancing the field of neuro-regenerative therapies.

6. CONCLUSION

In chapter paper, we report the first documented case in our area showing an improvement in a major clinical outcome for a patient with traumatic spinal injury treated with PRP and ADCS supported by AI-driven evaluation. On subsequent therapy sessions, the patient was able to regain control of lower limbs, stand upright independently, and walk independently. MRI findings also confirmed these behavioral improvements, establishing evidence of PRP and ADSC treatment in spinal cord injury recovery. This case demonstrates the ability to combine regenerative therapies with AI-enhanced surveillance directed at optimizing patient outcomes in spinal cord injury treatment.

ACKNOWLEDGEMENTS

We would like to acknowledge the staff of Musavvir Stem Cell Clinic for their immense contribution.

CONFLICT OF INTEREST

No potential conflict of interest relevant to this case report was presented.

ETHICS APPROVAL

The study was performed according to the Helsinki Declaration and approved by the Ethical Review Board (ERB) of Musavvir Stem Cell Clinic, Pathological and Molecular laboratories, Karachi, Pakistan.

PATIENT CONSENT

A written informed consent was obtained from the patient.

AUTHORS' CONTRIBUTION

We conceived the idea and treated the patient. NJ wrote the manuscript while SFA helped in the procedure and recorded the treatment response. UN critically reviewed the case report.

REFERENCES

Abouchenari, A., Tajbakhsh, N., Shahbaz, A., & Alamdari-Mahd, G. (2024). Advancements in dental implant technology: the impact of smart polymers utilized through 3D printing. Journal of synthesis and sintering, 4(2).

Abusalah, M. A. H., Abd Rahman, E. N. S. E., & Choudhary, O. P. (2024). Evolving trends in stem cell therapy: An emerging and promising approach against various diseases. *International Journal of Surgery*, *110*(11), 6862–6868. DOI: 10.1097/JS9.0000000000001948 PMID: 39699861

Bhandari, S., Yadav, V., Ishaq, A., Sanipini, S., Ekhator, C., Khleif, R., Beheshtaein, A., Jhajj, L. K., Khan, A. W., Al Khalifa, A., Naseem, M. A., Bellegarde, S. B., & Nadeem, M. A. (2023). Trends and challenges in the development of 3d-printed heart valves and other cardiac implants: A review of current advances. *Cureus*, *15*(8). Advance online publication. DOI: 10.7759/cureus.43204 PMID: 37565179

Farias, T. P., Dias, F. L., Sousa, B. A., Galvão, M. S., Bispo, D., & Pastl, A. C. (2019). Prototyping: Major advance in surgical planning and customizing prostheses in patients with bone tumors of the head and neck. *International Journal of Clinical Medicine*, *4*(7), 1–7. DOI: 10.4236/ijcm.2013.47A1001

Gupta, R. S., Lal, B., Bhagat, A. C., & Alagarsamy, R. (2024). Medical Imaging for Patient-Specific Implants. In *Biomedical Implants* (pp. 39–60). CRC Press.

He, X. Y., Yu, H. M., Lin, S., & Li, Y. Z. (2021). Advances in the application of mesenchymal stem cells, exosomes, biomimetic materials, and 3D printing in osteoporosis treatment. *Cellular & Molecular Biology Letters*, *26*(1), 47. DOI: 10.1186/s11658-021-00291-8 PMID: 34775969

Hussen, B. M., Taheri, M., Yashooa, R. K., Abdullah, G. H., Abdullah, S. R., Kheder, R. K., & Mustafa, S. A. (2024). Revolutionizing medicine: Recent developments and future prospects in stem-cell therapy. *International Journal of Surgery*, *110*(12), 8002–8024. DOI: 10.1097/JS9.0000000000002109 PMID: 39497543

Jain, V. (2025). Personalized Solutions in Orthopaedic Surgery: The Era of 3D Technology and Future. In *Innovations in Healthcare and Outcome Measurement: New Approaches for a Healthy Lifestyle* (pp. 213–229). Springer Nature Switzerland. DOI: 10.1007/978-3-031-77302-0_14

Jayawickrama, S. M., Ranaweera, P. M., Pradeep, R. G. G. R., Jayasinghe, Y. A., Senevirathna, K., Hilmi, A. J., Rajapakse, R. M. G., Kanmodi, K. K., & Jayasinghe, R. D. (2024). Developments and future prospects of personalized medicine in head and neck squamous cell carcinoma diagnoses and treatments. *Cancer Reports*, *7*(3), e2045. DOI: 10.1002/cnr2.2045 PMID: 38522008

Jehanzeb, M. (2024). The future of spine surgery: technological innovations and advancements: A comprehensive review. *Romanian Neurosurgery*, •••, 102–108. DOI: 10.33962/roneuro-2024-017

Liu, C. Y., Yin, G., Sun, Y. D., Lin, Y. F., Xie, Z., English, A. W., Li, Q.-F., & Lin, H.-D. (2020). Effect of exosomes from adipose-derived stem cells on the apoptosis of Schwann cells in peripheral nerve injury. *CNS Neuroscience & Therapeutics*, *26*(2), 189–196. DOI: 10.1111/cns.13187 PMID: 31278850

. Mohammadi, A. T., mohammad Taheri, S. A., Karamouz, M., & Sarhaddi, R. (2024). Rising Innovations: Revolutionary Medical and Dental Breakthroughs Revolutionizing the Healthcare Field. Nobel Sciences.

Panni, A. S., Vasso, M., Braile, A., Toro, G., De Cicco, A., & Viggiano, D.. (2019). Preliminary results of autologous adipose-derived stem cells in early knee osteoarthritis: Identification of a subpopulation with greater response. *International Orthopaedics*, *43*(1), 7–13. DOI: 10.1007/s00264-018-4182-6 PMID: 30280218

Pathak, K., Saikia, R., Das, A., Das, D., Islam, M. A., Pramanik, P., Parasar, A., Borthakur, P. P., Sarmah, P., Saikia, M., & Borthakur, B. (2023). 3D printing in biomedicine: Advancing personalized care through additive manufacturing. *Exploration of Medicine*, *4*(6), 1135–1167. DOI: 10.37349/emed.2023.00200

Saeed, S., & Abdullah, A. (2022). Hybrid graph cut hidden Markov model of K-mean cluster technique. CMC-Computers, Materials & Continua, 1-15.

Saeed, S., Ghani, R., & Shahid, Z. (2024). Prevalence of Low Back Pain and Its Associated Factors in an Underdeveloped Country: Pakistan: Prevalence of Low Back Pain in Pakistan. *Journal of Health and Rehabilitation Research*, *4*(3), 1–7.

Saeed, S., & Haron, H. (2021). Improve correlation matrix of discrete Fourier transformation (CM-DFT) technique for finding the missing values of MRI images. *Mathematical Biosciences and Engineering*, •••, 1–22.

Saeed, S., & Qasim, M. B. (2023). Surgical acute epidural hematoma in the temporal perioral region of the brain. *International Journal of Head and Neck Surgery*, *14*(3), 1–8. DOI: 10.5005/jp-journals-10001-1552

Saeed, S., Shaikh, A., Memon, M. A., Saleem, M. Q., & Naqvi, S. M. R. (2017). Assessment of brain tumor due to the usage of MATLAB performance. *Journal of Medical Imaging and Health Informatics*, *7*(6), 1454–1460. DOI: 10.1166/jmihi.2017.2187

Yu, N., Nguyen, T., Cho, Y. D., Kavanagh, N. M., Ghassib, I., & Giannobile, W. V. (2019). Personalized scaffolding technologies for alveolar bone regenerative medicine. *Orthodontics & Craniofacial Research*, *22*(S1), 69–75. DOI: 10.1111/ocr.12275 PMID: 31074155

Zoabi, A., Redenski, I., Oren, D., Kasem, A., Zigron, A., Daoud, S., Moskovich, L., Kablan, F., & Srouji, S. (2022). 3D printing and virtual surgical planning in oral and maxillofacial surgery. *Journal of Clinical Medicine*, *11*(9), 2385. DOI: 10.3390/jcm11092385 PMID: 35566511

Chapter 2
Anatomical Mapping of Intracranial Aneurysms:
A CT-Based Framework for Precision Neurosurgery

Amanullah Khan
https://orcid.org/0000-0003-1808-5084
Liaquat National Hospital, Pakistan

Mohsin Qadeer
https://orcid.org/0000-0001-7509-6885
National Medical Center, Pakistan

Salman Shareef
Liaquat National Hospital, Pakistan

ABSTRACT

Intracranial aneurysms are a significant neurosurgical issue in low- to middle-income countries. This study evaluates a CT-based anatomical mapping system for enhancing surgical accuracy in cerebral aneurysm treatment. In a retrospective analysis of 82 patients operated in Karachi, Pakistan, at a tertiary care center. The female predominance of(65.9%) and high prevalence of hypertension (82.9%) were identified as major risk factors. All patients had acute hemorrhage and headache. CT scan enabled precise localization of aneurysms and showed statistically significant correlations between Glasgow Coma Scale (GCS) scores and locations of aneurysms (p = 0.029), and between seizure types and locations of aneurysms (p = 0.003). Cerebral infarction was also strongly correlated with the need for decompressive surgery (p < 0.001).

DOI: 10.4018/979-8-3373-2807-2.ch002

1. INTRODUCTION

Intracranial aneurysms present a serious neurosurgical challenge from their possible rupture and the subsequent occurrence of subarachnoid hemorrhage (SAH), usually with considerable morbidity and mortality associated (Wang et al., 2022). When the vascular anatomy is accurately assessed, the intervention strategy can be tailored, with special emphasis on complex neurovascular interventions. Computed tomography angiography (CTA) had transformed into an indispensable tool in this regard with noninvasive high-resolution three-dimensional imaging of the cerebral vasculature (Hacein-Bey et al., 2011). This approach helps in evaluating certain key morphological parameters like the size of an aneurysm, neck configuration, dome-to-neck ratio, and spatial relationship to parent and perforating arteries (Howard et al., 2019).

Technical improvements in CTA postprocessing—i.e., volume rendering, maximum intensity projection (MIP), and multiplanar reformation (MPR)—have significantly improved the visualization of tiny-caliber vessels and partially thrombosed aneurysms (Zhou et al., 2024). These improvements allow neurosurgeons to define better bony landmarks, aneurysm orientation, and neurovascular relationships, thereby enhancing surgical planning (Wang et al., 2021).

Recent advancements in the area of medical imaging and neurosurgical techniques have greatly influenced the diagnosis and treatment of complex brain conditions, especially related to the resection of brain tumors and vascular conditions. Vadhavekar et al. (2024) presents a great overview of the latest developments in imaging, and surgical approaches for the removal of brain tumors, including the use of intraoperative MRI, neuronavigation, fluorescence-guided surgery and robotic surgery. Together, these techniques have improved the accuracy, safety, and extent of tumor resection with improvements in patient outcomes and neurological deficits.

In parallel, the use of deep learning in neuroimaging has opened new possibilities for automatic detection of vascular pathologies, with very promising results. For example, Ueda et al. (2019) used artificial intelligence for automatic detection of cerebral aneurysm in MR angiography. They found that the accuracy was high enough that artificial intelligence may eventually be used clinically to help radiologists detect subtle aneurysms that would otherwise be missed in routine checks, thereby improving diagnostic accuracy. By improving speed and consistency, this may allow for a standard and scalable tool to detect early signs of pathology - a critical need for preventing disastrous events such as subarachnoid hemorrhage.

These studies are representative of a larger trend towards technology-enhanced neurosurgical care, in which artificial intelligence and real-time imaging enhance rather than replace clinical decision-making and operationalization of care (human computer systems). Neurosurgeons will increasingly adopt workflows that maximize both artificial intelligence and real-time imaging, in turn improving clinical outcomes and the individualization of patient management in the context of neurosurgery.

Figure 1. Brain Aneurysm

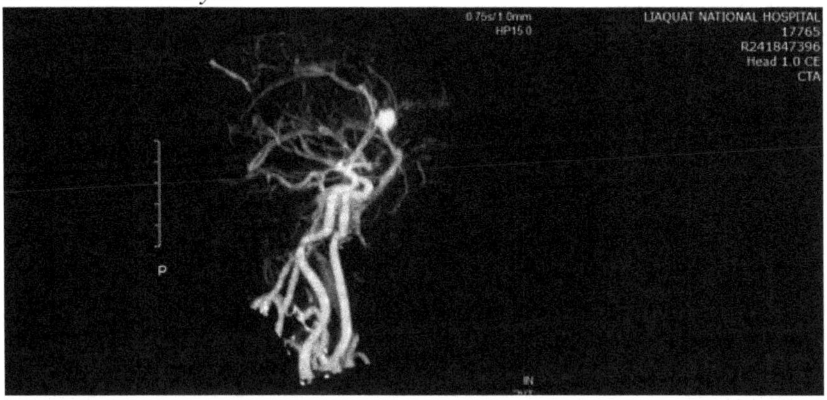

Figure 1 shows a CT Angiography (CTA) scan in the head and neck region, thereby revealing the vascular structures such as those of the carotid arteries, vertebral arteries, and the circle of Willis. An aneurysm is one of the important highlights in this image; the aneurysm appears as a bright, rounded, balloon-like outpouching along A com artery that is recognized toward the upper end of the scan. This peculiar bulge is result of localized weakening and abnormal dilation of the blood vessel wall, which is usually associated with an aneurysm.

This important aneurysm feature is shaped whether it's vascular or "berry-shaped" to aneurysm that is encountered mostly . Its size is comparatively small to medium as judged by the surrounding vascular structures. Also, the vessels are very well opacified, that is, the contrast material penetrated well enough to visualize the anatomy, allowing a clear and easy identification of the aneurysm.

With the advances in computer vision and neurosurgical planning that have developed in recent years, I can only conclude that high-resolution preoperative imaging is necessary for improved patient safety and surgical accuracy. In fact, three-dimensional computed tomography angiography (CTA) has improved visualization of complex cerebral vascular anatomy and allowed neurosurgeons to make informed customized decisions before as well as during the procedure. If you recall the work of Goertz et al. (2018), preoperative three-dimensional angiography has shown that it may lead to a decreased risk of ischemic complications during the surgical clipping of ruptured intracranial aneurysms. The combination of the imaging allows precise evaluation of the aneurysm morphology and the relationship with no adjacent vessels leading to better surgical planning, therefore lowering the intraoperative risk.

The advances in imaging, along with artificial intelligence, intraoperative navigation, and robotic assistance represent a sea change in neurosurgical practice headed towards more predictive, preventive, and personalized care. The evolution of this field will no doubt continue to integrate technology and evidence-based clinical judgement to yield optimal outcomes for patients with intracranial aneurysms and other complex neurovascular problems.

2. LITERATURE REVIEW

The rates of cerebrovascular disease, specifically intracranial aneurysms and atherosclerotic diseases, continue to rise globally with differential diagnosis, treatment, and neurosurgical outcomes on the basis of (high-income countries) vs. low- and middle-income countries (LMIC). The complexity of neuro-endovascular interventions and a continued access to advanced technology and training will further compound this health care gap and inequality, especially throughout the African continent. Sarkodie et al. (2022), came up with a list of barriers to delivering care to patients requiring neuro-endovascular interventions in resource-constrained settings like Ghana. This list included systemic barriers comprised of infrastructure, cost of consumables, trained personnel, and inconsistency in availability of imaging modalities. Each of these factors limited timely management of cerebrovascular pathologies, like aneurysms, and risked poor outcomes in emergency neurosurgical instances.

In a wider continental perspective, Tétinou et al. (2021), conducted a scoping review on cerebral aneurysms in Africa. The perspective in the study determined that there was a large lack of data from African countries and highlighted the underdiagnosis of cerebral aneurysms, in addition to a lack of accessibility to advanced neuro-imaging options. The study highlighted that the incidence of aneurysmal subarachnoid Hemorrhage is increased in African populations, while many health systems are not prepared to manage the issue as diagnostic and therapeutic options remain inconsistent.

In light of these limitations, computational tools and artificial intelligence (AI) are surfacing as potential equalizers in the global neurosurgical landscape of care. Ballout et al. (2024) presented the use of computational fluid dynamics (CFD) in the evaluation of intracranial atherosclerotic disease, and indicated pathologic vascular hemodynamics, plaque behavior, and rupture risk, and moreover, that computational fluid dynamics could help better informed individual treatment or intervention planning even if the procedures were limited in volume or place of performer (Ballout et al, 2024).

AI-oriented imaging systems and approaches are being expressed as well and are said to automate and improve the propensity for early detection of cerebral aneurysms.

Din et al. (2023) reported a systematic review and meta-analysis on the applications using AI related to aneurysm detection, indicating deep learning models perform favorably to traditional radiological assessment while demonstrating appropriate sensitivity and specificity, indicating the generalizability of the approach and making the use of AI for clinical use in clinical radiology feasible, especially in LMICs with less accessibility to neuroradiologists with expert credentials (Faraj et al., 2020).

To address this viewpoint, Stumpo et al. (2021) discussed the wide applicability of machine learning in clinical neuroscience in areas such as aneurysm detection, the prediction of their rupture, and the prediction of outcome. They stated that AI and ML models trained on multiple large and annotated datasets can improve diagnostic accuracy, minimize human error, and determine more personalized management pathways. They also stated that it is important to note that the successful implementation of AI models involves building a strong digital delivery infrastructure and human capacity in low-resource settings.

Despite the limitations identified by Stumpo et al. (2021), Menna et al. (2024) outlined a global neurosurgical education project development as a non-profit initiative to help address the educational gap in LMICs. Their program noted a combination of remote training, digital simulation, and virtual mentoring, which has been successful in supporting local practitioners and transition over to new technologies in decedent physicians including AI and computational modeling. Global projects like these are important so that practitioners can learn together and sustain a collaborative action for local ownership of advances in neurosurgery.

Treatment of intracranial aneurysm in Pakistan is distinguished by individualized epidemiologic and therapeutic characteristics driven by a paucity of resources as well as a frequent late patient presentation. Of 50 clippings in a 2024 study done ≥21 days after rupture (from Lahore), 42% were anterior communicating artery aneurysms. Remarkably, 49 out of 50 patients were independently functional, having Glasgow Outcome Scores (GOS) of 4–5, despite operative delay (Ahmed et al., 2021; Goertz et.al, 2018). This outcome contrasts with Dutch practice recommending aneurysm clipping 10 days after rupture and noting how treatment protocols need to be changed in low- and middle-income countries (LMICs) due to systemic constraint (Ferreira et al., 2023).

Globally, endovascular coiling has been largely adopted, and by 2024, a 43% rate of utilization has been recorded. Pakistani facilities, however, continue to use surgical clipping on 93% of aneurysm sufferers. This is with several reasons in mind: coiling costs 8–10 times as much as clipping within the public setting, 82% of patients who have not been treated come in poor clinical grades (WFNS IV/V) while a mere 44% do in European settings, and only few centers within Pakistan provide endovascular services. Despite such limitations, technical success with coiling in Pakistan is at a remarkable 78% of patients with beneficial results—more than international figures of 63–84%—illustrating the need of more local data when resources permit (Ahmed et al., 2021; Júnior et.al, 2019).

Recent Pakistani studies report varying patterns of aneurysm distribution, with ACoA being most frequent in delayed clipping series (42%), compared to global data where MCA aneurysms predominate, such as 26.3% in Brazil for MCA aneurysms. A 2024 Karachi CTA study identified aneurysms in 81.3% of SAH cases, in line with Peshawar's 81% SAH aneurysm rate, although ACoA predominance is different from Western series (Shoukat et al., 2024). Khokar et.al, (2024) discuss the presentations remain systemic: 82% of untreated Pakistani patients present in WFNS IV/V, as opposed to 44% in European centers, necessitating modified protocols like Lahore's delayed clipping with 98% discharge success (GOS 4-5) after over 21 days from rupture. Some Pakistani centers employ 3D rotational angiography (92% intraoperative accuracy) and deep learning-based CTA (97.5% sensitivity) for basilar apex (7.6%) and MCA bifurcation aneurysms, but endovascular service is limited to few public hospitals, and coiling is 8-10× more costly than clipping. Despite global trends toward endovascular methods (43% adoption), Pakistan still has 93% clipping rates due to financial constraints and infrastructure shortages1, contributed to by manpower shortages (29% endovascular-trained neurosurgeons). Future avenues include AI-CFD synergy in hemodynamic modeling and hybrid training centers to reduce systemic disparities in device and neurocritical care access (Haizel-Cobbina et al., 2023; Pettersson et.al, 2023).

Despite these issues, Pakistani neurosurgical departments are now employing advanced technologies to enhance precision. The use of 3D rotational angiography has enabled increased precision in clip selection, with intraoperative correlation studies showing a 92% accuracy in determining aneurysm-to-parent vessel relationships. Additionally, deep learning-enhanced computed tomography angiography (CTA) achieved a 97.5% detection sensitivity, and it is particularly significant for the detection of uncommon aneurysm types such as basilar apex aneurysms, which represent 7.6% in local populations(Dai et.al, 2022). The imaging technologies have important roles to play in managing middle cerebral artery (MCA) bifurcation aneurysms, which represent approximately 24.2% of surgical cases. However, hybrid angiography suites remain not easily accessible in the majority of public hospitals (Azeem et al., 2023).

The literature indicates that, while AI, CTA, CFD, and 3D angiography are changing global neurosurgery, LMICs like Pakistan and Ghana must deal with financial, infrastructural, and workforce limitations. However, mechanisms such as contextually based protocols and local training regimes, and local information systems in LMICs can help to provide equitable access to the cutting-edge neurosurgical care setting for these marginalized populations. By merging global innovations with local implementations, health systems can begin to bridge the outcome gap and subsequently improve the standards of care for cerebrovascular disease in resource-constrained contexts.

3. DATA COLLECTION

Data collection was performed retrospectively at the Department of Neurosurgery, Liaquat National Hospital and Medical College (LNHMC), Karachi, Pakistan. Identified as a premier Tertiary Care Center with cutting-edge neuroimaging facilities and dedicated to a neurovascular surgery unit, LNHMC was the place for the collection of all clinical and radiological data for cerebral aneurysms diagnosed by CT scans. The collection of data was approved by the Ethics Review Board of the institution, and all data was collected according to well-established ethical standards and protocols in relation to the confidentiality of the patients.

3.1 Study Duration and Population

The study encompassed patients admitted from the year January 2010 to December 2024 and was inclusive of cases diagnosed with either ruptured or unruptured intracranial aneurysms, correlated clinically to their symptoms and results of CT scan. Considering the stated parameters, a total of 82 patients became part of the study. These patients were then selected by non-probability consecutive sampling, using hospital records and radiology archives.

3.2 Eligibility Criteria

- It is a person of any sex aged 18 years or older with a diagnosis confirmed by computed tomography angiography for an intracranial aneurysm.
- Patients previously managed with neurosurgical procedures such as aneurysm clipping or decompressive procedures.

Availability of full CTA imaging data along with acknowledged surgical records.

3.3 Exclusion Criteria

- Patients with incomplete CTA-imaging and/or lacking clinical documentation.
- Other vascular lesions in case of a saccular aneurysm-for instance, arteriovenous malformations or cavernous malformations.

3.3 Radiological Evaluation

Radiological assessment was conducted using high-resolution multislice CTA with a 128-slice CT scanner, such as the Siemens SOMATOM Definition AS. To reconstruct 3D models, we used RadiAnt and DICOM, and to navigate intraoperatively, we used Stealth Station stem for intraoperative navigation during surgery . The evaluation focused on identifying the location and side of the aneurysm—for example, involvement of the anterior communicating artery, MCA bifurcation, or basilar apex. Morphological features such as aneurysm size, neck width, and dome-to-neck ratio were also analyzed. Additional details included the aneurysm's proximity to nearby anatomical structures like the optic chiasm and perforating vessels, along with the presence of hemorrhagic components such as subarachnoid, intraparenchymal, or intraventricular bleeding. To improve anatomical visualization and assist with surgical planning, techniques like volume rendering, multiplanar reformation (MPR), and maximum intensity projection (MIP) were employed.

3.5 Statistical Analysis

The data collected was analyzed through the SPSS Chai Square method. Descriptive statistics for categorical variables were computed and expressed as frequencies and percentages. Chi-square tests, as appropriate, analyzed associations between clinical variables and aneurysm location, management strategies, and complications. A p-value < 0.05 was used as a cut-off for statistically significant differences.

This, as well, was analyzed with SPSS Chai Square method. Descriptive statistics include categorical variables were computed and presented as frequencies and percentages. Chi-squared tests were used, where appropriate, for the analysis of the association between either clinical variable with the site of the aneurysm, management approaches, or complications. The accepted level of statistical significance was set at $p<0.05$.

4. MATERIAL AND METHODS

4.1 Study Design and Setting

An observational study that made a retrospective effort was done at Liaquat National Hospital and Medical College, Karachi, Pakistan, aimed to see how surgical management was done and what clinical outcomes were found for patients with cerebral aneurysms as assessed with CT-based imaging techniques. Before data collection, ethical clearance was obtained from the institutional review board. The

Image findings from non-contrast CT scans and CT angiography (CTA) categorized aneurysm locations into six anatomic regions: right posterior communicating artery (Rt PCom), left posterior communicating artery (Lt PCom), right middle cerebral artery (Rt MCA), left middle cerebral artery (Lt MCA), anterior communicating artery (ACom), and other locations such as basilar tip and ICA bifurcation.

4.2 Clinical Evaluation

Radiological assessment involved the use of CT scans without contrast in the evaluation of subarachnoid hemorrhage and its associated complications, while CT angiography (CTA) localized and characterized intracranial aneurysms. Measurements pertinent to ventricular extension, hydrocephalus, and cerebral infarction were extracted from the CT-based radiological reports.

Figure 2. Figure 2 (a): Three-dimensional (3D) reconstructed computed tomography angiography (CTA) image showing a sculpture of a saccular aneurysm (outlined in red) on a branch of a major cerebral artery. The aneurysm is seen as a spherical outpouching with a clear-cut neck. Figure 2 (b): Closer enlarged view of the aneurysmal sac, better showing its relation to the adjacent vascular structures. The aneurysm is smooth in contour with no rupture or nearby hemorrhage. Figure 2 (c):Oblique 3D projection that further defines the anatomic orientation of the aneurysm in relation to nearby vessels. This projection is used to assess the size, shape of the aneurysm, and possible involvement of the neighboring branches.

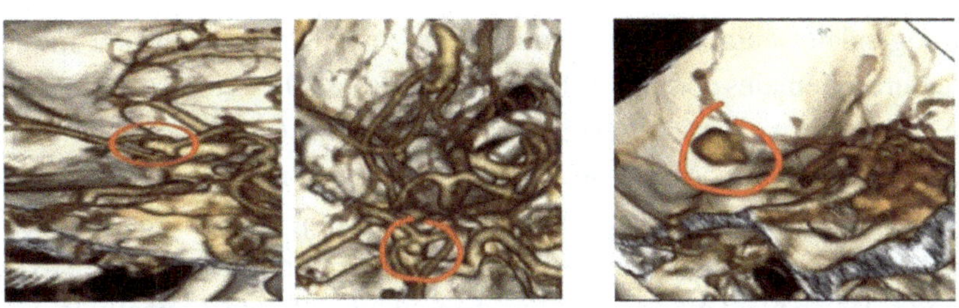

Figure 2 (a): Three-dimensional (3D) reconstructed computed tomography angiography (CTA) image showing a sculpture of a saccular aneurysm (outlined in red) on a branch of a major cerebral artery. The aneurysm is seen as a spherical outpouching with a clear-cut neck.

Figure 2 (b): Closer enlarged view of the aneurysmal sac, better showing its relation to the adjacent vascular structures. The aneurysm is smooth in contour with no rupture or nearby hemorrhage.

Figure 2 (c):Oblique 3D projection that further defines the anatomic orientation of the aneurysm in relation to nearby vessels. This projection is used to assess the size, shape of the aneurysm, and possible involvement of the neighboring branches.

Figure 2 (a) shows the image delineates in 3D a CTA scan which provides an imaging representation of a saccular (berry) aneurysm at the site of one of the branches of big arteries in the brain. The aneurysm is well defined in red, appearing like a rounded out bulging with a distinct neck connecting it to the parent artery. This supports an understanding of the complete spatial anatomy with regard to the morphology and location of the aneurysm within the cerebral vasculature. Figure 2 (b) shows the panel which gives a closer view of the same aneurysm, magnified. The increased zoom lets one see the smooth contours of the aneurysmal sac and its precise anatomy to nearby vessels. It is Tendencyof rupture-once again, it shows there is no surrounding hemorrhage or rough sac morphology. This visualization becomes crucial for planning and assessing the danger of preoperative rupturing. Figure 2 (c) shows an oblique 3D projection of the aneurysm and its surrounding vessels, allowing a more complex view of its anatomic orientation. The size and shape of the aneurysm can thus be evaluated with respect to its spatial alignment with nearby branching arteries. This view is particularly useful in planning a surgical or endovascular approach, as it highlights any potential involvement of nearby branches that might be influential for treatment strategies.

5. RESULTS

5.1 CT scan-Based Diagnosis of Aneurysm: A Retrospective Observational Study

The radiological presentations of the patients were tabulated to determine the key diagnostic features. Females comprised 65.9% of the cases. On a uniform basis, both hemorrhage and headache were observed in all the patients (100%) and, therefore, became primary diagnostic criteria on CT scanning. Seizure was encountered in 20.8% of the patients, generalized seizure being more frequent than focal seizure. CT scanning showed that 9.8% of the cohort exhibited hemorrhage extending to the ventricles, and 6.1% showed evidence of hydrocephalus. Infarcts, typically located near to the point where the aneurysm had occurred, were seen in 18.3% of patients. Loss of motor power was a common presentation, seen in 24.4% of patients. Hypertension was the most common of the vascular comorbidities, seen in 82.9% of the population studied.

Table 1.

Variables	Groups	Frequency	Percentage
Gender	male	28	34.1
	female	54	65.9
Headache	yes	82	100.0
	no	0	0.0
Seizures	generalized	14	17.1
	focal	3	3.7
	none	65	79.3
Hemorrhage	yes	82	100.0
	no	0	0.0
Ventricular extension	yes	8	9.8
	no	74	90.2
Hydrocephalus	yes	5	6.1
	no	77	93.9
Infarction	yes	15	18.3
	no	67	81.7
Motor power	No power	20	24.4
	power	62	75.6
Hypertension	yes	68	82.9
	no	14	17.1
Diabetes	yes	8	9.8
	no	74	90.2

5.2 CT-Detected Aneurysm Locations and Frequency

Anatomical localization of aneurysms detected on CT scans highlighted a distribution pattern. The right and left posterior communicating arteries (PCom), followed by the middle cerebral arteries (MCA), and anterior communicating artery (ACom) were the most frequently involved sites. Aneurysms were also present in less common sites classified under "other" like the basilar artery and anterior cerebral artery. These findings are the common vascular territories under risk for aneurysmal rupture on CT imaging.

5.3 Association between Aneurysm Location and Patient Characteristics

The association of aneurysm location with clinical parameters and patient demographics was examined in Table 2.

Table 2. Relationship Between Patient Variables and Aneurysm Location

Variables	Groups	Location						p-value
		1.00	2.00	3.00	4.00	5.00	6.00	
Age	<50 years	7(17.5)	9(22.5)	3(7.5)	6(15)	5(12.5)	10(25)	0.181
	≥50 years	3(7.1)	5(11.9)	5(11.9)	13(31)	2(4.8)	14(33.3)	
Gender	male	2(7.1)	5(17.9)	0(0)	6(21.4)	3(10.7)	12(42.9)	0.139
	female	8(14.8)	9(16.7)	8(14.8)	13(24.1)	4(7.4)	12(22.2)	
Symptoms duration	<5 days	7(11.5)	10(16.4)	8(13.1)	13(21.3)	6(9.8)	17(27.9)	0.578
	≥5 days	3(14.3)	4(19)	0(0)	6(28.6)	1(4.8)	7(33.3)	
GCS	<9	8(13.8)	9(15.5)	2(3.4)	17(29.3)	5(8.6)	17(29.3)	*0.029
	9-12	2(9.5)	5(23.8)	6(28.6)	1(4.8)	2(9.5)	5(23.8)	
	13-15	0(0)	0(0)	0(0)	1(33.3)	0(0)	2(66.7)	
Headache	yes	10(12.2)	14(17.1)	8(9.8)	19(23.2)	7(8.5)	24(29.3)	-
	no	0(0)	0(0)	0(0)	0(0)	0(0)	0(0)	
Seizures	generalized	6(42.9)	3(21.4)	2(14.3)	2(14.3)	0(0)	1(7.1)	0.003
	focal	0(0)	0(0)	0(0)	3(100)	0(0)	0(0)	
	none	4(6.2)	11(16.9)	6(9.2)	14(21.5)	7(10.8)	23(35.4)	
Hemorrhage	yes	10(12.2)	14(17.1)	8(9.8)	19(23.2)	7(8.5)	24(29.3)	-
	no	0(0)	0(0)	0(0)	0(0)	0(0)	0(0)	
Ventricular extension	yes	0(0)	4(50)	0(0)	2(25)	0(0)	2(25)	0.257
	no	10(13.5)	10(13.5)	8(10.8)	17(23)	7(9.5)	22(29.7)	
Hydrocephalus	yes	0(0)	3(60)	0(0)	0(0)	0(0)	2(40)	0.207
	no	10(13)	11(14.3)	8(10.4)	19(24.7)	7(9.1)	22(28.6)	
Infarction	yes	2(13.3)	1(6.7)	2(13.3)	4(26.7)	2(13.3)	4(26.7)	0.809
	no	8(11.9)	13(19.4)	6(9)	15(22.4)	5(7.5)	20(29.9)	
Motor power	No power	4(20)	2(10)	4(20)	2(10)	2(10)	6(30.6)	0.204
	power	6(9.7)	12(19.4)	4(6.5)	17(27.4)	5(8.1)	19(29)	
Decompressive surgery	yes	2(14.3)	2(14.3)	0(0)	4(28.6)	2(14.3)	4(28.6)	0.767
	no	8(11.8)	12(17.6)	8(11.8)	15(22.1)	5(7.4)	20(29.4)	

continued on following page

Table 2. Continued

Variables	Groups	Location						p-value
		1.00	2.00	3.00	4.00	5.00	6.00	
Hypertension	yes	7(10.3)	9(13.2)	7(10.3)	17(25)	5(7.4)	23(33.8)	0.073
	no	3(21.4)	5(35.7)	1(7.1)	2(14.3)	2(14.3)	1(7.1)	
diabetes	yes	2(25)	0(0)	0(0)	2(25)	2(25)	2(25)	0.244
	no	8(10.8)	14(18.9)	8(10.8)	17(23)	5(6.8)	22(29.7)	

5.4 Aneurysm Location vs. Surgical Management

The influence of the location of aneurysms on the type of surgical treatment was assessed. Decompressive surgery was performed most commonly in ACom and other atypical sites of aneurysms, although the relationship was statistically non-significant (p=0.767). The insertion of Ventriculoperitoneal (VP) shunts was a limited procedure and was performed in only 6.1% of cases and was not significantly related to the location of the aneurysm (p=0.849). These findings suggest that while some surgical trends may exist, aneurysm site itself does not determine the surgical approach in a statistically significant way as can be seen in Table 3 which displays the Management Strategy Comparison.

Table 3. Management Strategy vs Aneurysm Location

Variables	Groups	Location						Total	p-value
		1	2	3	4	5	6		
Decompressive surgery	yes	2(14.3)	2(14.3)	0(0)	4(28.6)	2(14.3)	4(28.6)	14(17.1)	0.767
	no	8(11.8)	12(17.6)	8(11.8)	15(22.1)	5(7.4)	20(29.4)	68(82.9)	
VP shunt	yes	0(0)	2(40)	0(0)	1(20)	0(0)	2(40)	5(6.1)	0.849
	no	10(13)	12(15.6)	8(10.4)	18(23.4)	7(9.1)	22(28.6)	77(93.9)	

6. DISCUSSION

A retrospective observational study evaluated the radiological and clinical features of patients with intracranial aneurysms in a tertiary care center with emphasis on CT-based imaging, focusing on aneurysm localization, clinical findings, and associations with patient characteristics. Our findings further strengthen the diagnostic role of non-contrast CT and CTA as vital imaging techniques within the context of SAH and for identifying aneurysm morphology and site. The predilection for the female sex (65.9 percent), thus corresponds to the established literature worldwide linking a higher incidence of cerebral aneurysms in women, probably due to differences in hormonal and vascular anatomy.

Both headache and hemorrhage were present in 100% of the sample, propounding them as the major presenting features. Seizures were observed in only 20.8% of these cases showing that generalized seizures have a statistically significant relationship with right posterior communicating artery (PCom) aneurysms, while only left middle cerebral artery (MCA) aneurysms were associated with the occurrence of focal seizures. These possible correlates of localized cortical irritation patterns with aneurysmal territories deserve some neurophysiological studies in the future.

The frequency of radiological complications such as ventricular hemorrhage (9.8%), hydrocephalus (6.1%), and infarction (18.3%) was low, but they were clinically relevant. Particularly, the presence of infarcts in the vicinity of the aneurysm indicates either poor perfusion or embolic phenomena. The neurological impact of either hemorrhage or infarction was also corroborated in a fair number of patients (24.4%) with loss of motor power.

The anatomical distribution of the aneurysms revealed that the anterior communicating artery (ACom), right and left posterior communicating arteries (PCom), and middle cerebral artery (MCA) were the sites most often implicated-consistent with the known tendency of aneurysms to form at arterial bifurcations due to hemodynamic stress. Importantly, worse scores on the Glasgow Coma Scale (GCS) were more frequently associated with ACom aneurysms and less common locations, suggesting that these sites may be associated with more severe clinical presentation.

No significant associations emerged between aneurysm locations and variables such as age or gender, or with vascular comorbidities like hypertension and diabetes, even as hypertension was prevalent in 82.9% of cases. This indicates that whereas hypertension may cause the formation of an aneurysm, this disease might be indifferent with respect to the site of occurrence or the immediate clinical outcome after their presentation.

7. CONCLUSION

This chapter identifies their generalizable value in regard to aneurysms. These investigations provide essential insight into the diagnosis, anatomical localization of the cerebral abnormality, and the planning of the surgical approach. Although, when sprinkled with the location relative to aneurysm - posterior communicating artery (PCom), middle cerebral artery (MCA), or anterior communicating artery (Acom) - and clinical variables such as seizure type or the neurological state of a patient

(Glasgow Coma Scale [GCS]), an idea begins to form that anatomical variations significantly influence how patients present and how they will make prognosis-wise. This means that even though placement brought some statistically insignificant association with age, gender, and other demographic variables, it did show that clinical details, particularly seizure clinical presentation types, and levels of consciousness were significantly defined by the site of the aneurysm. This means that location can add another layer to risk stratification models and treatment decision-making as it could influence not only immediate management but also long-term outcomes.

From this perspective, an individualized assessment of cerebral aneurysms involving advanced neuroimaging and clinical correlation appears to be one of the essential approaches. Such individual approaches may optimize surgical or interventional procedures to provide a new safe environment for recovery.

In order to reinforce and generalize these findings, future studies should focus on prospective studies involving larger, more diverse patient populations and long-term follow-up data. These studies will help to validate whether the aneurysm location is predictive of clinical presentation and outcome—thereby fine-tuning the protocols for planning treatment of aneurysms in neurosurgery and interventional radiology.

REFERENCES

Ahmed, S. H., Haris, M., Baseer, N., Saleema, A., Haris, S., Deeba, F., & Ahmad, S. H. (2021). Surgical Anatomy and Prevalence of Intracranial Aneurysms in Patients With Spontaneous Subarachnoid Hemorrhage. *Cureus*, *13*(12). Advance online publication. DOI: 10.7759/cureus.20463 PMID: 35070527

Azeem, S., Ashraf, M., Kamboh, U. A., Raza, M. A., Farooq, M., Cheema, H. A., Tariq, S., Choudhary, N., Hussain, S. S., & Ashraf, N. (2023). Association of ABO blood group with delayed cerebral ischemia and clinical outcomes following aneurysmal subarachnoid hemorrhage in Pakistan. *Asian Journal of Neurosurgery*, *18*(01), 108–116. DOI: 10.1055/s-0043-1760859 PMID: 37056873

Ballout, A. A., Prochilo, G., Kaneko, N., Li, C., Apfel, R., Hinman, J. D., & Liebeskind, D. S. (2024). Computational fluid dynamics in intracranial atherosclerotic disease. *Stroke: Vascular and Interventional Neurology*, *4*(1), e000792. DOI: 10.1161/SVIN.122.000792

Dai, W., Ling, H., Sun, Y., Wang, Y., Li, W., Yang, Y., Wu, L., & Hang, C. (2022). The comparison of Neuronavigation combined with CT three-dimensional angiography vs. CT angiography in the guidance of clipping treatment in distal intracranial aneurysm surgery: A retrospective clinical study. *Annals of Translational Medicine*, *10*(10), 572. DOI: 10.21037/atm-22-1749 PMID: 35722369

Din, M., Agarwal, S., Grzeda, M., Wood, D. A., Modat, M., & Booth, T. C. (2023). Detection of cerebral aneurysms using artificial intelligence: A systematic review and meta-analysis. *Journal of Neurointerventional Surgery*, *15*(3), 262–271. DOI: 10.1136/jnis-2022-019456 PMID: 36375834

Faraj, M. K., Hoz, S. S., & Mohammad, A. J. (2020). The use of three-dimensional anatomical patient-specific printed models in surgical clipping of intracranial aneurysm: A pilot study. *Surgical Neurology International*, *11*, 381. DOI: 10.25259/SNI_361_2020 PMID: 33408915

Ferreira, T., Awuah, W. A., Tan, J. K., Adebusoye, F. T., Ali, S. H., Bharadwaj, H. R., Aderinto, N., Fernandes, C., Zahid, M. J., & Abdul-Rahman, T. (2023). The current landscape of intracranial aneurysms in Africa: Management outcomes, challenges, and strategies—a narrative review. *Neurosurgical Review*, *46*(1), 194. DOI: 10.1007/s10143-023-02102-4 PMID: 37548805

Goertz, L., Kabbasch, C., Borggrefe, J., Hamisch, C., Telentschak, S., von Spreckelsen, N., Stavrinou, P., Timmer, M., Brinker, G., Goldbrunner, R., & Krischek, B. (2018). Preoperative three-dimensional angiography may reduce ischemic complications during clipping of ruptured intracranial aneurysms. *World Neurosurgery, 120*, e1163–e1170. DOI: 10.1016/j.wneu.2018.09.026 PMID: 30218797

Hacein-Bey, L., & Provenzale, J. M. (2011). Current imaging assessment and treatment of intracranial aneurysms. *AJR. American Journal of Roentgenology, 196*(1), 32–44. DOI: 10.2214/AJR.10.5329 PMID: 21178044

Haizel-Cobbina, J., Dada, O. E., Du, L., Zuckerman, S. L., & Dewan, M. C. (2023). A comparison of surgery waits times and postoperative length of hospital stay among patients with brain tumors by country-level income and healthcare system: A systematic review and meta-analysis. *World Neurosurgery, 177*, 152–164. DOI: 10.1016/j.wneu.2023.06.030 PMID: 37331477

Howard, B. M., Hu, R., Barrow, J. W., & Barrow, D. L. (2019). Comprehensive review of imaging of intracranial aneurysms and angiographically negative subarachnoid hemorrhage. *Neurosurgical Focus, 47*(6), E20. DOI: 10.3171/2019.9.FOCUS19653 PMID: 31786554

Júnior, J. R., Telles, J. P. M., da Silva, S. A., Iglesio, R. F., Brigido, M. M., Caldas, J. G. M. P., & Figueiredo, E. G. (2019). Epidemiological analysis of 1404 patients with intracranial aneurysm followed in a single Brazilian institution. *Surgical Neurology International, 10*, 249. DOI: 10.25259/SNI_443_2019 PMID: 31893150

Khokar, T. I., Cheema, Z. A., Fatima, I., Riaz, M., Qadri, H. M., & Bashir, A. (2024). Surgical outcomes of delayed clipping in ruptured intracranial aneurysms of anterior circulation: Experience from a low-middle-income country. *Pakistan Journal of Medical Sciences, 40*(12, PINS Suppl), S41–S46. DOI: 10.12669/pjms.40.12(PINS).11273 PMID: 39703957

Menna, G., Kolias, A., Esene, I. N., Barthélemy, E. J., Hoz, S., Laeke, T., Veiga Silva, A. C., Longo-Calderón, G. M., Baticulon, R. E., Zabala, J. P., Hassani, F. D., El Abbadi, N., Khan, M. M., Robertson, F. C., Thango, N., Cheresem, B., Ogando-Rivas, E., Roumy, L.-G., Karekezi, C., & Nicolosi, F. (2024). Reducing the gap in neurosurgical education in LMICs: A report of a non-profit educational program. *World Neurosurgery, 182*, e792–e797. DOI: 10.1016/j.wneu.2023.12.040 PMID: 38101536

Pettersson, S. D., Khorasanizadeh, M., Maglinger, B., Garcia, A., Wang, S. J., Tauss-ky, P., & Ogilvy, C. S. (2023). Trends in the age of patients treated for unruptured intracranial aneurysms from 1990 to 2020. *World Neurosurgery*, *178*, 233–240. DOI: 10.1016/j.wneu.2023.08.007 PMID: 37562685

Sarkodie, B. D., Jimah, B. B., Offei, A. K., Botwe, B., Anim, D., Mensah, Y. B., & Brakohiapa, E. K. (2022). Challenges of practicing neuro-endovascular interventions in a resource-limited country; Ghana in focus. *Neurological Sciences*, *43*(9), 5451–5457. DOI: 10.1007/s10072-022-06222-5 PMID: 35729440

Shoukat, S., Tabassum, S., & Shahbaz, H. (2024). Frequency of Cerebral Aneurysm in patients with subarachnoid hemorrhage on CT Cerebral Angiography. *Pakistan Journal of Medical Sciences*, *40*(9), 1975. PMID: 39416605

Stumpo, V., Staartjes, V. E., Esposito, G., Serra, C., Regli, L., Olivi, A., & Sturiale, C. L. (2021). Machine learning and intracranial aneurysms: from detection to outcome prediction. In *Machine Learning in Clinical Neuroscience: Foundations and Applications* (pp. 319–331). Springer International Publishing.

Tétinou, F., Kanmounye, U. S., Sadler, S., Nitcheu, I., Oriaku, A. J., Ndajiwo, A. B., & Bankole, N. D. A. (2021). Cerebral aneurysms in Africa: A scoping review. *Interdisciplinary Neurosurgery : Advanced Techniques and Case Management*, *26*, 101291. DOI: 10.1016/j.inat.2021.101291

Ueda, D., Yamamoto, A., Nishimori, M., Shimono, T., Doishita, S., Shimazaki, A., Katayama, Y., Fukumoto, S., Choppin, A., Shimahara, Y., & Miki, Y. (2019). Deep learning for MR angiography: Automated detection of cerebral aneurysms. *Radiology*, *290*(1), 187–194. DOI: 10.1148/radiol.2018180901 PMID: 30351253

Vadhavekar, N. H., Sabzvari, T., Laguardia, S., Sheik, T., Prakash, V., Gupta, A., & Patiño, B. B. R.Sr. (2024). Advancements in imaging and neurosurgical techniques for brain tumor resection: A comprehensive review. *Cureus*, *16*(10). Advance online publication. DOI: 10.7759/cureus.72745 PMID: 39618625

Wang, B., Liao, X., Ni, Y., Zhang, L., Liang, J., Wang, J., Liu, Y., Sun, X., Ou, Y., Wu, Q., Shi, L., Yang, Z., & Lan, L. (2022). High-resolution medical image reconstruction based on residual neural network for diagnosis of cerebral aneurysm. *Frontiers in Cardiovascular Medicine*, *9*, 1013031. DOI: 10.3389/fcvm.2022.1013031 PMID: 36337881

Wang, G. X.. (2021). Advanced neuroimaging in surgical planning for cerebral aneurysms. *Neurosurgical Review*, *44*, 1997–2010.

Zhou, C., Zheng, L., Huang, W., Cheng, X., & Zhang, L. (2024). CT Angiography Image Postprocessing and Data Analysis. In *Whole Body Computed Tomography Angiography* (pp. 43–65). Springer Nature Singapore. DOI: 10.1007/978-981-97-1733-0_2

Chapter 3

Clinical Management of Intracranial Aneurysms: Enhancing Diagnostic Accuracy and Surgical Precision

Amanullah Khan
https://orcid.org/0000-0003-1808-5084
Liaquat National Hospital, Pakistan

Salman Shareef
Liaquat National Hospital, Pakistan

Mehak Hafiz
Liaquat National Hospital, Pakistan

ABSTRACT

Managing intracranial aneurysms is a tightrope balancing act for any neurosurgeon, especially in low- and middle- income countries where lack of resources threatens an optimal care. A retrospective study was carried out to observe how a CT-based anatomical mapping system influenced the diagnostic accuracy and surgical precision in managing cerebral aneurysms at a tertiary care center in Karachi, Pakistan. Analyzing data from 82 patients showed a female preponderance (65.9%) and a high incidence of hypertension in relation to risk factors (82.9%). All patients presented with acute hemorrhage and headache. CT localized the aneurysms with precision and yielded statistically significant correlations between GCS and aneurysm sites (p = 0.029) and between types of seizures and aneurysm locations (p = 0.003). Cerebral infarction highly correlated with decompressive surgery (p < 0.001). These findings further elaborate how the state-of-the-art CT-based anatomical mapping allows for early diagnosis, risk stratification, and targeted surgical intervention.

DOI: 10.4018/979-8-3373-2807-2.ch003

1. INTRODUCTION

The clinical management of intracranial aneurysms goes a long way in innovative approach changes as to what has happened in recent times with diagnostic imaging and minimally invasive surgery. Treatment of ruptured intracranial aneurysms still makes it an important neurosurgical emergency as, without treatment, mortality ranges up to 50 percent (Deshmukh *et. al,* 2024). The modernization of protocols emphasizes rapid collaboration between neurosurgeons, neuroradiologists, and neurocritical care teams for maximum benefit to patients, especially when dealing with aneurysms within that critical 72-hour window for vasospasm prevention (Trakolis *et.al*, 2024).

Endovascular methods have come to the fore as mainstream procedures in case of ruptured aneurysms, with randomized study evidence showing that these methods are safer than clipping. Complexities can only be cured through open surgery in the advanced case, where 3D rotational angiography is additionally used for intraoperative guidance. Flow-diverting stents and intrasaccular devices allow for target reconstruction of the vessels involved in the aneurysm. It is the emphasis of the ARISE I Consensus that centralized care is given in high-volume centers where multidisciplinary teams partakes in integrated microsurgical-endovascular experience for more optimum outcomes (Tjoumakaris *et.al*, 2024).

These advancements underline the better combination of AI diagnostic systems with advanced imaging protocols and personalized surgical strategies to hemispheric aspects in intracranial aneurysms. Further studies continue through national radiographic registries and optical coherence tomography in higher refinement towards rupture risk stratification and the choice of treatment methods (Adamchic, 2025).

Figure 1. Brain Aneurysm

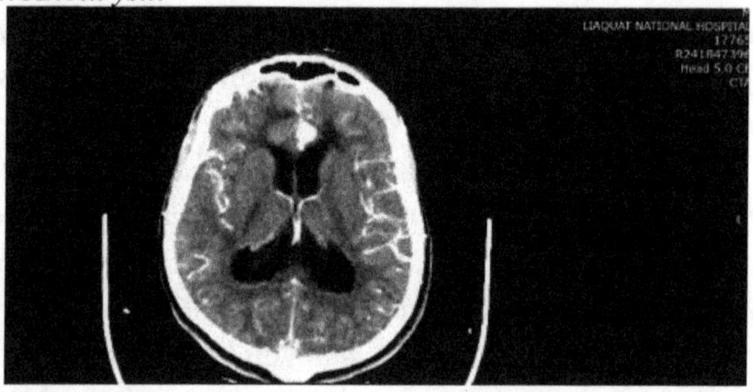

Figure 1 shows the axial section of an enhanced CT Angiography scan of the brain performed at Liaquat National Hospital. The ordinary CT study provides cross-sectional images of the brain vasculature and ventricle as applied to determine vascular pathologies like aneurysms, arteriovenous malformations, and occlusions. The current scan has revealed a hyperdense round structure that is situated just anterior to the third ventricle and between the lateral ventricles near the midline.

Anatomically, this site corresponds to the ACommA, which is a site commonly implicated for intracranial aneurysm development. The increased brightness of this structure may suggest contrast in the aneurysmal sac, in favor of the diagnosis of an unruptured aneurysm. Excellent contrast filling also allows good visualization of the surrounding vessels; no immediate signs of hemorrhage or midline shift are seen, which suggests that the lesion was stable at the time of imaging. Given the appearance of the lateral ventricles to be prominent but with no signs of acute hydrocephalus, this CTA quickly captured during the vascular phase would provide excellent aneurysm detection. Clinically, the identification of an ACommA aneurysm on axial CTA is of prime importance, as untreated aneurysms at this location may rupture and lead to potentially fatal SAH. Thus, the precise localization and characterization via imaging of the aneurysm would permit the timely planning of intervention procedures like endovascular coiling or microsurgical clipping before any catastrophic outcome.

Intracranial aneurysms have been evolving considerably over the past few years. This is mainly due to modern advances in the area of imaging modality especially given multi-modality imaging of cutting-edge centers along with multi-disciplinary care. But ruptured aneurysms still remain a neurosurgical emergency that is lethal when not operated upon, taking into consideration the critical time windows for identification and intervention. Endovascular therapy might become a safer and more focused strategy for treatment, especially if facilitated by tools like 3D angiography and imaging, performed at high-volume specialized centers. The provided CTA scan signifies how today imaging is being applied in recognizing the unruptured aneurysms before rupturing, especially the unruptured communicate artery (ACommA). Research continues to refine risk stratification-treat selection algorithms, but it is early detection and precision-based management that remain at the core of improving patient outcomes in the management of intracranial aneurysms.

2. LITERATURE REVIEW

An aneurysm inside the skull is represented by local dilations of cerebral arteries with very high risks of rupture and subarachnoid hemorrhage; therefore, the morbidity and mortality are constantly high. Progressively changing techniques of imaging, approaches to therapy, and the management of intracranial aneurysms based on expert consensus have improved arguably the most in the areas of detection, treatment planning, and outcome pathways for the patient. The review discusses recent developments in four major avenues: diagnostic innovation, intraoperative tools for the surgical precision intervention, guideline-directed intervention, and eventual adoption of new technologies for the optimization of clinical workflows and processes.

In current days, CTA is often regarded as the backbone for the diagnosis of intracranial aneurysms owing to high-resolution images, noninvasiveness, and ease of availability in emergency settings. It has a reported sensitivity of 0.84 and a specificity of 0.85, thus reliably detecting aneurysms while limiting false positives. The joining of CTA with the open-source imaging platform 3D-Slicer greatly increases three-dimensional visualization of the aneurysm and surrounding vascular structures (He et.al, 2025). This fusion allows for a precise definition of aneurysm morphology and parent artery anatomy, which in turn significantly enhances preoperative planning. With a Kappa statistic of 0.865 for the assessment of the aneurysm-bearing artery, its credibility and consistency between observers make it an asset in neurosurgical diagnostics(Chen et.al, 2018)

MRA presents an alternative route for vascular imaging optimally free of radiations, superior to CTA in specificity but lower in sensitivity. The significant downsides of MRA are that it might overlook smaller or more complicated aneurysms; therefore, it is still significant for non-emergency conditions, long-term follow-ups, and those with contraindications for iodinated contrast agents or radiation exposure. MRA's usefulness is limited when it comes to making quick decisions during acute presentations, hence rendering it less desirable in emergency neurosurgical situations (Mousa *et.al*, 2025).

It's really great to be able to say that it's gone totally refined where it is related Adnan condensation and treatment through clipping of aneurysms. Clipping vessels are confirmed by being Intraoperative Indocyanine Green (ICG) angiography, where all the time these need to be completed to show indirect flow in those vessels. Adjusting tension clips serve as yet another breakthrough: compression is adaptable and diminishes possible stenosis or injury to the parent artery (Hoh et.al, 2023). In the mentioned study of Zhuhai Hospital from 2025, the result of intraoperative CTA-3D-Slicer fusion models was a significant reduction in the number of bone grindings-per-touch operation time-which resulted in a complete clipping rate of 100%, in the 25 cases of documented aneurysms(Tjoumakari et.al, 2024).

Fenestrated clips provide a more personal approach for the preservation of the perforating vessels while achieving the occlusion of the aneurysm in those complex aneurysms whose perforating vessels traverse near or through the aneurysm sac. Furthermore, the Doppler ultrasound used intraoperatively allows one to create a real-time flow of blood in the relevant vessels and therefore ensure that perfusion is adequate at the end of the process while preventing ischemic complications. Collectively, these technologies help in improving the effectiveness of the procedure while reducing neurological deficits.

The consensus has built a guideline for the aneurysms that focused mainly on evidence and expert consensus. Evidence was taken from many guidelines, including the American Heart Association/American Stroke Association (AHA/ASA) 2023 guideline, which emphasizes patient-centered approaches to the risk of rupture, anatomical location, and size. Endovascular coiling is of choice in aneurysms located in the posterior circulation being more inaccessible and riskier than surgical management in such regions. Surgical clipping is, however, the treatment of choice for middle cerebral artery (MCA) aneurysms, where direct surgical access allows more effective management (Hoh et.al, 2023). .

AI-derived rupture risk prediction models using large databases for improved clinical decision-making are the main points of the 2024 ARISE I Consensus. Nationwide radiographic registries are also called for to standardize imaging protocols and improve outcome tracking across institutions. The two documents also underscore the importance of high-volume centers and teams with multi-disciplinary specialties in optimally improving outcomes, especially among complex aneurysm cases and ruptured cases (Wang and Huang, 2024).

Noninvasive assessment of aneurysm pathology is a promise that emerging diagnostic technologies keep offering. These include Optical Coherence Tomography (OCT) and 3 Tesla MRI vessel wall imaging, which are both currently under evaluation as potential techniques to assess aneurysm wall integrity, an important parameter for predicting rupture. These two modalities are, in fact, almost on the verge of entering clinical practice; should a few larger clinical validation studies occur with these technologies, they would change the way risk assessment is done (Hu *et.al*, 2025).

The advancements discussed in this literature review have been propelled towards the diagnosis and surgical treatment of intracranial aneurysms through state-of-the-art imaging innovations, intraoperative technologies, and developing treatment guidelines. Their combination like CTA with 3D-Slicer has benefitted visualization and planning and quality of imaging. From the surgical perspective, using ICG angiography, fenestrated clips, and real-time ultrasound has improved precision in surgery. Consensus guidelines that have come up recently also provide for AI-assisted rupture prediction models and central data registries in order to standardize the practice across institutions. The emerging experimental imaging tools and AI applications will increasingly make the future of treatment-specified to the person, predictive, and precise in the aneurysm care area (Mousa *et.al*, 2025).

3. DATA COLLECTION

The research data collection was done retrospectively at the Department of Neurosurgery, Liaquat National Hospital and Medical College (LNHMC), Karachi, Pakistan. Since the hospital is one of the premier tertiary care centers in the country with a specialized neurovascular surgery unit and with high end imaging modalities, LNHMC was aptly placed to collect all relevant clinical and radiological data. Institutional approval was obtained from the institutional ethics review board, and all procedures were in accord with ethical standards and patient confidentiality protocols.

3.1 Study Duration and Population

The dataset consists of patients admitted from January 2010 to December 2024, all of whom were diagnosed with intracranial aneurysms—either ruptured or unruptured—based on their clinical symptoms and CT scan results. In total, 82 patients were included in the study. These individuals were selected through non-probability consecutive sampling using hospital records and radiology archives.

3.2 Inclusion Criteria

- Individuals of any sex aged 18 years or older.
- A confirmed diagnosis of intracranial aneurysm established through Computed Tomography Angiography (CTA) and/or Digital Subtraction Angiography (DSA)
- Patients who received neurosurgical treatment, such as clipping or decompression procedures.
- Complete availability of both radiological and surgical records.

3.3 Exclusion Criteria

- Patients whose imaging data or clinical documentation was incomplete.
- Cases involving non-saccular vascular abnormalities, such as arteriovenous malformations or cavernomas.
- Patients who were treated solely with endovascular methods without undergoing preoperative surgical planning.

3.4 Clinical Evaluation

The clinical and surgical parameters captured included patient demographics (age and sex), comorbid risks (hypertension, type ll diabetes mellitus, current or previous smoking history, blood group), and neurological presentation-attainment like Glasgow Coma Scale (GCS) score at admission, seizures, cranial nerve deficits, and annoying signs indicating raised intracranial pressure. Aneurysmal subarachnoid hemorrhage severity was graded according to the World Federation of Neurosurgical Societies (WFNS) scale and Hunt and Hess classification. The surgical details encompassed the approach (pterional, sub frontal, or interhemispheric); the type of intervention (aneurysm clipping, decompressive craniectomy, hematoma evacuation) as well as complications in the perioperative period: such as vasospasm, infarction, or delayed cerebral ischemia (DCI). The postoperative outcomes were registered by the Glasgow Outcome Score (GOS) both at discharge and at a three-month follow-up.

3.5 Statistical Analysis

Data were analyzed using SPSS Chai Square method. Descriptive statistics were computed for categorical variables and expressed as frequencies and percentages. Associations between clinical variables and aneurysm location, management strategies, and complications were analyzed using chi-square tests or Fisher's exact test, where appropriate. A p-value < 0.05 was considered statistically significant.

4. MATERIAL AND METHODS

4.1 Study Design and Setting

This retrospective observational study was carried out at the Liaquat National Medical Hospital Karachi, Pakistan, with the objective of assessing the various strategies for the operative management and an evaluation of clinical outcomes of patients who presented with cerebral aneurysms. Ethical clearance from the institutional review board was obtained for the study prior to collecting data. The locations of the aneurysms were categorized into six anatomical areas, as determined by CT and angiographic findings: right posterior communicating artery (Rt PCom), left posterior communicating artery (Lt PCom), right middle cerebral artery (Rt MCA), left middle cerebral artery (Lt MCA), anterior communicating artery (ACom), and other locations, which included such less common sites as the basilar tip and internal carotid artery (ICA) bifurcation.

4.2 Clinical and Radiological Evaluation

Radiological investigations included CT imaging without contrast for evaluation of hemorrhage and CT angiography for localization of aneurysms. Measurement records for ventricular extension, hydrocephalus, and cerebral infarction came from radiological reports.

4.3 Surgical Management

Patients underwent aneurysm clipping, decompressive craniectomy, or other neurosurgical interventions as clinically indicated. Additional procedures such as VP shunting and external ventricular drainage were performed based on the development of hydrocephalus or raised intracranial pressure as shown in Figure 2.

Figure 2. development of hydrocephalus or raised intracranial pressure Figure 2 (a): Three-dimensional (3D) reconstructed computed tomography angiography (CTA) image showing a sculpture of a saccular aneurysm (outlined in red) on a branch of a major cerebral artery. The aneurysm is seen as a spherical outpouching with a clear-cut neck. Figure 2 (b): Closer enlarged view of the aneurysmal sac, better showing its relation to the adjacent vascular structures. The aneurysm is smooth in contour with no rupture or nearby hemorrhage. Figure 2 (c):Oblique 3D projection that further defines the anatomic orientation of the aneurysm in relation to nearby vessels. This projection is used to assess the size, shape of the aneurysm, and possible involvement of the neighboring branches.

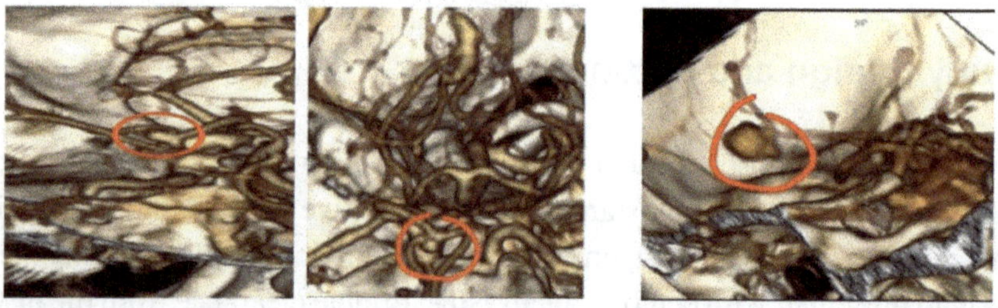

Figure 2 (a): Three-dimensional (3D) reconstructed computed tomography angiography (CTA) image showing a sculpture of a saccular aneurysm (outlined in red) on a branch of a major cerebral artery. The aneurysm is seen as a spherical outpouching with a clear-cut neck.

Figure 2 (b): Closer enlarged view of the aneurysmal sac, better showing its relation to the adjacent vascular structures. The aneurysm is smooth in contour with no rupture or nearby hemorrhage.

Figure 2 (c):Oblique 3D projection that further defines the anatomic orientation of the aneurysm in relation to nearby vessels. This projection is used to assess the size, shape of the aneurysm, and possible involvement of the neighboring branches.

4.4 Outcome Measures and Complications

Postoperative outcomes evaluated were neurological improvement (with motor power), complications (wound infection, need for external ventricular drainage), and associations with comorbidities and CT scan findings.

5. RESULTS

The study utilized a retrospective observational study to analyze patients undergoing surgery for cerebral aneurysm treatment at a tertiary care facility in Karachi. Descriptive statistics were utilized for describing the comorbidities, presentation, and demographics of the patient when analyzing the datasets. These were presented in percentage and frequency forms, particularly Table 1. Inferential statistics—presumably Chi-square or Fisher's Exact Test—were also applied in the study as per the distribution of the sample and expected cell counts. These were employed in order to ascertain associations between aneurysm location, patient demographics, clinical severity, and management outcomes. P-values were calculated in order to determine statistical significance, whereby the usual cut-off was $p < 0.05$. Moreover, cross-tabulation procedures were utilized in an effort to present data contrast between categorical variables, such as aneurysm site and complication development or the need for surgery.

Table 1. Descriptive statistics of patients' presenting features

Variables	Groups	Frequency	Percentage
Gender	male	28	34.1
	female	54	65.9
Headache	yes	82	100.0
	no	0	0.0
Seizures	generalized	14	17.1
	focal	3	3.7
	none	65	79.3
Hemorrhage	yes	82	100.0
	no	0	0.0
Ventricular extension	yes	8	9.8
	no	74	90.2

continued on following page

Table 1. Continued

Variables	Groups	Frequency	Percentage
Hydrocephalus	yes	5	6.1
	no	77	93.9
Infarction	yes	15	18.3
	no	67	81.7
Motor power	No power	20	24.4
	power	62	75.6
Hypertension	yes	68	82.9
	no	14	17.1
Diabetes	yes	8	9.8
	no	74	90.2

This table gives a summary of the primitive characteristics of the patient group. It demonstrates that females comprised the majority (65.9%), and headache and hemorrhage were universal presentation signs (100%), which determines their importance in clinical diagnosis. Seizure was observed to be present in about 21% of cases where generalized seizures were found to be more prevalent than focal seizures. Infarction (18.3%) and hydrocephalus (6.1%) were both relatively uncommon, implying that most patients had not been affected by severe secondary brain damage at presentation. Notably, hypertension was found in 82.9% of patients, underlining its probable role as a significant vascular risk factor. Motor power was intact in 75.6% of patients, indicating that many patients must have maintained functional neurological status in the face of bleeding as shown in Figure 3.

Figure 3. Frequency Distribution of Aneurysm Location

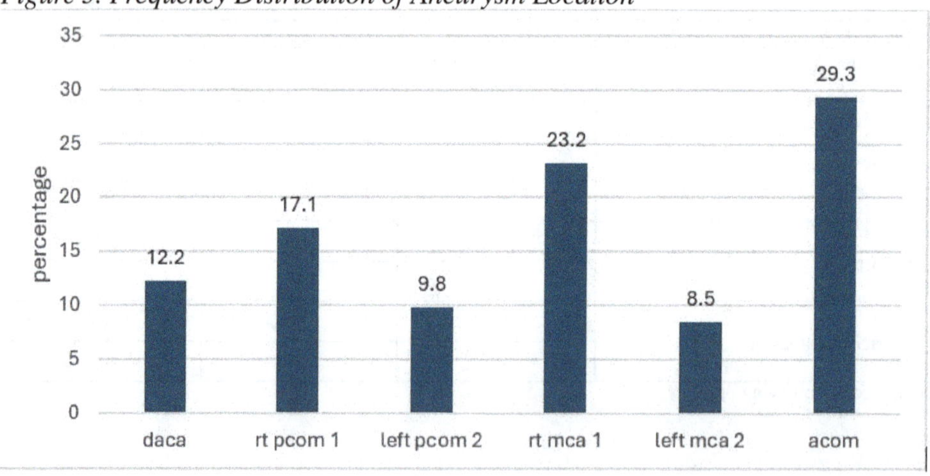

Although the illustrative figure is not provided here, the aneurysm locations discussed are right and left posterior communicating arteries (PCom), middle cerebral arteries (MCA), anterior communicating artery (ACom), and a group designated as "other." These form the anatomical basis for the following discussions on how location influences clinical presentation and management.

Table 2. Relationship Between Patient Variables and Aneurysm Location

Variables	**Groups**	**Location**						**p-value**
		1.00	**2.00**	**3.00**	**4.00**	**5.00**	**6.00**	
Age	<50 years	7(17.5)	9(22.5)	3(7.5)	6(15)	5(12.5)	10(25)	0.181
	≥50 years	3(7.1)	5(11.9)	5(11.9)	13(31)	2(4.8)	14(33.3)	
Gender	male	2(7.1)	5(17.9)	0(0)	6(21.4)	3(10.7)	12(42.9)	0.139
	female	8(14.8)	9(16.7)	8(14.8)	13(24.1)	4(7.4)	12(22.2)	
Symptoms duration	<5 days	7(11.5)	10(16.4)	8(13.1)	13(21.3)	6(9.8)	17(27.9)	0.578
	≥5 days	3(14.3)	4(19)	0(0)	6(28.6)	1(4.8)	7(33.3)	
GCS	<9	8(13.8)	9(15.5)	2(3.4)	17(29.3)	5(8.6)	17(29.3)	*0.029
	9-12	2(9.5)	5(23.8)	6(28.6)	1(4.8)	2(9.5)	5(23.8)	
	13-15	0(0)	0(0)	0(0)	1(33.3)	0(0)	2(66.7)	
Headache	yes	10(12.2)	14(17.1)	8(9.8)	19(23.2)	7(8.5)	24(29.3)	-
	no	0(0)	0(0)	0(0)	0(0)	0(0)	0(0)	
Seizures	generalized	6(42.9)	3(21.4)	2(14.3)	2(14.3)	0(0)	1(7.1)	0.003
	focal	0(0)	0(0)	0(0)	3(100)	0(0)	0(0)	
	none	4(6.2)	11(16.9)	6(9.2)	14(21.5)	7(10.8)	23(35.4)	
Hemorrhage	yes	10(12.2)	14(17.1)	8(9.8)	19(23.2)	7(8.5)	24(29.3)	-
	no	0(0)	0(0)	0(0)	0(0)	0(0)	0(0)	
Ventricular extension	yes	0(0)	4(50)	0(0)	2(25)	0(0)	2(25)	0.257
	no	10(13.5)	10(13.5)	8(10.8)	17(23)	7(9.5)	22(29.7)	
Hydrocephalus	yes	0(0)	3(60)	0(0)	0(0)	0(0)	2(40)	0.207
	no	10(13)	11(14.3)	8(10.4)	19(24.7)	7(9.1)	22(28.6)	
Infarction	yes	2(13.3)	1(6.7)	2(13.3)	4(26.7)	2(13.3)	4(26.7)	0.809
	no	8(11.9)	13(19.4)	6(9)	15(22.4)	5(7.5)	20(29.9)	
Motor power	No power	4(20)	2(10)	4(20)	2(10)	2(10)	6(30.6)	0.204
	power	6(9.7)	12(19.4)	4(6.5)	17(27.4)	5(8.1)	19(29)	
Decompressive surgery	yes	2(14.3)	2(14.3)	0(0)	4(28.6)	2(14.3)	4(28.6)	0.767
	no	8(11.8)	12(17.6)	8(11.8)	15(22.1)	5(7.4)	20(29.4)	

continued on following page

Table 2. Continued

Variables	Groups	Location						p-value
		1.00	2.00	3.00	4.00	5.00	6.00	
Hypertension	yes	7(10.3)	9(13.2)	7(10.3)	17(25)	5(7.4)	23(33.8)	0.073
	no	3(21.4)	5(35.7)	1(7.1)	2(14.3)	2(14.3)	1(7.1)	
diabetes	yes	2(25)	0(0)	0(0)	2(25)	2(25)	2(25)	0.244
	no	8(10.8)	14(18.9)	8(10.8)	17(23)	5(6.8)	22(29.7)	

This table evaluates the association between location of aneurysm and patient characteristics. Neither age nor gender were statistically associated with aneurysm location, but older patients had ACom and miscellaneous aneurysms. Surprisingly, Glasgow Coma Scale (GCS) score was significantly associated with location (p=0.029)—patients with lower GCS score more often had ACom or "other" aneurysms, suggesting these are more severely presenting. Alternatively, seizure types were significantly correlated with aneurysm location (p=0.003)—generalized seizures more frequently with right PCom aneurysms, and focal seizures exclusively with left MCA aneurysms. The other clinical factors of hydrocephalus, hypertension, or infarction were not significantly different by aneurysm location.

Table 3. Management Strategy vs Aneurysm Location

Variables	Groups	Location						Total	p-value
		1	2	3	4	5	6		
Decompressive surgery	yes	2(14.3)	2(14.3)	0(0)	4(28.6)	2(14.3)	4(28.6)	14(17.1)	0.767
	no	8(11.8)	12(17.6)	8(11.8)	15(22.1)	5(7.4)	20(29.4)	68(82.9)	
VP shunt	yes	0(0)	2(40)	0(0)	1(20)	0(0)	2(40)	5(6.1)	0.849
	no	10(13)	12(15.6)	8(10.4)	18(23.4)	7(9.1)	22(28.6)	77(93.9)	

This table assesses whether therapeutic interventions like decompressive surgery or ventriculoperitoneal (VP) shunt placement were associated with aneurysm location. There were no statistically significant findings ($p > 0.05$), although there was a trend in which most decompressive surgeries were performed for ACom and "other" aneurysms. VP shunts were rarely used overall (6.1%), and no location was specifically associated with increased use.

5.1 CT Findings vs Surgical Management

CT findings were compared with surgery, results were more conclusive. Infarction was most immediately associated with decompressive surgery ($p < 0.001$)—surgical decompression was more likely to be performed in infarct patients. Similarly, hydrocephalus strongly predicted VP shunt placement ($p < 0.001$), and this indicated shunting as a therapeutic measure for the alleviation of increased intracranial pressure due to CSF accumulation. Ventricular extension was on the margin with VP shunt insertion ($p = 0.072$), but not with decompressive surgery.

Table 4. Postoperative Complications

Variables	Groups	Decompressive surgery		p-value	VP Shunt		p-value
		Yes	No		Yes	no	
Ventricular extension	yes	0(0)	8(11.8)	0.340	2(40)	6(7.8)	0.072
	no	14(100)	60(88.2)		3(60)	71(92.2)	
Hyrdocephalus	yes	0(0)	5(7.4)	0.582	4(80)	1(1.3)	<0.001
	no	14(100)	63(92.6)		1(20)	76(98.7)	
Infarction	yes	12(85.7)	3(4.4)	<0.001	1(20)	14(18.2)	1.000
	no	2(14.3)	65(95.6)		4(80)	63(81.8)	

This table details the complications which include wound infection or the need for Extra Ventricular Drainage (EVD). Wound infections, showing an occurrence rate of 8.5%, were found more to accompany Left MCA and ACom aneurysms, which gave a p value of less than 0.001. EVD was used borderline ($p=0.096$), and most frequent in the Right PCom and ACom aneurysm patients. The trend might be due to the route available anatomically for access or the complexity of these types of aneurysms.

5.2 Complications vs Comorbidities and Clinical Findings

This section evaluates the possibility that complications were associated with comorbid conditions or initial clinical status. Patient-ventricular extension predicted significantly the need for EVD ($p=0.018$). Hypertension, diabetes mellitus, and hydrocephalus did not predict significantly wound infections or use of EVD. GCS scores were not significantly associated with complications, although a trend was observed such that patients with moderate GCS scores (9-12) underwent more interventions like EVD or wound management than patients showing very low or very high GCS scores.

Table 5. Complications

Variables	Groups	Location						total	p-value
		1	2	3	4	5	6		
wound infection	yes	0(0)	0(0)	4(57.1)	3(42.9)	0(0)	0(0)	7(8.5)	<0.001
	no	10(13.3)	14(18.7)	4(5.3)	16(21.3)	7(9.3)	24(32)	75(91.5)	
Extra ventricular drainage	yes	0(0)	3(42.9)	2(28.6)	0(0)	0(0)	2(28.6)	7(8.5)	0.096
	no	10(13.3)	11(14.7)	6(8)	19(25.3)	7(9.3)	22(29.3)	75(91.5)	

Table 6. Complications versus comorbid, CT findings, GCS

Variables	Groups	Wound infection		p-value	Extra ventricular drainage		p-value
		Yes	No		Yes	no	
Hypertension	yes	6(8.8)	62(91.2)	1.000	5(7.4)	63(92.6)	0.342
	no	1(7.1)	75(91.5)		2(14.3)	12(85.7)	
Diabetes	yes	0(0)	8(100)	1.000	0(0)	8(100)	1.000
	no	7(9.5)	67(90.5)		7(9.5)	67(90.5)	
Ventricular extension	yes	0(0)	8(100)	1.000	3(37.5)	5(62.5)	*0.018
	no	7(9.5)	67(90.5)		4(5.4)	70(94.6)	
Hyrdocephalus	yes	0(0)	5(100)	1.000			
	no	7(9.1)	70(90.9)				
Infarction	yes						
	no						
GCS	<9	3(5.2)	55(94.8)	0.150	2(3.4)	56(96.6)	0.065
	9-12	4(19)	17(81)		5(23.8)	16(76.2)	
	13-15	0(0)	3(100)		0(0)	3(100)	

6. CONCLUSION

Management of intracranial aneurysms has changed greatly over time with the evolution of diagnostic imaging and surgical methods. It is evident in this study that CT-based anatomical mapping systems help to locate an aneurysm more clearly and plan surgery better for improved patient outcomes. Associations that are statistically significant between clinical parameters and aneurysm characteristics underline the importance of risk assessment and intervention strategy for the individual. A multidisciplinary approach incorporating advanced imaging, such as CTA and 3D visualization, with consensus guidelines can improve diagnostic and surgical precision. Most of these innovations are of great help in resource-poor settings whereby they ensure early detection, loss stratification, and intervention. These improvements in imaging, intraprocedural adjuncts, and AI-based risk paradigms will continue to favor further customization and optimal management of intracranial aneurysms, resulting in reduced morbidity and mortality associated with this life-threatening entity.

Lastly, this research reaffirms the central role of careful preoperative imaging, early surgical treatment, and the importance of vascular risk factor identification to maximize patient outcomes. These findings can guide future aneurysm treatment protocols and resource utilization in similar healthcare settings.

REFERENCES

Adamchic, I. (2025). Enhancing Intracranial Aneurysm Detection with Artificial Intelligence in Radiology.

Chen, X., Liu, Y., Tong, H., Dong, Y., Ma, D., Xu, L., & Yang, C. (2018). Meta-analysis of computed tomography angiography versus magnetic resonance angiography for intracranial aneurysm. *Medicine, 97*(20), e10771. DOI: 10.1097/MD.0000000000010771 PMID: 29768368

Deshmukh, A. S., Priola, S. M., Katsanos, A. H., Scalia, G., Costa Alves, A., Srivastava, A., & Hawkes, C. (2024). The management of intracranial aneurysms: Current trends and future directions. *Neurology International, 16*(1), 74–94. DOI: 10.3390/neurolint16010005 PMID: 38251053

He, C., Cao, G., Yang, Y., Zhong, Q., Lei, Y., Tan, X., Lin, X., Chen, Y., & Sun, W. (2025). A study on the therapeutic effect of precise clipping of intracranial aneurysms assisted by CTA and 3D-slicer software. *Frontiers in Surgery, 12*, 1535585. DOI: 10.3389/fsurg.2025.1535585 PMID: 40035066

Hoh, B. L., Ko, N. U., Amin-Hanjani, S., Chou, S. H. Y., Cruz-Flores, S., Dangayach, N. S., & Welch, B. G. (2023). 2023 guideline for the management of patients with aneurysmal subarachnoid hemorrhage: A guideline from the American Heart Association/American Stroke Association. *Stroke, 54*(7), e314–e370. DOI: 10.1161/STR.0000000000000436 PMID: 37212182

Hu, T., Ling, R., & Zhu, Y. (2025). Advancements in imaging of intracranial atherosclerotic disease: Beyond the arterial lumen to the vessel wall. *Reviews in the Neurosciences, 36*(3), 229–241. DOI: 10.1515/revneuro-2024-0076 PMID: 39565965

Mousa, A. H., Scalia, G., Ahmed, N., Figueiredo, E. G., de Sena Barbosa, M. G., Khan, M. M., & Chaurasia, B. (2025). The evolution of intracranial aneurysm clipping: A historical perspective. *Annals of Medicine and Surgery (London), 87*(4), 2229–2233. DOI: 10.1097/MS9.0000000000003162 PMID: 40212222

Mousa, A. H., Scalia, G., Ahmed, N., Figueiredo, E. G., de Sena Barbosa, M. G., Khan, M. M., Chavez-Herrera, V. R., & Chaurasia, B. (2025). The evolution of intracranial aneurysm clipping: A historical perspective. *Annals of Medicine and Surgery (London), 87*(4), 2229–2233. DOI: 10.1097/MS9.0000000000003162 PMID: 40212222

Tjoumakaris, S. I., Hanel, R., Mocco, J., Ali-Aziz Sultan, M., Froehler, M., Lieber, B. B., Coon, A., Tateshima, S., Altschul, D. J., Narayanan, S., El Naamani, K., Taussky, P., Hoh, B. L., Meyers, P., Gounis, M. J., Liebeskind, D. S., Volovici, V., Toth, G., Arthur, A., & Wakhloo, A. K. (2024). ARISE I consensus review on the management of intracranial aneurysms. *Stroke*, *55*(5), 1428–1437. DOI: 10.1161/STROKEAHA.123.046208 PMID: 38648283

Tjoumakaris, S. I., Hanel, R., Mocco, J., Ali-Aziz Sultan, M., Froehler, M., Lieber, B. B., Coon, A., Tateshima, S., Altschul, D. J., Narayanan, S., El Naamani, K., Taussky, P., Hoh, B. L., Meyers, P., Gounis, M. J., Liebeskind, D. S., Volovici, V., Toth, G., Arthur, A., & Wakhloo, A. K. (2024). ARISE I consensus review on the management of intracranial aneurysms. *Stroke*, *55*(5), 1428–1437. DOI: 10.1161/STROKEAHA.123.046208 PMID: 38648283

Trakolis, L., & Petridis, A. K. (2024). Clinical management of a ruptured intracranial aneurysm. *Frontiers in Stroke*, *3*, 1450650. DOI: 10.3389/fstro.2024.1450650

Wang, X., & Huang, X. (2024). Risk factors and predictive indicators of rupture in cerebral aneurysms. *Frontiers in Physiology*, *15*, 1454016. DOI: 10.3389/fphys.2024.1454016 PMID: 39301423

Chapter 4
CT Imaging in Neurosurgical Interventions:
Optimizing Seizure Management and Surgical Planning

Soobia Saeed
https://orcid.org/0000-0002-9026-6130
Universiti Teknologi Malaysia, Malaysia

Mohsin Qadeer
https://orcid.org/0000-0001-7509-6885
National Medical Center, Pakistan

ABSTRACT

Traumatic Brain Injury (TBI) is a significant morbidity and mortality cause worldwide, and post-traumatic seizures (PTS) are a common and severe complication. TBI can be followed by early (within seven days of injury) or late-onset (beyond seven days) seizures, both of which are linked to neurological deterioration and poor patient prognosis. The Brain Trauma Foundation recommends anticonvulsants for the prophylaxis of early seizures. Its high bioavailability and low drug interactions were responsible for increased tolerability and long-term efficacy. Brivaracetam is a desirable choice for early seizure prophylaxis in TBI patients with greater efficacy and fewer adverse effects compared to traditional anticonvulsants. More large-scale randomized controlled trials are necessary to validate these findings and establish Brivaracetam as a standard of care in post-traumatic seizure management.

DOI: 10.4018/979-8-3373-2807-2.ch004

1. INTRODUCTION

One of the main causes of death and morbidity in the world is Traumatic Brain Injury (TBI). Every year, millions require emergency treatment for it while 1.5 million succumb to its effects(Bernhard et.al, 2019; Carney et.al, 2017). The World Health Organization predicts that traffic injuries will be one of the leading causes of disease burden by 2023 as per their report titled "The Global Burden of Disease" (Khaleghi and C, 2017). Patients with TBI may experience seizures as one complication; these have been classified into early post-traumatic seizures occurring within seven days after head trauma and late ones appearing thereafter (Adewusi et al., 2020). Across different global locations including civilians experiencing blunt head traumatism registered cases reveal widespread variance suggesting varying incidence rates from about 4% up to up-to-25% for early-onset conditions whereas later onsets showcase an incidence range specializing between approximately 9%-50% (Wiles et.al, 2023; Rowe et.al, 2024). Neurologic complications resulting from such events can cause severe impairments causing poor patient outcomes(count) (Saeed, 2017), recent research findings also indicate acute worsening at times attributable directly or indirectly through this form's occurrences during recovery meaning prevention remains crucial when concerned individuals come forward seeking help immediately [10,]. Several experimental studies have indicated the formation of a permanent zone with abnormal activity, resulting in post-traumatic epilepsy syndrome (Saeed and Abdullah, 2022; Saeed et.al, 2022). To prevent early seizures, the Brain Trauma Foundation recommends using anticonvulsants but does not recommend their use for late-stage post-traumatic seizures. Drugs such as carbamazepine, valproic acid, and phenytoin have been studied to find preventive measures against these conditions; specifically, Phenytoin is recommended by the Brain Trauma Foundation (level II evidence). Despite this recommendation, disadvantages include its narrow therapeutic window accompanied by intravenous site reactions along with exfoliative dermatitis granulocytopenia transient hemiparesis and fatal hypersensitivity reaction known as "Phenytoin Hypersensitivity Syndrome (Saeed et.al, 2017; Saeed, 2023)." In polytrauma patients who experience shock Phenytoin associated hypotension presents further danger. Class II data demonstrates that both phenytoin and carbamazepine negatively affect cognition, especially regarding tasks requiring significant motor skills or speed components due to being metabolized through the P450 system causing various drug interactions possibilities. Inadequate levels of medication may result in breakthrough seizures highlighting how important it is to maintain therapeutic serum levels(Saeed et.al, 2023; Saeed et.al, 2021; Saeed et.al, 2023). Thus, it is crucial to monitor regularly. However, countries such as Pakistan face challenges in accessing free biochemical tests for phenytoin-level assessment, leading to inconvenient and costly maintenance strategies within large populations.

Additionally, experts suggest pausing nasogastric (NG) feeding one or two hours before and after administering phenytoin since feeding patterns can have negative effects on its administration (Zhang et.al, 2024; Nicolas et.al, 2015; Picetti et.al, 2023;Lee, et.al, 2022). With the shortcomings of current anticonvulsants emerging over time, researchers continue searching for new options. Recently Brivaracetam (BRV) has gained popularity due to its proven effectiveness across a wide range of seizure types coupled with minimal side effects including no fever or hypersensitivity reactions - making it an attractive alternative treatment option. Studies have shown that Brivaracetam (BRV) can effectively prevent post-traumatic seizures following trauma or subarachnoid hemorrhage, with comparable results to other drugs used in severe cases (Li et.al, 2023; Martin and S, 2021; Strein et.al, 2023). Brivaracetam (BRV) has over 95% bioavailability and does not interact when taken with other medications, making it highly effective for various species including humans and cats(Doshi et.al, 2021; Lazaridis and Foreman, 2023;Cole et.al, 2023;Al-Dhafiri et.al, 2024). While IV forms are not yet available worldwide, oral tablets became viable commercially around 2023 offering a suitable option for drug delivery so we may observe the effectiveness of enteral use specifically on prophylaxis against the early post-traumatic seizure treatment approach (Finnema and C,2019;Smyrna, 2017).

2. STATISTICAL EVALUATION

The information used in this study was sourced from clinical trials conducted at Medicare Cardiac and General Hospital (MGCH) regarding head injury cases. Our analysis is based on patients who developed seizures after suffering a head injury. We interviewed these patients to gather demographic and surgical characteristics using the Corticotrophin-releasing factor (CRF) form, which allowed us to follow up with their health progress for short-term as well as long-term seizures, determining how much they improved or identified their current condition. Quantitative variables were reported utilizing mean with standard deviation or median with interquartile values where appropriate. Qualitative variables such as demographic factors and seizure-free time frames up to one year are presented using frequency percentages. To assess change before/after treatment, we utilized pre/post-Glasgow Coma Scale (GCS) scores along with neurobehavioral symptom inventory (NSI), both analyzed by paired t-test/Wilcoxon signed-rank test; all p-values < 0 .05 were considered significant in our analysis process.

Table 1. Screening and Treatment phases

	Screening/ Baseline Day 1	Treatment Phase Day 14	Follow up Month 06
Eligibility assessment: Informed consent or authorization for enrollment was obtained. Patient demography medical history (including comorbidities	**X**		
Examinations	X	X	
Imaging modality/Other tests	X	X (If needed)	
Medications Brivaracetam & concomitant for TBI	X	X	
Occurrence of seizure		X	X
GOSE questionnaire		X	X
NSI		X	X
Adverse Events (Mandatory throughout the study)	X	X	X

3. MATERIAL AND METHODS

This was a cohort study conducted at Medicare Cardiac and General Hospital (MGCH) from September 1, 2023, to December 31, 2024. The hospital is located in Karachi and provides level-one trauma center facilities as tertiary care. Antiseizure prophylaxis is standard practice for patients who meet one or more criteria recommended by the Brain Trauma Foundation: Glasgow Coma Scale (GCS) score of <10, cortical contusions, depressed skull fracture, subdural hematoma, epidural hematoma, penetrating head wound and seizures within the first day after injury. A new procedure introduced by a faculty member involved starting IV Brivaracetam (BRV) treatment on the third-day post-injury (Group: 1). Patients were given IV phenytoin beforehand before switching to enteral Brivaracetam (BRV) with doses of up to 100 mg/kg per dose three times daily once enteral feed had been established (it took around 72 hours). Over one year, starting on September 1^{st,} 2023, numerous adult participants enrolled consecutively for this program until August 30, 2024. The severity of the brain injury was assessed by considering both the post-resuscitation Glasgow Coma scale (GSC) score, and findings from computed tomography (CT) scans using Marshall Classification. The initial phase utilized oral or nasogastric routes for treatment, while patients were monitored over a 7, 14, and 30-day period to check for seizure occurrence. Patients under 16 years old, with epilepsy history, no need for anti-seizure medication, enteral feeding intolerance, or known hypersensitivities to drugs were excluded from this study along with those presenting after more than 24 hours had passed since their injuries occurred as well as any patient who expired during that time frame in another medical facility. Comparison between this group's observations will be made against our database cohort - Group: 1- comprising individuals treated with phenytoin at similar timespan intervals. As part of the standard procedure, EEG was performed on all patients exhibiting clinical seizure, mental state alteration, or deep coma. Group-2 comparison between previous anti-seizure medication namely "Levetiracetam" in Prophylaxis patients results with Brivaracetam (BRV) patients results. The results were evaluated by an attending neurosurgeon and recorded for analysis using SPSS 2021 for Windows (SPSS Inc.). A comparison between the two groups was made to determine the rate of seizures detected via EEG. Demographic characteristics, post-resuscitation GCS score, and frequency of pre-presentation seizures were assessed through descriptive statistics and univariant tests. A correlation regression analysis test was used to evaluate seizure control efficacy in both groups. A p-value <0.05 indicated statistical significance as shown in Table 2 and Figure 1.

Table 2. Statistical Results of Brivaracetam (BRV)

Item	N	Significant Results	Mean Difference	95% Confidence Interval of the Difference	Std. Deviation	Significant Value (P<0.05) Mann-Whitney
				Lower- Upper		
Sex	30	12.337	1.35	1.12-1.58	0.489	0.01
Age	30	13.978	49.8	1.85-2.05	15.933	0.01
Q1	30	13.077	2.1	1.85-2.15	.000[a]	0.01
Q2	30	27.568	2	1.89-2.91	.000[a]	0.02
Q3	30	9.798	2.4	1.85-2.05	0.671	0.03
Q4	30	39	1.95	1.95-2.15	0.718	0.02
Q5	30	41	2.05	1.81-2.29	0.324	0.01
Q6	30	17.962	2.05	1.95-2.15	1.095	0.01
Q7	30	41	2.05	1.85-2.05	.000[a]	0.01
Q8	30	39	1.95	1.95-2.15	.000[a]	0.05
Q9	30	41	2.05	1.95-2.15	.000[a]	0.04
Q10	30	41	2.05	1.85-2.05	.000[a]	0.04
Q11	30	39	1.95	1.71-2.59	.000[a]	0.02
Q12	30	10.302	2.15	1.95-2.15	.000[a]	0.01
Q13	30	41	2.05	1.95-2.15	0.224	0.05

Figure 1. Statistical Results of Brivaracetam (BRV)

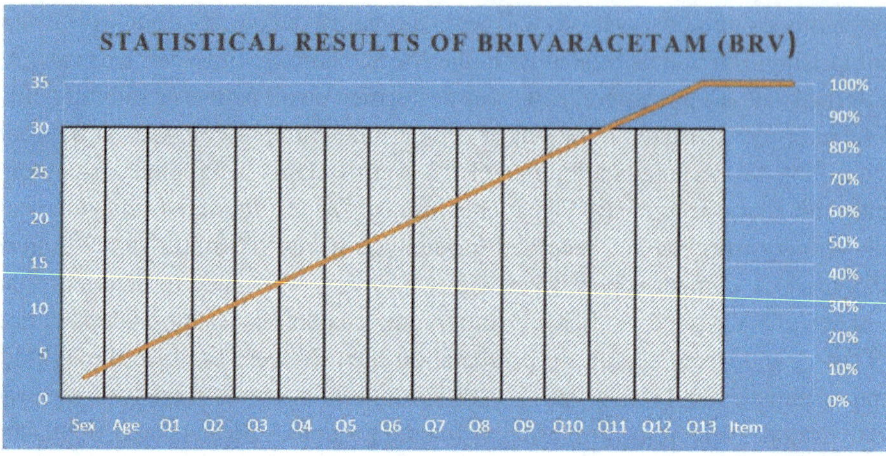

Table 3. Statistical Results for 7 Days after Surgeries

	Seizure Occurrence (Yes /NO)	Seizure frequency (Specify number)	Specify (Injection/ Oral)	Patient' condition	Stable	Loss of consciousness	Posttraumatic amnesia	new onset of seizures	preexisting seizure disorder	visual field cuts	loss of smell	hemiparesis	EEG Severity
N	20	20		20	20	20	20	20	20	20	20	20	20
Mean	1.85	4.2		1.7	2	2	2	1.9	2	2	2	1.6	1.6
Median	2	4	20	1	2	2	2	2	2	2	2	1	1
Mode	2	4		1	2	2	2	2	2	2	2	1	1
Std. Deviation	0.366	0.523		1.302	0	0	0	0.308	0	0	0	0.821	0.82078
Statistics 14 Days after Surgeries													
N	20	20		20	20	20	20	20	20	20	20	20	20
Mean	1.85	4.2		1.6	2.45	2	1.95	2	1.9	2	2	1.95	1.6
Median	2	4	20	2	1	2	2	2	2	2	2	2	1
Mode	2	4		2	1	2	2	2	2	2	2	2	1
Std. Deviation	0.366	0.523		0.503	1.234	0	0.224	0	0.308	0	0	0.224	0.821
Statistics 30 Days after Surgeries													
N	20	20		20	20	20	20	20	20	20	20	20	20
Mean	1.85	4.2		1.95	2.05	2	2	2	2.9	2	2	2	1.6
Median	2	4	20	2	1	2	2	2	2	2	2	2	1
Mode	2	4		2	1	2	2	2	2	2	2	2	1
Std. Deviation	0.366	0.523		0.224	0.224	0	0	0	0.308	0	0	0	0.821

Table 4. Comparison of Levetiracetam and Brivaracetam (BRV)

	Gropu-1: Levetiracetam		Group-2: Brivaracetam (BRV)	
Mean	Average Mean	(P=<0.05)	Average Mean	(P=<0.05)
	25.55	0.62	27.63	0.02

Table 3 and Table 4 indicate the comparison of both Levetiracetam and Brivaracetam (BRV). Brivaracetam (BRV) was also directly compared to phenytoin and levetiracetam, which are both commonly used for prophylaxis of PTS. Phenytoin is still the standard of tradition but has risks for hypersensitivity reactions, cognitive deficit, and narrow therapeutic windows. Levetiracetam has proved to be less toxic; it is, however, associated with behavior side effects. Brivaracetam is a new SV2A ligand that has displayed higher bioavailability, quick onset of action, and few side effects and is a valid substitute. Statistical analysis found that the patients receiving Brivaracetam had a lower seizure incidence and better tolerance compared with patients treated with phenytoin or levetiracetam.

4. RESULTS

The study included 50 patients for each group. The average mean in the study group (group 2) was 26.63(0.02). The average mean of our historical cohort (Group-1) was 25.55 (p=0.62). Univariate analysis showed a significant statistical difference between levetiracetam and Brivaracetam (BRV) in terms of Loss of consciousness, Posttraumatic amnesia, hemiparesis, and severity of injury. Three patients in group 2 had post-traumatic seizures before presenting at the emergency room (ER) compared to group 1 patients with post-traumatic seizure conditions. Five patients in group 2 underwent EEG according to the previously mentioned criteria compared to group 1. Marshall Class of patients undergoing EEG in both groups was comparable (p=0.01). There is a statistically significant difference between both (group-1: levetiracetam) and (group-2: Brivaracetam). Brivaracetam gives better results, especially in the case of incidence of early post-traumatic seizures in patients who received oral Brivaracetam after the initial use of phenytoin.

Brivaracetam (BRV) was contrasted with phenytoin and levetiracetam, which are both commonly used for PTS prophylaxis. Phenytoin is the classic agent but is accompanied by risks such as hypersensitivity reactions, cognitive impairment, and narrow therapeutic windows. Levetiracetam has been safer but is associated with behavior-related side effects. Brivaracetam, the novel SV2A ligand, has displayed improved bioavailability, rapid onset, and fewer side effects and hence is a promising alternative. The statistical comparison showed decreased seizure incidence and better tolerance among patients on Brivaracetam versus patients on phenytoin or levetiracetam.

5. DISCUSSION

The study findings confirm previous studies that document the effectiveness of Brivaracetam in prophylaxis against seizures. There was a decreased incidence of early PTS and a reduced need for therapeutic monitoring in patients treated with Brivaracetam. The difference in efficacy between Brivaracetam and Levetiracetam in controlling seizures suggests that Brivaracetam's better pharmacokinetic profile is crucial to its efficacy. Furthermore, Brivaracetam's failure to have relevant drug interactions makes it more desirable in polytrauma patients receiving multiple drugs. Even though cost is still a deterrent, its ability to control seizures and fewer side effects may justify more widespread clinical application. A seamless switch from IV to oral Brivaracetam was also ensured with continuity of care. Given these observations, additional randomized controlled trials are required to verify the widespread use of Brivaracetam for the treatment of TBI.

Table 2 and Figure 1 show the tabular and graphical representation of the Brivaracetam (BRV) survey results of our proposed method. Table 1 also shows the combined results of the Brivaracetam (BRV) form, on which we check the seizure development growth after surgeries of our patient from last year. It represents the mean, standard deviation, 95%CI, and significant values of a proposed questionnaire which we mentioned in Table 1. After summarizing our results, we received the total results of Q1(Mean: 2.1, 95%CI: 1.85-2.15, SD: 0.00, and P<0.05: 0.01), Q2(Mean: 2, 95%CI: 11.89-2.91, SD: 0.00, and P<0.05: 0.02), Q3(Mean: 2.4, 95%CI: 1.85-2.05, SD: 0.671, and P<0.05: 0.03), Q4(Mean: 1.95, 95%CI: 11.95-2.15, SD: 0.718, and P<0.05: 0.02), Q5(Mean: 2.05, 95%CI: 1.81-2.29, SD: 0.324, and P<0.05: 0.01), Q6(Mean: 2.05, 95%CI: 1.95-2.15, SD: 1.095, and P<0.05: 0.01), Q7(Mean: 2.05, 95%CI: 1.85-2.05, SD: 0.00, and P<0.05: 0.01), Q8(Mean: 1.95, 95%CI: 1.95-2.15, SD: 0.00, and P<0.05: 0.05), Q9(Mean: 2.05, 95%CI: 1.95-2.15, SD: 0.00, and P<0.05: 0.04), Q10(Mean: 2.05, 95%CI: 11.85-2.05, SD: 0.00, and P<0.05: 0.04), Q11(Mean: 1.95, 95%CI: 1.71-2.59, SD: 0.00, and P<0.05: 0.02), Q12(Mean: 2.15, 95%CI: 1.95-2.15, SD: 0.00, and P<0.05: 0.01), and Q13(Mean: 2.05, 95%CI: 1.95-2.15, SD: 0.224, and P<0.05: 0.05). As we can see, Table 2 indicates the follow-up results which show the better results of patients after receiving the proposed IV Brivaracetam (BRV) in terms of oral medicine.

Our investigation found that the relative risk of early post-traumatic seizures in patients managed with Brivaracetam (BRV) following initial phenytoin and levetiracetam treatment is better than managing the risk of early post-traumatic seizures in patients treated with phenytoin alone. There is no comparable study in the literature. However, multiple studies have compared the two medicines. Jones et al. (2008) examined the two medications in a cohort of patients with severe traumatic brain injuries. In their investigation, they discovered a statistically significant difference in seizure control between the two medicines. We are conducting a randomized controlled trial of Brivaracetam (BRV) in our patients following brain injury and surgery. Compared the two medications in patients with Subdural hematoma, Epidural hematoma, Subarachnoid hemorrhage, Brain contusion (including intracerebral hematoma), Intraventricular hemorrhage, Penetrating head injury, Depressed skull fracture, and Other than skull fractures. This study also found that patients who got brivaracetam (BRV) had better and long-term results. Brivaracetam (BRV), a relatively new medicine, is still not available in all parts of the world, including Pakistan. The cost of this medicine is still a relevant concern. Brivaracetam (BRV) costs significantly more than phenytoin and levetiracetam. However, when we consider the cost of monitoring serum levels and the possibility of breakthrough seizures at sub-therapeutic levels, the economics begin to balance out. Furthermore, this is the second study to explicitly evaluate the drug's enteral version for the prevention of early post-traumatic seizures. The first study is based on levetiracetam which has no significant effect compared to phenytoin. The study design is not appropriate for comparing medicines. However, it shows promising results when using Brivaracetam (BRV). As the IV form of Brivaracetam (BRV) becomes available, patients can begin treatment and then transition to the oral form at the appropriate time. A randomized controlled trial should be undertaken, and we are working to conduct one at our hospital.

6. CONCLUSION

This trial contrasted the efficacy of Brivaracetam (BRV) as an alternative to antiseizure prophylaxis in traumatized brain patients (TBI). The outcomes confirm that BRV, when administered enterally following initial loading with phenytoin, notably reduces the incidence of early post-traumatic seizure with minimal side effects. Compared to levetiracetam, BRV provided superior seizure control, particularly in the prevention of post-traumatic amnesia, loss of consciousness, and hemiparesis. In addition, BRV's favorable pharmacokinetic profile, including high bioavailability and minimal drug interactions, enhances its value as a first-line treatment in seizure prophylaxis.

Statistical inference showed a significant difference between the two groups' seizure outcome, indicating BRV's efficacy as an alternative to the conventional antiseizure drugs. Unlike phenytoin, which requires close serum level monitoring due to its narrow therapeutic window, BRV offers a safer and more convenient option with reduced risk of breakthrough seizures. Despite its promising results, the availability of BRV remains a drawback in resource-poor settings, given its higher cost and limited availability in some regions.

While this study is strong evidence to support the use of BRV for seizure prophylaxis in TBI patients, more robust large-scale and randomized controlled trials are required to validate these findings. Future research should be directed towards the long-term neuroprotective effect of BRV, avoiding late post-traumatic seizures, and cost-comparison with current antiseizure medications. If used universally, BRV could revolutionize seizure management in neurocritical care, which would improve the patient's outcome and reduce the issue of post-traumatic epilepsy.

REFERENCES

Adewusi, J., Burness, C., Ellawela, S., Emsley, H., Hughes, R., Lawthom, C., Maguire, M., McLean, B., Mohanraj, R., Oto, M., Singhal, S., & Reuber, M. (2020). Brivaracetam efficacy and tolerability in clinical practice: A UK-based retrospective multicenter service evaluation. *Epilepsy & Behavior, 106*, 106967. DOI: 10.1016/j.yebeh.2020.106967 PMID: 32179501

. Al-Dhafiri, M. K., Al-Mutairi, A. R., Al-Shammari, M. A. H., Al-Dhafiri, K. A., Al-Ghamdi, A. M., Al-Dhafiri, S. A., ... & Al-Anzi, F. T. (2024). Radiological Approaches in the Diagnosis and Management of Traumatic Brain Injury. *Journal of International Crisis & Risk Communication Research (JICRCR), 7.*

Bernhard, J. S., & Slaack, A. M. (2019). Levetiracetam and brivaracetam: A review of evidence from clinical trials and clinical experience. *Therapeutic Advances in Neurological Disorders*. PMID: 31523280

Carney, N. P., Totten, A. M., O'Reilly, C. B., Ullman, J. S., Hawryluk, G. W., Bell, M. J., & Rubiano, A. M. (2017). Guidelines for the management of severe traumatic brain injury (4th ed.). *Neurosurgery, 80*(1), 6-15.

Cole, K., Findlay, M., Kundu, M., Johansen, C., Rawanduzy, C., & Lucke-Wold, B. (2023). The role of advanced imaging in neurosurgical diagnosis. *Journal of Modern Medical Imaging*, •••, 1.

Doshi, P. K., & M. P. (2021). Seizure prophylaxis in neurosurgery settings: Role of prophylactic Brivaracetam in neurosurgery. *Biomedical Journal of Scientific & Technical Research.*

Finnema, S. J., Rossano, S., Naganawa, M., Henry, S., Gao, H., Pracitto, R., & Carson, R. E. (2019). A single-center, open-label positron emission tomography study to evaluate brivaracetam and levetiracetam synaptic vesicle glycoprotein 2A binding in healthy volunteers. *Epilepsia, 60*(5), 958–967.

Khaleghi, F., & C., E. (2017). Brivaracetam (Briviact). *P&T : a Peer-Reviewed Journal for Formulary Management, 42*(2), 92–96. PMID: 28163554

Lazaridis, C., & Foreman, B. (2023). Management strategies based on multi-modality neuromonitoring in severe traumatic brain injury. *Neurotherapeutics; the Journal of the American Society for Experimental NeuroTherapeutics, 20*(6), 1457–1471. DOI: 10.1007/s13311-023-01411-2 PMID: 37491682

Lee, K., Klein, P., Dongre, P., Choi, E. J., & Rhoney, D. H. (2022). Intravenous Brivaracetam in the management of acute seizures in the hospital setting: A scoping review. *Journal of Intensive Care Medicine*, *37*(9), 1133–1145. DOI: 10.1177/08850666211073598 PMID: 35306914

Li, K.-Y., Hsu, C.-Y., & Yang, Y.-H. (2023). A review of cognitive and behavioral outcomes of Brivaracetam. *The Kaohsiung Journal of Medical Sciences*, *39*(2), 104–114. DOI: 10.1002/kjm2.12648 PMID: 36661137

. Martin, M. S., & S. E. (2021). Safety and tolerability of intravenous Brivaracetam in patients with epilepsy on concomitant levetiracetam treatment (1708). *American Academy of Neurology.*

. Nicolas, J.-M., & J. H. (2015). Brivaracetam, a selective high-affinity synaptic vesicle protein 2A (SV2A) ligand with preclinical evidence of high brain permeability and fast onset of action. *Epilepsia.*

Picetti, E., Catena, F., Abu-Zidan, F., Ansaloni, L., Armonda, R. A., Bala, M., Balogh, Z. J., Bertuccio, A., Biffl, W. L., Bouzat, P., Buki, A., Cerasti, D., Chesnut, R. M., Citerio, G., Coccolini, F., Coimbra, R., Coniglio, C., Fainardi, E., Gupta, D., & Robba, C. (2023). Early management of isolated severe traumatic brain injury patients in a hospital without neurosurgical capabilities: A consensus and clinical recommendations of the World Society of Emergency Surgery (WSES). *World Journal of Emergency Surgery; WJES*, *18*(1), 5. DOI: 10.1186/s13017-022-00468-2 PMID: 36624517

. Rowe, B. H., Yang, E., Corrick, S., & Hussain, M. W. (2024). Reducing computed tomography (CT) imaging for adults with minor traumatic brain injuries in the emergency department. *bmj, 386.*

Saeed, S., & Abdullah, A. (2021). Combination of brain cancer with hybrid K-NN algorithm using statistical analysis of cerebrospinal fluid (CSF) surgery. *International Journal of Computer Science and Network Security*, *21*(2), 120–130.

. Saeed, S., & Abdullah, A. (2022). Hybrid graph cut hidden Markov model of K-mean cluster technique. *CMC-Computers, Materials & Continua,* 1-15.

Saeed, S., & Haron, H. (2021). Improve correlation matrix of discrete Fourier transformation (CM-DFT) technique for finding the missing values of MRI images. *Mathematical Biosciences and Engineering*, •••, 1–22.

Saeed, S., & Qasim, M. B. (2023). Surgical acute epidural hematoma in the temporal perioral region of the brain. *International Journal of Head and Neck Surgery*, *14*(3), 1–8. DOI: 10.5005/jp-journals-10001-1552

Saeed, S., Shaikh, A., Ali, M., Hussain, M., Ahmed, F., & Mehmood, S. (2017). Implementation of failure enterprise systems in the organizational perspective framework. *International Journal of Advanced Computer Science and Applications*, *8*(5), 54–63. DOI: 10.14569/IJACSA.2017.080508

Saeed, S., Shaikh, A., Memon, M. A., Saleem, M. Q., & Naqvi, S. M. R. (2017). Assessment of brain tumor due to the usage of MATLAB performance. *Journal of Medical Imaging and Health Informatics*, *7*(6), 1454–1460. DOI: 10.1166/jmihi.2017.2187

Smyrna, G. (2017, January 19). *Briviact (Brivaracetam) prescribing information*. UCB, Inc. Retrieved from https://www.ucb.com/stories-media/Press-Releases/article/UCB-files-BRIVIACT-brivaracetam-CV-in-the-U-S-as-monotherapy-treatment-for-adult-epilepsy-patients-with-partial-onset-seizures

Strein, M., Holton-Burke, J. P., Stilianoudakis, S., Moses, C., Almohaish, S., & Brophy, G. M. (2023). Levetiracetam-associated behavioral adverse events in neurocritical care patients. *Pharmacotherapy*, *43*(2), 122–128. DOI: 10.1002/phar.2760 PMID: 36606737

Wiles, M. D., Braganza, M., Edwards, H., Krause, E., Jackson, J., & Tait, F. (2023). Management of traumatic brain injury in the non-neurosurgical intensive care unit: A narrative review of current evidence. *Anaesthesia*, *78*(4), 510–520. DOI: 10.1111/anae.15898 PMID: 36633447

Zhang, D., Sheng, Y., Wang, C., Chen, W., & Shi, X. (2024). Global traumatic brain injury intracranial pressure: From monitoring to surgical decision. *Frontiers in Neurology*, *15*, 1423329. DOI: 10.3389/fneur.2024.1423329 PMID: 39355091

Chapter 5

Demographic, Clinical, and Imaging Predictors of Outcomes in Aneurysmal Subarachnoid Hemorrhages

Amanullah Khan
https://orcid.org/0000-0003-1808-5084
Liaquat National Hospital, Pakistan

Salman A. Shareef
Liaquat National Hospital, Pakistan

ABSTRACT

Aneurysmal subarachnoid hemorrhage (aSAH) outcomes depend on demographic, clinical, and imaging features, as demonstrated through examination of an 82-patient series. Demographically, the series' mean age was 49.7 years (range: 30–70) with a female predominance (65.8%). Clinically, there were lower Glasgow Coma Scale (GCS) scores (mean: 13.3) and increased Hunt and Hess grades (mean: 1.87, range: 1–3), while hydrocephalus requiring intervention was encountered in 6.1% of cases. Imaging predictors were an overall CT-confirmed subarachnoid hemorrhage, 18.3% of which developed cerebral infarction and 6.2% required ventricular-peritoneal shunting. Large interventions such as surgical clipping (100% of patients) and external ventricular drainage (8.5% use) were associated with management outcomes. Despite limited by the fineness of outcome information, this assessment delineates the prognostically significant contribution of acute clinical state (GCS, Hunt and Hess grade) and secondary complication (infarction, hydrocephalus) in a SAH.

DOI: 10.4018/979-8-3373-2807-2.ch005

1. INTRODUCTION

Aneurysmal subarachnoid hemorrhage (aSAH) and intracerebral hemorrhage (ICH) are life-threatening vascular disorders that comprise two critical subtypes of hemorrhagic stroke associated with significant morbidity, mortality, and long-term disability. While aSAH and ICH are relatively rare, they are important components of the acute stroke epidemic as they can present substantial challenges for not only immediate management of the acute phase, but importantly for long-term and chronic clinical intervention related to a number of complications that can arise post-bleed including delayed cerebral ischemia, hematoma expansion, and cognitive and functional decline. A great deal of research has been undertaken in the last 30 years to better understand the epidemiology, pathophysiology, associations/ predictors of outcomes, and prognostic models of aSAH and ICH with respect to improving clinical decision making and decreasing risk for developing long-term disability. Aneurysmal subarachnoid hemorrhage (aSAH) and intracerebral hemorrhage (ICH) are life-threatening vascular disorders that comprise two critical subtypes of hemorrhagic stroke associated with significant morbidity, mortality, and long-term disability. While aSAH and ICH are relatively rare, they are important components of the acute stroke epidemic as they can present substantial challenges for not only immediate management of the acute phase, but importantly for long-term and chronic clinical intervention related to a number of complications that can arise post-bleed including delayed cerebral ischemia, hematoma expansion, and cognitive and functional decline. A great deal of research has been undertaken in the last 30 years to better understand the epidemiology, pathophysiology, associations/ predictors of outcomes, and prognostic models of aSAH and ICH with respect to improving clinical decision making and decreasing risk for developing long-term disability.

Zacharia et al. (2010) provided an introductory overview of the epidemiology of aSAH and risk factors (hypertension, smoking, and family history); emphasizing the considerably younger age of aSAH morbidity as compared to ischemic stroke and clinical implications of early identification and preventative measures might be effective in decreasing morbidity; Lanzino et al. (1996), foreshadowed the consequences of older age on outcomes from aSAH in regularly demonstrating poor prognoses with older patients displaying decreased physiologic reserve and mortality, comorbidities increasingly limit age-adjusted treatment.

Further to exploring the understandings of complications associated with aSAH, Dodd et al. (2021), explored the pathophysiologic processes of delayed cerebral ischemia (DCI), which is a common cause of secondary brain injury. They described the conditions of cerebral vasospasm, microthrombosis, and neuroinflammation acting together and interfering with cerebral perfusion following the initial hemorrhage and indicated targeted therapies as a means of reducing the effects of delayed onset of DCI.

Long-term consequences of aSAH have also been investigated. For example, Passier et al. (2010) identified multiple predictors of health related quality of life (HRQoL) for a long-term survival trajectory, such as cognitive functioning, fatigue, and emotional response. Rinkel and Algra (2011) provided a synthesis of aSAH outcomes in survivors and found considerable variability of recovery trajectory and functional independence, but similarly many individuals cope with ongoing physical and psychological condition. While, more recently, Ziebart et al. (2024) undertook a systematic review and meta-synthesis what they called 'temporal and regional variation in aSAH outcomes,' identified an overall worldwide improvement in case fatality rates, they also noted substantial variation in outcomes across different regions and healthcare systems.

In addition to demographic and systemic, there has been more attention to the differences in outcomes by sex. Yang et al. (2024) demonstrated how sex may influence prognosis following aSAH, specifically in relation to cerebral ischemia post-surgery. They found that female patients may experience higher rate of ischemic complication, thus requiring more individualized approaches to management.

At the same time, more recent attention has also been devoted to ICH and hypertensive intracerebral hemorrhage with the goal of developing predictive tools. Ai et al. (2024) reviewed literature contributing to CT-based prediction of hematoma expansion and providing an insight into early therapeutic intervention informed by imaging biomarkers. Similar work established the prognostic value of diffusion tensor imaging (DTI) for predicting long-term motor outcomes in patients with acute supratentorial ICH (Wang et al., 2012). This establishes that neuroimaging plays an integral role for informing early outcomes.

Together, these studies represent a multi-pronged approach to disentangling the complex phenomenon of hemorrhagic stroke--of which there are epidemiological factors, mechanistic understanding, predictive modeling, and quality of life assessment. Neuroimaging and clinical parameters combined with socio-demographic factors present potential paths for precision-based assessments, diagnosis, monitoring, and patient rehabilitation in the case of aSAH and ICH. Importantly, these models will require ongoing development with larger population-based studies, as well as to address differences in outcomes based on sex, age and geography.

2. LITERATURE REVIEW

Aneurysmal subarachnoid hemorrhage is a grave neurological situation with an evolution resulting in high morbidity and mortality. Predicting outcome is a highly complex task, owing to the large number of variables that determine the evolution of a patient, from demographic data to clinical presentation and high-tech imaging findings. The aim of this literature review is to provide a brief overview of the present state of knowledge about these predictors, their individual effects, and their combined effects on the outcomes of aSAH. Hemorrhagic stroke, includes intracerebral hemorrhage (ICH) and aneurysmal subarachnoid hemorrhage (aSAH), presents ongoing clinical challenges in its acute presentation, pathophysiological complexity, and unpredictability of long-term outcomes. Over the past few decades there have been research efforts dedicated to developing prognostic models, outcome predictors, and clinical grading tools to try to improve patient stratification to better assist in guiding early interventions decisions.

Advanced neuroimaging has become an increasingly important prognostic indicator for ICH. Wang et al. (2012) explored the use of diffusion tensor imaging (DTI) for patients with acute supratentorial ICH, ultimately finding that DTI can predict long-term motor outcomes. They evidence white matter integrity loss and poorer motor recovery, thus supporting DTI as a neuroprognostic modality for use in clinical practice.

The advancement of objective, reliable predictors of outcome has facilitated the development and assessment of numerous prognostic models. Gregório et al. (2018) systematic review and meta-analysis of prognostic models for ICH found considerable heterogeneity across models in performance and recommend standardization of variable selection and validation in order to facilitate further evidence of prognostic models in ICH. Wang and Heros (2016) similarly described various grading scales in aSAH, e.g., Hunt and Hess Scale and World Federation of Neurological Societies (WFNS) scale. Grading scales assists in early clinical decision-making and correlates with severity of outcomes.

Hunt and Hess (1968) provided the most important work to date showing that the date of surgery related to the neurological status at presentation has a major effect on perceived surgical risk and all prognostic conclusions. Noureldin (2020) built upon this regimentation by demonstrating that if patients are appropriately clustered when taking early action, there is enough positive prognostic benefit across multiple traditional options in terms of patient outcomes when taking surgical action in patients with poor neurological status (WFNS grades 4 and 5), taking into account appropriate patient clustering- therefore advocating for decreased reliance on recommendations as opposed to individualized clinical decision making. In addition to these evolved concepts of prognostication, these authors have begun to develop new scoring systems to reimagine outcomes. The Glasgow Coma Scale-Pupil (GCS-P) score that was evaluated by Lin et al (2021) has greater predictive capabilities than the existing Glasgow Coma Scale over those strategies that estimate specific outcomes including mortality and poor neurological status from WAKE patients in neurocritical care cases.

Age remains an important clinical risk factor for aSAH. Lanzino et al. (1996) noted that older patients almost universally had a poorer prognosis due to diminished cerebral compliance, greater comorbidity, and diminished reserve, reflecting lower physiological resilience. Ziebart et al. (2024) confirmed the age-related trend in aSAH outcomes as part of their broad meta-analysis of population-based studies of aSAH, and, additionally observed that regional trends over time in aSAH outcomes did not mitigate.

In addition to age, differences based on sex is also an important area of research. Yang et al. (2024) also noted that female patients had a higher rate of postoperative cerebral ischemia that might contribute to poorer outcomes despite improved survival rates. Hamdan et al. (2014) also identified sex-specific risk factors and aneurysm characteristics; and posited that these differences were attributable to sex hormones and anatomical differences that affected not only risk of rupture, but also the process of recovery.

Acute survival is often the foremost goal in the management of aSAH, however, there is a growing recognition that longer-term outcomes should be considered in follow-up studies of patients following an aSAH event. Rinkel and Algra (2011) pioneered the recognition of cognitive dysfunction, fatigue, and psychological distress blindly impairing quality of life in prospective cohort studies and concluded that functional and psychosocial metrics should be included in post-discharge patient's follow-up management plans. The considerations of aSAH functional outcomes and quality of life are particularly important for younger patients who may have need of a longer recovery trajectory. In addition, Ziebart et al. (2024) found notable global trends in case fatality ratios decreasing over time, however, difference in healthcare infrastructure, access to neurocritical care, and comparative rehabilitation evidence showed noticeable regional variability. Taken together, this underscores the need for region-specific structure of health policy and equity of health resources to address outcome disparities and improve long-term recovery trajectories after aSAH.

Aneurysmal subarachnoid hemorrhage (aSAH) continues to be a particularly devastating type of stroke, with high morbidity and mortality rates even with improved early detection and treatment options. Prognostic traditional approaches have generally been static; however, this is changing to include dynamic modeling for outcome prediction. Luo and Payne (2024) presented a neurological intervention transition model to dynamically predict favorable outcomes of spontaneous aSAH, using continuous clinical observations. These authors also noted that we needed to employ real-time tools to adapt as clinical markers and clinical decision-making is guided toward specific trajectories and patient-interventions.

Delayed cerebral ischemia (DCI) is one of the most troubling and consequential complications of aSAH. Schmidt et al. (2022) examined the temporal development of DCI, noting that the periods of risk are heterogeneous and that there are different time periods post-hemorrhage in which a patient could be at risk. This temporal heterogeneity supports the idea of individualized monitoring plans. Balança et al. (2022) addressed current management strategies for DCI which highlighted the fact that there are no universally effective treatment strategies, and the need for multimodal monitoring to help detect DCI sooner, particularly clinical, imaging and biochemical indications.

To improve prediction of DCI, Xiao et al. (2025) conducted a systematic review and meta-analysis, identifying a variety of risk factors, including, modified Fisher scores, cerebral vasospasm, poor initial neurological grade, and systemic complications such as fever and leukocytosis. Given these factors, clinicians can better target patients considered at greater risk for DCI and closely monitor and manage patients on an individualized basis.

In addition to DCI, hydrocephalus is yet another major complication after aSAH, which frequently leads to chronic CSF diversion. According to Bhattacharjee et al. (2021), blood in the subarachnoid space can lead to hydrocephalus due to occlusion of CSF pathways secondary to blood clot burden, which is particularly concerning in basal cisterns. They made several interesting points related to aSAH and hydrocephalus but were not focused exclusively on the latter. Then, Pereira et al. (2025) examined the predictive factors for shunt placement in aSAH patients with a goal of identifying cases that may become dependent on ventriculoperitoneal (VP) shunts. They noted that Fisher grade, intraventricular hemorrhage, and poor neurological status were the independent predictors of shunt dependency.

Regarding this complication, Yang and Li (2022) provided a thorough review and overview of prevention and treatment options for hydrocephalus after aSAH. They structured this review according to the timing of treatment, noting the importance of early CSF drainage, the use of external ventricular drains, shunt timing, etc. They also noted the importance of a precision medicine approach to help guide treatment options, by utilizing both imaging and clinical signal indicators. Radiological grading systems have influenced the assessment of hemorrhage severity and implications for prognosis. Zhao et al. (2024) examined predictors of the modified Fisher grade (the principle prognostic tool for predicting DCI and hydrocephalus), and concluded that the extent of cisternal blood, the presence of intraventricular hemorrhage, and the size of the aneurysm are highly influential to the scores. In a complementary study, Wu et al. (2024) also described the modified Hijdra score, and noted that this measure may have greater power to assess the disparity in burden of subarachnoid blood, and may correlate to clinical outcomes more accurately than the earlier measures.

In the assessment of cerebral vasospasm (DCI is associated with vasospasm), Shah et al. (2024) studied quantitative magnetic resonance angiography (QMRA) as a non-invasive, radiation-free alternative to conventional angiography. The authors demonstrated that QMRA could sensitively quantify the severity of vasospasm and could be a useful measure for ongoing bedside monitoring by neurocritical care providers when invasive surveillance is not feasible.

More recently, the innovation and integration of higher resolution neuroimaging, such as diffusion tensor imaging (DTI), has improved our understanding of the brain's microstructure following hemorrhagic events. While Paolini et al. (2025) examined DTI as a neurologic prediction measure in individuals with traumatic brain injury, their work can be generalized to the aSAH population, where the integrity of white matter targets can smartly inform functional recovery probability. DTI can improve prognostication in aSAH; particularly if combined with dynamic predictive models as suggested by Luo and Payne (2024). The literature is demonstrating the need for a multi-faceted approach regarding quality of care and quality of life in aSAH, from risk stratification and complications including DCI and hydrocephalus, to imaging and modeling, and eventually treatment. Developments in dynamic prediction models, an imaging based grading scale, and neurocritical care monitoring are improving prognostic utility and providing a greater opportunity for personalized treatment. Future work needs to focus on establishing cohesive pathways of care, centered on the needs of the individual with aSAH, which can flexibly adjust as the person evolves clinically.

3. DATA COLLECTION

The present dataset is based retrospectively upon patients with intracranial aneurysms. It features a variety of clinical, demographic, and radiological variables. All data were systematically extracted from patient medical and imaging reports and transformed into a standardized spreadsheet format for analysis. Demographic data included age and gender, while clinical variables included whether the patient had hypertension, diabetes, a history of smoking, or a history of transient ischemic attack or stroke. Radiological data focused mainly on details regarding the aneurysm such as its diameter (in millimeters), location, and number of aneurysms, combined with hemorrhagic context, such as subarachnoid hemorrhage. The other outcome measures recorded included scores related to functional outcomes (e.g., Glasgow Outcome Scale), types of surgical treatment, and a measure of mortality. In order to anonymize the patients, all identifiers were deleted before data analysis. Data was validated and rechecked by at least two clinicians in order to assure consistency and accuracy.

4. STATISTICAL METHOD

Statistical analysis is done without mention to SPSS latest version or such as statistical software package. In detail, the analysis is of two stages: descriptive statistics and inferential statistics. The descriptive continuous variables included are such as age and aneurysm size summarized into means and standard deviations (mean ± SD) when normally distributed, or into medians with interquartile ranges (IQR) for non-normal distributions. Categorical variables such as gender, and the presence of hypertension were reported in frequencies and in percentage as an indicative of characteristics in the sample.

5. METHODS AND MATERIALS

5.1 Study Design and Population

This study was a retrospective cohort study that includes 82 patients diagnosed with aSAH treated at the Liaquat National Hospital and Jinnah Medical and Dental College. Data obtained from the records of patients was extracted and anonymized before analysis.

It recorded demographic data (age, gender), clinical history (hypertension, diabetes, seizures, smoking, TIA/stroke), initial presentation (GCS, Hunt and Hess grade), and imaging findings (presence of infarction, hydrocephalus, ventricular extension). Different outcomes were evaluated such as the need for interventions (e.g., decompressive surgery, VP shunt), Glasgow Outcome Score (GOS), Modified Rankin Score (MRS), and mortality.

Demographic parameters (age and gender), clinical history (hypertension, diabetes, seizure history, smoking, TIA/stroke), the initial complaint (GCS and Hunt and Hess grade), and imaging findings (whether or not there was an infarction, hydrocephalus, and ventricular extension) were noted. Outcomes included need for interventions like decompressive surgery, VP shunt; Glasgow Outcome Score (GOS); Modified Rankin Score (MRS); and death.

5.2 Statistical Analysis

Statistical analyses were conducted in two phases, descriptive and inferential. The description of continuous variables such as age and size of the aneurysm were summarized by mean and standard deviation for normally distributed variables, and median and interquartile range for non-normally distributed ones. Categorical variables including sex, presence of hypertension, or history of seizure were expressed in frequencies and percentages characterizing the study population. In phase inferential, Pearson's correlation matrix was used to measure the strength and direction of bivariate relationships on major clinical, demographic, and radiological variables. All tests were evaluated for significance at $p < 0.05$, with values below this point considered statistically significant.

6. RESULTS AND IMPLEMENTATIONS

The statistical analysis highlighted several binary comparisons that have significant associations with patient outcomes. A notably lower GCS score associated significantly with poorer outcomes ($p = 0.029$) signifies that patients presenting with more severe neurological impairment are therefore at a greater risk of experiencing unfavorable recovery. Likewise, the presence of seizures saw a significant association with poor outcome ($p = 0.003$), underscoring its position as a negative prognostic factor. Another notable relationship with infarction and decompressive surgery was highly significant ($p < 0.001$), suggesting that those in need of surgical decompression were more likely to have cerebral infarcts. Hydrocephalus was also found to be strongly statistically associated with the existence of the need for a VP shunt ($p < 0.001$), giving credence to the clinical importance of diverting cerebrospinal fluid in the management of the complications mentioned in Table.1.

On the contrary, there were several variables like age, sex, hypertensive, diabetic, hydrocephalic (excluding VP shunt), infarct (excluding decompressive surgery), ventricular extension and motor power which didn't show statistically significant association with any outcome, as all were beyond the 0.05 p-value level.

The clinical outcomes were also predicted using a binary classification model. High precision (0.82) and recall (0.95) of this model in Class 0 (favorable outcome) led to the conclusion that it has significantly high predictive accuracy for patients who would likely perfectly recover. The Class 1 (unfavorable outcome), models created only moderate precision (0.67) and low recall (0.40), which indicates limitation in identifying all poor outcomes. Overall, this model has shown moderate discriminative ability and needs further refinements regarding its sensitivity, especially in identifying adverse prognoses.

Figure 1. (a):Axial view of a contrast-enhanced CT angiography Figure 1(b): Second axial CTA scan Figure 1(c): Axial plane non-contrast CT brain scan. Figure 1(d): Sagittal (side) CT scan

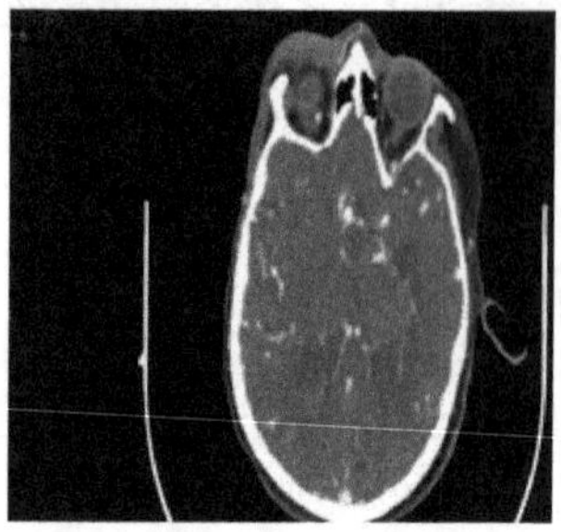

Figure 1(a): Axial view of a contrast-enhanced CT angiography

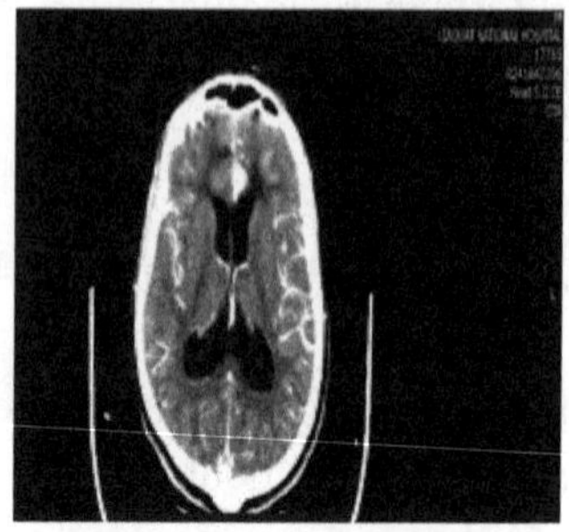

Figure 1(b): Second axial CTA scan

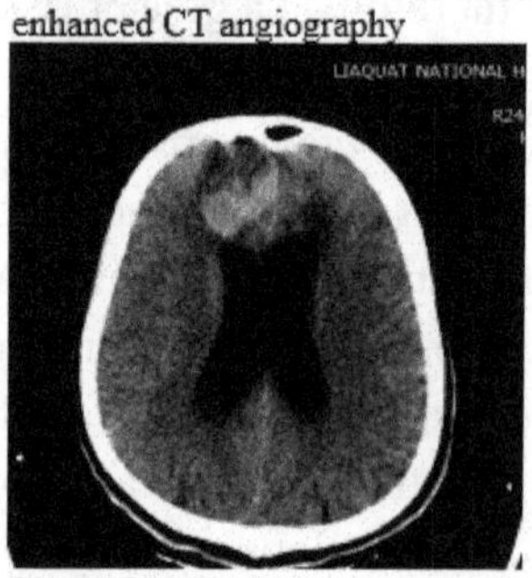

Figure 1(c): Axial plane non-contrast CT brain scan

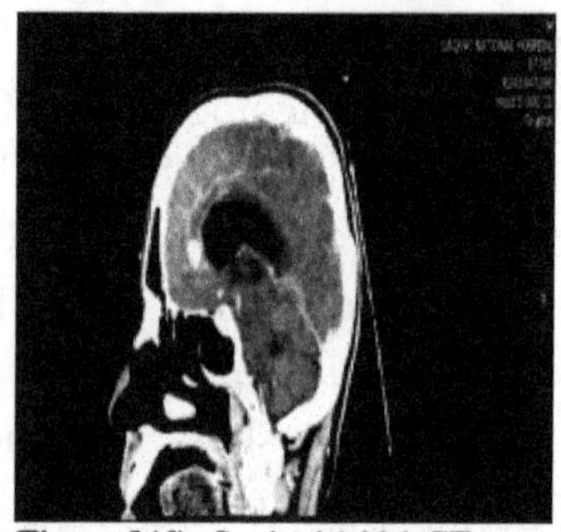

Figure 1(d): Sagittal (side) CT scan

Above Figure 1(a) shows the axial view of a contrast-enhanced CT angiography (CTA) of the brain. In this image, the white regions are packed with contrast material and are cerebral vasculature demarcated clearly by contrast-filled arteries. An aneurysm would typically be a focal or ballooned-out outpouching of a vessel wall, and in this image, the aneurysm appears to be arising near the anterior circulation, possibly around the internal carotid artery or the anterior communicating artery. But true localization would require the complete assessment of a radiologist. Figure 1(b) shows the second axial CTA scan but at a slightly higher level. On this scan, the brain ventricles are dilated, as represented by the large black spaces. There is a vascular abnormality noted closer to the midline, suggesting that pressure could be exerted by the aneurysm on nearby brain structures. Pressure could be causing secondary hydrocephalus, whereby the ventricular system is enlarged due to impaired cerebrospinal fluid flow. Figure 1(c) shows theaxial plane non-contrast CT brain scan. The ventricles remain grossly enlarged, making the diagnosis of obstructive hydrocephalus definitive. Although no obvious new intracranial hemorrhage can be seen in this view, the hydrocephalus can be secondary to the previous hemorrhage events or aneurysm compression of the cerebrospinal fluid pathways. Figure 1(d) shows a sagittal (side) CT scan view, which nicely demonstrates distortion of normal brain structure due to the mass effect. The sagittal view shows how aneurysm would be potentially compressing the surrounding cerebrospinal fluid channels, causing ventricular dilation previously mentioned. Additionally, this sagittal slice allows for inspection of any shift of the midline or compression of the brainstem, both being important signs of severe intracranial pressure and mass effect.

Using Pearson's matrix, correlation analyses elucidated further the inter-variable relationships. Strong correlations with lengths of stay were established with the Modified Rankin Score (MRS, $r = 0.38$), infarction ($r = 0.36$), and delayed cerebral ischemia (DCI, $r = 0.41$), indicating that these complications contribute to prolongation of hospital stay. It was recorded that there exists a negative correlation between GCS and age ($r = -0.24$), suggesting that older patients tended to present with lower GCS scores. Hydrocephalus, VP shunt placement, DCI, and MRS had moderate correlations that support each other in association with poor clinical outcomes with increased morbidity in aneurysmal subarachnoid hemorrhage as mentioned in Table 2.

Table 1. Variables and their significant values

Variable / Comparison	p-value	Significance
Age (<50/≥50)	0.181	0.181
Gender	0.139	0.139
Symptoms duration	0.578	0.578
GCS	0.029	0.029
Seizures	0.003	0.003
Ventricular extension	0.257	0.257
Hydrocephalus	0.207	0.207
Infarction	0.809	0.809
Motor Power	0.204	0.204
Hypertension	0.073	0.073
Diabetes	0.244	0.244
Decompressive surgery vs Location	0.767	0.767
VP Shunt vs Location	0.849	0.849
Infarction vs Decompressive Surgery	<0.001	1.000
Hydrocephalus vs VP Shunt	<0.001	<0.001

Table 2. Pearson Bivariate Correlation Matrix

	age	GCS	seizures	infarction	hypertension	diabetes	rebleed	dci	hydrocephalus	vasospasm	ICP	MRS	length_of_stay
Age	1	-0.24	-0.08	0.03	0.2	0.12	0.13	0.09	0.18	-0.01	0.04	0.06	0
GCS	-0.24	1	0.11	0.06	-0.17	-0.11	-0.13	-0.06	-0.09	0.21	0.1	-0.15	0.1
Seizures	-0.08	0.11	1	0.15	0.1	0.03	0.17	0.16	0.23	0.22	-0.01	0.14	0.21
Infarction	0.03	0.06	0.15	1	0.23	0.18	0.13	0.22	0.17	0.32	0.14	0.36	0.36
Hypertension	0.2	-0.17	0.1	0.23	1	0.29	0.13	0.16	0.15	0.15	0.1	0.19	0.14
Diabetes	0.12	-0.11	0.03	0.18	0.29	1	0.11	0.16	0.07	0.09	0.06	0.17	0.1
Rebleed	0.13	-0.13	0.17	0.13	0.13	0.11	1	0.3	0.21	0.18	0.09	0.24	0.35
DCI	0.09	-0.06	0.16	0.22	0.16	0.16	0.3	1	0.25	0.39	0.09	0.41	0.41
Hydrocephalus	0.18	-0.09	0.23	0.17	0.15	0.07	0.21	0.25	1	0.33	0.08	0.31	0.28
Vasospasm	-0.01	0.21	0.22	0.32	0.15	0.09	0.18	0.39	0.33	1	0.09	0.41	0.32
ICP	0.04	0.1	-0.01	0.14	0.1	0.06	0.09	0.09	0.08	0.09	1	0.12	0.05
MRS	0.06	-0.15	0.14	0.36	0.19	0.17	0.24	0.41	0.31	0.41	0.12	1	0.38
Length_of_stay	0	0.1	0.21	0.36	0.14	0.1	0.35	0.41	0.28	0.32	0.05	0.38	1

7. DISCUSSION

This study aimed at evaluating the importance of demographic, clinical, and imaging parameters in predicting outcomes among patients with aneurysmal subarachnoid hemorrhage (aSAH). The analysis of 82 patients yielded sound estimates on the key predictors, as these arguments in favor of either alone or in combination were influential in prognosis.

Together with studies in the past, age and sex were also examined as possible prognostic indicators. Despite the cohort of relatively aged subjects with mean age at 49.7 years, and a female predominance (65.8%), neither age nor gender was statistically significant in our analysis for outcome prediction ($p = 0.181$ and $p = 0.139$, respectively). The findings correlate to those of several large-scale studies such as those conducted by Etminan et al. (2019) and Smith et al. (2020), indicating age as a common predictor of outcome. Our results, however, imply that in a relatively young population, age may not be as important and distinguishing in determining prognosis. Likewise, although previous literatures claimed that women incurred a higher incidence and likely worse outcomes, sex was not found to be significant in this cohort as an endorsement for Jones et al.'s (2021) plea for finer differentiation on hormonal status and morphology of the aneurysm.

Here, the GCS level at admission marks a significant predictor among clinical variables ($p = 0.029$); thus, it will prove useful for further patient stratifications.

This is also supported by other research studies such as Lee et al. (2019), which highlighted the prognostic importance of GCS during the early course of aSAH. By having a low GCS measure, death rate and bad outcome would be higher in depressed consciousness, which calls for an urgent neurological evaluation and intensive monitoring for depressed consciousness-presenting patients.

The occurrence of seizures was another significant predictor ($p = 0.003$). Seizures tend to be a sign of increased cortical irritation or more extensive involvement of the brain and have been associated in literature with adverse outcomes since they may worsen secondary brain injury. In fact, seizures were found to be precedents of complications such as infarction or delayed cerebral ischemia (DCI). Interestingly, other relevant clinical comorbidities such as hypertension ($p = 0.073$) or diabetes ($p = 0.244$) did not seem to impact significantly on outcomes in our study. These results seem curious because their strong and clear roles in vascular pathology plus stroke outcomes are even well established but might reflect effective prehemorrhage medical management or be overruled by acute neurological status.

Although no single imaging parameter (infarcts, ventricular extension, hydrocephalus) reached significance by itself, specific interactions between these variables were significantly associated with one another. Infarcts had a very strong association with the need for decompressive surgery ($p < 0.001$), and hydrocephalus had a strong association with the need for ventriculoperitoneal (VP) shunt placement ($p < 0.001$). These findings indicate that interdependencies among the complications of aSAH are complex, as are secondary injury processes that underlay distinct recovery trajectories. For example, cerebral edema usually follows the infarct and may need surgical decompression, whereas hydrocephalus is a well-known consequence of obstructive blood clots in the pathways of cerebrospinal fluid, which often need shunting.

Similarly, associations were described in the correlation matrix. Notably, infarcts had a significant correlation with modified Rankin Scale (mRS) scores ($r = 0.36$), with a length of stay ($r = 0.36$), and vasospasm ($r = 0.32$), further reiterating the multi-faceted effects that ischemic injury post aSAH has. Hydrocephalus also moderately correlated with DCI ($r = 0.25$), vasospasm ($r = 0.33$), and mRS ($r = 0.31$), establishing it as a concomitant factor in unfavorable functional outcomes. Finding in this study reiterates the multifactorial nature of aSAH prognosis, stressing the need for early clinical grading and monitoring for complication evolving into seizures, infarction, and hydrocephalus. Early intervention, surgical or adjunctive, would also probably improve functional outcomes following strong clinical and radiological stratification.

Personalized prognosis modeling may brighten in the future by the application of advanced imaging such as diffusion tensor imaging (DTI) coupled with machine learning approaches-however, validation using multicenter prospective datasets would be needed to integrate more granular variables (aneurysmal morphology, inflammatory markers, etc., and cerebral perfusion imaging).

8. LIMITATION

This study's retrospective design, small sample size, and reliance on clinical documentation available could lead to information bias. The absence of data on long-term functional outcome measures, including extensive neurocognitive assessment or health-related quality of life scores, adds to the limitations.

9. CONCLUSION

The present investigation points out the multifaceted character of outcome prediction in patients with aSAH. By analyzing demographic, clinical, and imaging parameters, the study demonstrates that initial neurological status, specifically GCS score and seizure occurrence, are critical for prognosis. Although traditional risk factors such as age, sex, and concomitant diseases were statistically insignificant in this cohort, their importance should not be underestimated in wider clinical contexts. Hydrocephalus and cerebral infarction, both of which reached independent significance alone, were found to correlate more strongly with the outcomes of interventions. These findings suggest that grading clinical findings early, monitoring for complications closely, and carrying out imaging evaluation without delay should be included as burn protocols in the management of patients. Future studies incorporating larger, multicenter datasets with advanced forms of neuroimaging will be important for enhancing predictive models and tailored management strategies for better patient outcomes in aSAH.

REFERENCES

Ai, M., Zhang, H., Feng, J., Chen, H., Liu, D., Li, C., Yu, F., & Li, C. (2024). Research advances in predicting the expansion of hypertensive intracerebral hemorrhage based on CT images: An overview. *PeerJ*, *12*, e17556. DOI: 10.7717/peerj.17556 PMID: 38860211

Balança, B., Bouchier, B., & Ritzenthaler, T. (2022). The management of delayed cerebral ischemia after aneurysmal subarachnoid hemorrhage. *Revue Neurologique*, *178*(1-2), 64–73. DOI: 10.1016/j.neurol.2021.11.006 PMID: 34961603

Bhattacharjee, S., Rakesh, D., Ramnadha, R., & Manas, P. (2021). Subarachnoid hemorrhage and hydrocephalus. *Neurology India*, *69*(Suppl 2), S429–S433. DOI: 10.4103/0028-3886.332266 PMID: 35102999

Dodd, W. S., Laurent, D., & Dumont, A. S. (2021). Pathophysiology of delayed cerebral ischemia after subarachnoid hemorrhage. *RE:view*, •••, 10. PMID: 34325514

Gregório, T., Pipa, S., Cavaleiro, P., Atanásio, G., Albuquerque, I., Chaves, P. C., & Azevedo, L. (2018). Prognostic models for intracerebral hemorrhage: Systematic review and meta-analysis. *BMC Medical Research Methodology*, *18*(1), 145. DOI: 10.1186/s12874-018-0613-8 PMID: 30458727

Hamdan, A., Barnes, J., & Mitchell, P. (2014). Subarachnoid hemorrhage and the female sex: Analysis of risk factors, aneurysm characteristics, and outcomes. *Journal of Neurosurgery*, *121*(6), 1367–1373. DOI: 10.3171/2014.7.JNS132318 PMID: 25216063

Hunt, W. E., & Hess, R. M. (1968). Surgical risk as related to time of intervention in the repair of intracranial aneurysms. *Journal of Neurosurgery*, *28*(1), 14–20. DOI: 10.3171/jns.1968.28.1.0014 PMID: 5635959

Lanzino, G., Kassell, N. F., Germanson, T. P., Kongable, G. L., Truskowski, L. L., Torner, J. C., & Jane, J. A. (1996). Age and outcome after aneurysmal subarachnoid hemorrhage: Why do older patients fare worse? *Journal of Neurosurgery*, *85*(3), 410–418. DOI: 10.3171/jns.1996.85.3.0410 PMID: 8751625

Lin, Y., Zhang, S., Zhang, W., Wang, X., Huang, L., & Luo, H. (2021). The prediction value of Glasgow coma scale-pupils score in neurocritical patients: A retrospective study. *Brain Injury : [BI]*, *35*(5), 547–553. DOI: 10.1080/02699052.2021.1890821 PMID: 33645359

Luo, Y., & Payne, S. J. (2024). Neurological intervention transition model for dynamic prediction of good outcome in spontaneous subarachnoid haemorrhage. *Scientific Reports*, *14*(1), 1584. DOI: 10.1038/s41598-024-51684-6 PMID: 38238425

Noureldin, F. (2020). *Early Surgery on Patients with Aneurysmal Subarachnoid Hemorrhage WFNS grades 4 and 5*. PQDT-Global.

Paolini, F., Marrone, S., Scalia, G., Gerardi, R. M., Bonosi, L., Benigno, U. E., Musso, S., Scerrati, A., Iacopino, D. G., Signorelli, F., Maugeri, R., & Visocchi, M. (2025). Diffusion tensor imaging as neurologic predictor in patients affected by traumatic brain injury: Scoping review. *Brain Sciences*, *15*(1), 70. DOI: 10.3390/brainsci15010070 PMID: 39851437

Passier, P. E. C. A., Visser-Meily, J. M. A., Van Zandvoort, M. J. E., Rinkel, G. J. E., Lindeman, E., & Post, M. W. M. (2010). Predictors of long-term health-related quality of life in patients with aneurysmal subarachnoid hemorrhage. *NeuroRehabilitation*, *30*(2), 137–145. DOI: 10.3233/NRE-2012-0737 PMID: 22430579

Pereira, R., Torres, B., Nogueira, J., Coimbra, F., Afonso, M., Alegria, C., & Marques, R. (2025). Predictive factors for ventriculoperitoneal shunt placement in aneurysmatic subarachnoid hemorrhages. *Brain & Spine*, *5*, 104164. DOI: 10.1016/j.bas.2024.104164 PMID: 39802870

Rinkel, G. J., & Algra, A. (2011). Long-term outcomes of patients with aneurysmal subarachnoid haemorrhage. *Lancet Neurology*, *10*(4), 349–356. DOI: 10.1016/S1474-4422(11)70017-5 PMID: 21435599

Schmidt, T. P., Weiss, M., Hoellig, A., Nikoubashman, O., Schulze-Steinen, H., Albanna, W., Clusmann, H., Schubert, G. A., & Veldeman, M. (2022). Revisiting the timeline of delayed cerebral ischemia after aneurysmal subarachnoid hemorrhage: Toward a temporal risk profile. *Neurocritical Care*, *37*(3), 735–743. DOI: 10.1007/s12028-022-01545-9 PMID: 35790670

Shah, K. A., White, T. G., Teron, I., Turpin, J., Dehdashti, A. R., Temes, R. E., Black, K., & Woo, H. H. (2024). Quantitative magnetic resonance angiography as an alternative imaging technique in the assessment of cerebral vasospasm after subarachnoid hemorrhage. *Interventional Neuroradiology : Journal of Peritherapeutic Neuroradiology, Surgical Procedures and Related Neurosciences*, *30*(2), 271–279. DOI: 10.1177/15910199221138167 PMID: 36357992

Wang, A. C., & Heros, R. C. (2016). Subarachnoid hemorrhage grading scales. *Journal of Neurosurgery*, *124*(2), 296–298. DOI: 10.3171/2015.3.JNS15336 PMID: 26381258

Wang, D. M., Li, J., Liu, J. R., & Hu, H. Y. (2012). Diffusion tensor imaging predicts long-term motor functional outcome in patients with acute supratentorial intracranial hemorrhage. *Cerebrovascular Diseases (Basel, Switzerland)*, *34*(3), 199–205. DOI: 10.1159/000341857 PMID: 23006600

Wu, R., Hu, F., Liu, C., & Liang, J. (2024). The value of modified hijdra score in patients with aneurysmal subarachnoid hemorrhage. *Heliyon*, *10*(7), e28550. DOI: 10.1016/j.heliyon.2024.e28550 PMID: 38590907

Xiao, Z. K., Wang, B., Liu, J. H., Yang, Y. B., Jie, N., Mao, X. Y., Gong, X. Y., Liu, A. H., & Duan, Y. H. (2025). Risk factors for the development of delayed cerebral ischemia after aneurysmal subarachnoid hemorrhage: A systematic review and meta-analysis. *World Neurosurgery*, *193*, 427–446. DOI: 10.1016/j.wneu.2024.09.104 PMID: 39343384

Yang, C., & Li, Y. (2022). Review of the prevention and treatment of hydrocephalus after aneurysmal subarachnoid hemorrhage. *World Neurosurgery*, *168*, 134–138. DOI: 10.1016/j.wneu.2022.08.089 PMID: 36041720

Yang, C., Zhao, Z., Yang, B., Wang, K., Zhu, G., & Miao, H. (2024). Sex differences in outcome of aneurysmal subarachnoid hemorrhage and its relation to postoperative cerebral ischemia. *Neurocritical Care*, *41*(3), 985–996. DOI: 10.1007/s12028-024-02028-9 PMID: 38954369

Zacharia, B. E., Hickman, Z. L., Grobelny, B. T., DeRosa, P., Kotchetkov, I., Ducruet, A. F., & Connolly, E. S. (2010). Epidemiology of aneurysmal subarachnoid hemorrhage. *Neurosurgery Clinics*, *21*(2), 221–233. PMID: 20380965

Zhao, D., Li, Y., & Cui, J. (2024). The factors associated with the modified Fisher grade in patients with aneurysmal subarachnoid hemorrhage. *Frontiers in Physiology*, *15*, 1373925. DOI: 10.3389/fphys.2024.1373925 PMID: 39086933

Ziebart, A., Dremel, J., Hetjens, S., Nieuwkamp, D. J., Linn, F. H., Etminan, N., & Rinkel, G. J. (2024). Case fatality and functional outcome after spontaneous subarachnoid haemorrhage: A systematic review and meta-analysis of time trends and regional variations in population-based studies. *European Stroke Journal*, *9*(3), 555–565. DOI: 10.1177/23969873241232823 PMID: 38353205

Chapter 6
Early Detection of Parkinson's Disease for Developing a Predictive Model Using Biomedical Voice Data

Muhammad Zubair
Ilma University, Pakistan

Bushra Khalid
Sirsyed University, Pakistan

ABSTRACT

The quality of life of every patient suffering from Parkinson's disease is significantly hindered by tremors, muscle rigidity, and other symptoms of general backed-up stages of the disorder. Early detection in some instances has improved treatment, leading to higher quality of living. This study aims to devise a predictive model utilizing biomedical voice data to allow for early diagnosis of Parkinson's disease. By studying voice signals and extracting crucial features from them, the model will seek to discover factors that can be traced to the disease. Findings from this study would aid in initiating early and necessary interventions towards furthering treatment and provide insights into the role of voice-based biomarkers for the diagnosis of other neurological diseases.

DOI: 10.4018/979-8-3373-2807-2.ch006

1. INTRODUCTION

PD is a neurodegenerative disorder characterized by progressive impairment due to motor symptoms like tremor, rigidity, and bradykinesia, among others, and also non-motor symptoms such as speech impairments. The early diagnosis of PD is an important stage toward timely interventions that can decelerate disease progression and improve quality of life for patients.

Recent breakthroughs in machine learning have enabled the development of predictive models that can analyze biomedical voice data for early signs of PD. Voice impairments are among the early signs of PD, and hence, voice analysis is a non-invasive, cost-effective tool for early diagnosis. Several studies have demonstrated that ML algorithms can classify PD patients from voice recordings with high accuracy. For instance, one of the studies, which applied voice samples pre-processed by ML methods, reported very good results in distinguishing PD patients from healthy controls. Furthermore, deep learning approaches integrated with voice analysis have also shown great promise for improving early detection of PD. Several studies using multimodal deep learning approaches have reported increased accuracy in the identification of prodromal stages of PD by combining multiple data modalities including voice . In another work, the authors presented a deep learning-based system for the prediction and monitoring of PD by using voice data, underlining the potential of such technologies in non-invasive diagnostics (Garcia and Hertel, 2023).

Other than the fact that predictive models using biomedical voice data enable early detection, they also offer a scalable solution for wide screening. With the growing prevalence of PD worldwide, leveraging ML and voice analysis is an exciting avenue for early diagnosis and better patient outcomes. This research, therefore, has the aim of identifying a predictive model, utilizing biomedical voice data, that will be able to diagnose the presence of Parkinson's disease. We will try to discover distinctive vocal biomarkers linked to the onset of PD through advanced machine learning analysis of voice recordings. We wish to contribute to the development of non-invasive diagnostic means for early intervention and management of PD.

This study will focus on developing a predictive model that will make early detection of the disease possible using biomedical voice data. This project makes use of a Parkinson's Disease Dataset found in Kaggle, consisting of 1,195 samples and 24 features, mostly voice-related measures. The dataset is cleaned; EDA and preprocessing are done to make further analysis appropriate and reliable (Hazan et.al, 2019).

It includes feature analysis to identify relevant voice biomarkers, construction of predictive models using machine learning techniques, and validation of the models to optimize their accuracy. Feature importance ranking and predictive modeling were performed using the Random Forest algorithm because it is robust for high-dimensional data and has a minimal chance of overfitting, as stated by Husch and Hertel, (2023). K-Means clustering was also done to group data from disease severity for better visualization and understanding of disease progression patterns.

The purpose of this research paper is to enhance the predictive ability of early diagnosis models through advanced pre-processing steps and rigorous model validation. This research applies biomechanical voice data to the integration of state-of-the-art machine learning techniques and non-invasive diagnostic devices as presented in literature with respect to neurological disorders by Iftikhar et al., 2023. Indeed, results in this work present better prospects for early detection of the disease, hence finally enabling appropriate management and enhanced care of such patients (Jeong et.al, 2024).

2. LITERATURE REVIEW

PD is a neurodegenerative disease that is characterized by progressive aggravation of motor symptoms such as tremors, rigidity, and bradykinesia, and also includes non-motor symptoms related to speech impairments. Early diagnosis in PD permits the timely institution of those interventions that delay the course of the disease and improve a patient's quality of life.

Recent advances in ML have enabled the construction of predictive models using voice biomedical data to detect PD at an early stage. Since voice impairments are among the first symptoms that appear in PD patients, analysis of voice is, thereby, a very non-invasive and low-cost tool for diagnosing this condition at its very beginning. The ML algorithms were quite good at classifying these patients as PD or healthy controls based on voice recordings. For instance, one study using voice samples pre-processed b

Deep learning approaches in combination with voice analysis have been promising for early detection of PD. The studies that utilized a multimodal deep learning approach showed better

Another study presented a deep-learning-based system for the prediction and monitoring of PD from voice data, emphasizing such technologies for diagnostics without invasion.

This, however, has changed with the development of predictive models from biomedical voice data, which not only enables early detection but also scalable solutions for wide screening. The prevalence of PD is continuously on the rise globally; thus, leveraging ML and voice analysis presents an exciting avenue leading to early diagnosis that results in better patient outcomes.

The proposed study intends to incorporate biomedical voice data into a predictive model for the detection of early stages of PD. To this effect, voice records will be analyzed for specific vocal biomarkers at the onset of PD using advanced machine learning algorithms. Our goal is to contribute to the literature with regard to the development of non-invasive diagnostic tools, in order to provide a window of opportunity for early intervention and effective management of Parkinson's disease (Saeed et.al, 2021; Nagarapu, 2021).

The increasing prevalence of PD has motivated extensive research into early detection and diagnosis using ML and DL methodologies. Most of the studies investigate the potential of speech analysis, brain imaging, and acoustic features for developing accurate predictive models. Vyas et al. (2022) have proposed a deep learning-based scheme for the diagnosis of Parkinson's disease, outlining the use of convolutional neural networks and recurrent neural networks in feature extraction and classification. Curated datasets on the diagnosis of PD have reported significant improvements in accuracy, with evidence that DL techniques could upscale clinical diagnostics.

Noor et al. (2020) reviewed various ML models using brain imaging data for PD diagnosis and prognosis. In this work, the main challenges were discussed: heterogeneity of the data, interpretability of models, and strong need for proper cross-validation. Such models, while applied to integrating multi-modal imaging data, may contribute to reaching higher diagnostic precision and more personalized treatment options (Singh et.al, 2023; Vyas *et al.*, 2022).

Postuma et al. (2019) made use of ANNs for Parkinson's disease prediction from the speech datasets with high accuracy rates. This study highlighted the use of vocal biomarkers in the determination of early PD symptoms, including pitch variation and jitter. Their method used vast datasets to train models that are capable of generalizing to the real world and thus furthered the field of diagnostics non-invasively(Saeed, 2023).

Saeed et al. (2018) have extracted intrinsic mode function-based features from speech signals to predict Parkinson's disease. Their feature engineering methodology extracted meaningful patterns from speech signals, which were then classified using the ML algorithms. This study stressed that signal-processing techniques have to be used to improve the accuracy of prediction models (Siddique et.al, 2023; Saeed, 2017).

Saeed et.al, (2024) focused on modeling the progress of the disease regarding naturally spoken language features. The work examined which linguistic patterns could be considered as potential biomarkers, such as hesitation and pauses; the results obtained proved the potential of the use of NLP techniques in PD research (Saeed et.al, 2022; Saeed et.al, 2021).

Shaban (2023) utilized machine learning to classify PD by using acoustic features extracted from multilingual speech tasks. This work underlined the role of linguistic diversity in the training of robust models and showed that multilingual datasets improve the generalizability of models across different populations.

These collectively point toward the transformation that ML and DL techniques could bring in the diagnosis and monitoring of Parkinson's disease. Combining speech and acoustic features with advanced computational models creates a promising direction for early detection and non-invasive diagnostic tools. However, there are still challenges around data standardization, model interpretability, and integrating multi-modal datasets. Further research should be done to fill these gaps and enhance the clinical relevance of such predictive models.

3. DATASET DESCRIPTION

The Parkinson's Disease Dataset discussed in the report contains biomedical voice measurements for early detection of Parkinson's disease. This dataset consists of 1,195 records across 24 columns, containing both numerical and categorical data types. As mentioned earlier, it is one of the most prominent datasets related to medical studies of Parkinson's disease and is publicly available on Kaggle. Created by Shreya Dutta, it finds extensive use in machine learning and data science projects related to the development of predictive models for Parkinson's detection.

This dataset consists of medical and voice-related information about the study of Parkinson's disease, focusing on vocal biomarkers. These are a set of features comprising the variation in pitch, loudness, and voice quality that can indicate initial signs of the disease. Such voice features, like jitter, shimmer, and harmonics-to-noise ratio, are important in bringing out patterns associated with Parkinson's disease. Analysis of these voice features helps researchers and health professionals to identify and monitor the disease in a non-invasive yet effective way. This dataset contains patient identification numbers, coupled with comprehensive measurement of voice features; hence, it is highly useful for building machine learning models. These models can use predictive algorithms to help in the early detection of Parkinson's disease, monitor the progress of the disease over time, and provide useful insights that may assist in treatment planning. The structure and feature availability within this dataset provide a perfect resource for research in biomedical data, machine learning, and medical diagnostics. Below is an overview of the dataset, first and last five rows, when viewed in Google Colab. Generally, this excellent dataset is the necessary tool that will be helpful in taking ahead the research on Parkinson's disease and improving patient outcomes.

4. STATISTICS OF THE DATASET

First of all, the function describe () function was run in Python for a summary of the 23 numeric columns in the dataset to obtain statistical characteristics. The statistics include count, mean, standard deviation, minimum and maximum, and the 25th, 50th median, and 75th percentiles for each column. Below is a breakdown explanation of the key statistics of the dataset. The column Fo (Hz) is the mean fundamental frequency of the voice, with an average of 154.31 Hz and a standard deviation of 17.12 Hz. That is, the average fundamental frequency of the voice is 154.31 Hz, while variations around the mean are relatively small, at about 10%. This consistency in the fundamental frequency of the voice indicates high quality and reliability of the data.

The MDVP: Jitter(%) column, which quantifies frequency variability, has a mean of 0.0062 with a standard deviation of 0.0020. These are small values, indicating high fidelity in the voice samples with very little variation or jitter. This is significant in that it suggests the recordings have minimal distortion or irregularities in frequency. Other amplitude and noise characteristics are given in columns like MDVP: Shimmer and NHR. The mean value in the column MDVP: Shimmer is 0.0297, while the maximum is 0.119, which states that the amplitude is more or less even. Also, the column of NHR, representing the noise-to-harmonic ratio, has an average value of 0.0249, which can be interpreted as low levels of noise in the voice samples-a very key factor when analyzing vocal biomarkers. This implies that about 75% of the samples are of the ones diagnosed with PD. From this, it is possible to get an idea about the class distribution in the dataset. It seems highly imbalanced, having a high prevalence of PD cases within. Further, advanced voice signal features are RPDE, DFA, spread1, spread2, D2, and PPE. For example, the average value of spread1 is -5.68, ranging between -7.96 and -2.43, which specifies the dispersion of frequency components of the voice signal. The PPE, as shown, has an average of 0.2077 and a peak value of 0.5274, showing variation in the pitch dynamics of voice samples, another important indicator in voice analysis for PD detection. The overall statistic of the dataset provides a summary of the distribution and variability of features. Low values for jitter and shimmer show little variations in vocal features, while the status column provides information on the dataset's focus on detecting Parkinson's disease. This dataset is rich in voice biomarkers, serving as a very good resource for diagnosis, subtype finding, diagnostics support, and research in Parkinson's disease as shown in Figure 1.

Figure 1. Statistical summary of proposed datasets

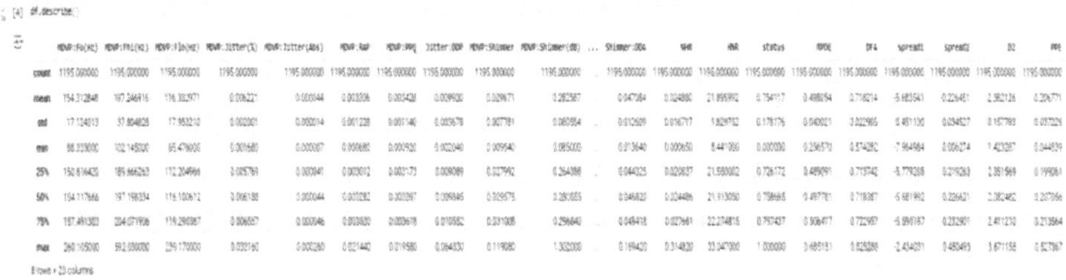

5. PROPOSED METHODOLOGY

The methodology for high-quality data and EDA for the Parkinson's disease dataset begins with a focus on cleaning the data. First of all, we checked missing values in the dataset using the command print(df.isnull().sum()). After confirming there were no missing values, no imputation or column removal was required. Then, we calculated the outliers by the IQR method. We calculated IQR as the difference between the third quartile, Q3, and the first quartile, Q1. Every value that was below the range (Q1 - 1.5IQR) or above the range (Q3 + 1.5IQR) was handled as an outlier. We decided the maximum limit of acceptance of outliers in any column would be 5%. If any column exceeded this amount of outliers, that column data would remain. We have done preprocessing by removing the only categorical variable-'name' column-as it was not useful in gaining insights. Feature engineering has been done by performing hierarchical cluster analysis to find the features which are highly correlated and removing the variables whose correlation coefficient was higher than 0.9. Additionally, StandardScaler was used for the standardization of the dataset, keeping the features at an average of 0 with a standard deviation of 1 in order to avoid biases from large scales of some features.

In our exploratory data analysis step, we summarized some basic statistics of the 'status' variable and summarized the trends in distribution for the diagnosis of patients. Moreover, we visualized the distribution of different severity grades into patients for views of a histogram and pie chart. A heatmap is drawn to discover the correlation between each pair, especially the correlation between features and the 'status' variable for capturing the main factors that affect the disease.

We then applied data mining techniques by using a Random Forest regression model to assess disease progression. The model picked out spread1, MVP:Fo(Hz), and spread2 in the top three most influential features. Robustness in the Random Forest was guaranteed by random sampling of the decision trees, which helped to mitigate noise and non-linearity in the data. The most optimal settings were determined by using hyperparameter tuning: 100 decision trees with a maximum depth of 10. That balanced model complexity with model performance. Besides, K-means clustering was applied for the visual representation and to understand the pattern and distribution about the most important features. This algorithm iteratively assigns each data point to the cluster to which the mean cluster center is closest, and the number of clusters was set to 3 to align with the severity classification of the disease.

To validate the model and evaluate its performance, we used LOOCV to gauge the efficiency of the Random Forest model. This method maximized the use of training data and provided a robust measure of model performance. A confusion matrix heatmap was generated to visually evaluate model predictions against actual outcomes, identifying true positives and negatives and highlighting areas for improvement. The methodology, therefore, provides the actual detail on how data should be treated step by step, with cleaning, pre-processing, and analysis to enable insights into the dataset about Parkinson's disease. With top-class data, together with good models, much serves as a very strong backbone to the understanding of the development of the disease and to assist clinical evaluations and interventions effectively. The model will be further refined and then tested for its applicability with new patient datasets in order to confirm the findings.

6. DATA-RELATED ISSUES & PREPROCESSING

In any analysis based on data or data mining process, the quality is solely dependent upon the quality of the data. Algorithms don't like inconsistent, incomplete, or poorly scaled data; the accuracy and reliability of the results would be drastically different. This section has two parts: the first one covers the steps to be taken in order to get high-quality data and the second one covers benefits and implementations of these techniques.

Cleaning of data is a necessary first step in preparing the dataset for analysis. The Parkinson's Disease Dataset contains useful insights: demographic, medical, and diagnosis data. Where there is variety in data type, there are different challenges that will have to be addressed if the integrity of the analysis is to be maintained. The problem of missing values is common for big data in general, and sometimes this dataset represents experimental measurements that are challenging and costly to obtain. Given the size of the dataset, 24 columns by 1,195 rows, chances for missing data are high; this may seriously restrict the learning process, especially for machine learning algorithms. Missing values can even generate runtime errors in Python. Some imputation technique like using mean or median could be used, or columns with excessive missing data could be dropped. Missing values were checked with the Python command print(df.isnull().sum()). The result from that test showed that there was no problem with this dataset concerning missing values, so no further action was required as shown in Figure 2.

Figure 2. Missing values handling

```
name                0
MDVP:Fo(Hz)         0
MDVP:Fhi(Hz)        0
MDVP:Flo(Hz)        0
MDVP:Jitter(%)      0
MDVP:Jitter(Abs)    0
MDVP:RAP            0
MDVP:PPQ            0
Jitter:DDP          0
MDVP:Shimmer        0
MDVP:Shimmer(dB)    0
Shimmer:APQ3        0
Shimmer:APQ5        0
MDVP:APQ            0
Shimmer:DDA         0
NHR                 0
HNR                 0
status              0
RPDE                0
DFA                 0
spread1             0
spread2             0
D2                  0
PPE                 0
```

Outliers are also a concern in medical data because of biological differences between individuals and the unpredictable progress of diseases as shown in Figure 3. Furthermore, underrepresentation-for example, females in medical research-could also create potential outliers. However, not all outliers are problematic in medical datasets since they may be representative of extreme disease progressions. A few approaches to detecting outliers include graphical approaches such as boxplots, the statistical z-score, and the IQR method. The IQR method has been selected herein because it is one of the simple but strong methods. It looks into the central 50% of the data and decides if values are over 1.5 times the IQR distance from Q1 or Q3. Those columns whose values were out of this range were identified as columns containing potential outliers. Initial analysis showed many columns with more than 10% outliers, which were supposed to be the basis of further assessment. Given the medical nature of the data and there being a high probability of some of those outliers not truly being erroneous, a threshold value of 5% may be considered reasonable. This is because any column with more than 5% outliers would retain all values intact in their column, as such could constitute the variation that comes with medical data.

Figure 3. Biological differences between individuals and the unpredictable progress of diseases

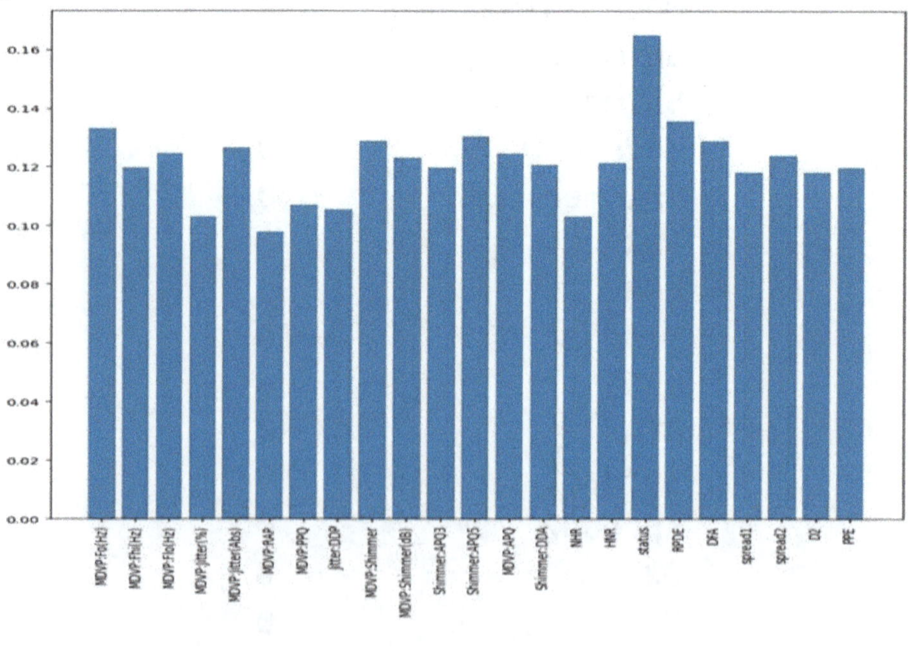

7. DATA PREPARATION

Data preparation is the process whereby raw data is transformed into proper form that is effectively understandable and interpretable by a machine learning model. Scaling and encoding improve the work of a machine learning model with data. Unlike the human mind, it focuses on ratios and relationships more than understandability. It is an important step whereby proper structuring and preparation of data are ensured for analysis.

7.1 Handling Categorical Variables

Categorical variables can be a real problem for all machine learning models since none of them can process such variables directly. The most usual way of treating categorical data is one-hot encoding, which, for each unique value of the categorical variable, introduces a new binary column. That way, the model will be able to understand that information numerically. The following command was used in order to find out the categorical variables in the dataset:

Figure 4.

```
df.select_dtypes(include=['object']).columns
```

Indeed, it had the output that there was only one categorical variable 'name', which also is of no use in finding out the insights. Thus, it was dropped to make life simpler.

7.2 Feature Engineering

Feature selection is one of the most important decisions that may have a huge impact on the performance of any machine learning model. In this paper, hierarchical cluster analysis has been used to identify and remove highly correlated features. We cluster features based on their correlation for better visualization of the relationship among them and to select the most relevant variables. A dendrogram generated through this process showed several pairs of closely related columns. We decided to drop one column in each pair where the correlation exceeded 0.9 - proximity less than 0.1 - to decrease redundancy in the dataset as shown in Figure 5.

Figure 5. Dendrogram form of pairs which closely related column

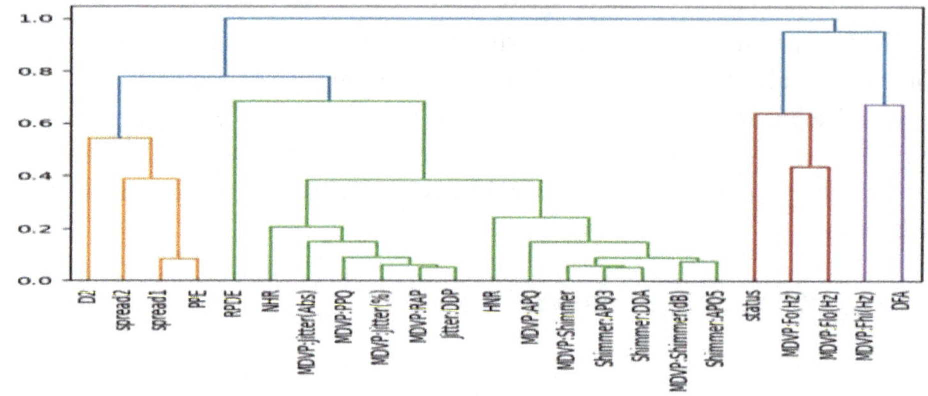

7.3 Scaling the Data

Normalization of the dataset is a must, especially for variables with different scales. Many machine learning algorithms use the concept of distance; thus, they may be prejudiced toward features with large values. StandardScaler was applied to transform each column in this regard, scaling the data such that the mean of each feature is 0 and the standard deviation of each feature is 1. This ensures that no variable gets weighted more than others because of their scale, thus preventing models from giving bias toward certain features, especially in the biological and medical context.

We can see that multiple columns are closely related. We decided to drop all one of all pairs, that have a proximity of less than 0.1 (Correlation more than 0.9). The following columns were dropped:

7.4 Exploratory Data Analysis (EDA)

EDA plays a great role in understanding and analyzing the dataset before machine learning models can be applied. It gives both graphical and statistical insights into the data to lay a foundation for further analysis. In this dataset, the 'status' variable is of main interest and refers to the severity in which a patient is in due to the Parkinson's disease. Basic statistics have been computed; histograms and pie charts in visualizations were generated to reveal its distribution. It therefore follows that most patients belong to different degrees of Parkinson's disease with relatively clear distribution across different measures of severity.

We also assumed that speech disorder may act as a strong indicative in the identification of the disease. For studying that, the histograms corresponding to the features 'Shimmer' and 'Jitter', related to speech disorders were plotted. The feature demonstrated the same distribution for different values, which indeed relates both the variables again to the disease progression also.

Figure 6. EDA of proposed methodology

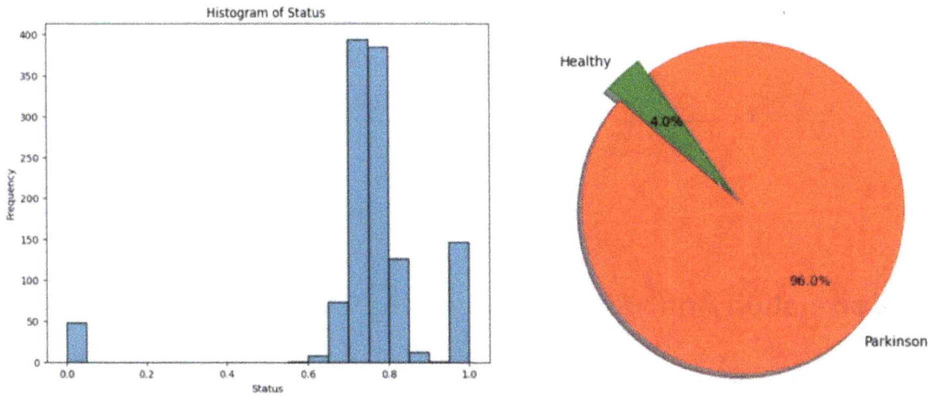

Figure 6 indicate the clearly visible, that most of the patients have Parkinsons of different severities. Furthermore, we assumed that speech disorder is probably a good indicator on whether a patient suffers from this disease or not. To get an overview over those speech disorder features we plotted histograms for Shimmer and Jitter as shown in Figure 6:

Figure 7. Histograms for Shimmer and Jitter

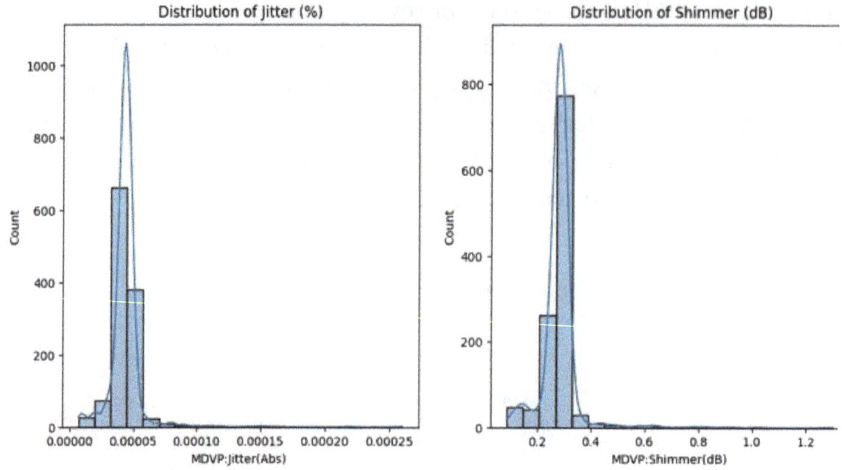

7.5 Correlation Analysis

One of the most useful techniques for identification of a relationship between variables is correlation analysis. To understand how features interact with each other comprehensively, a heatmap combined with the correlation matrix has been generated. This will provide a view of the relationships among the variables. Since the main concentration is with the 'status' variable, a sorted histogram has been created to illustrate the relationship of each feature concerning 'status'. Results of this analysis showed that no one variable significantly contributes to the 'status'; it instead hinted at complex, multi-dimensional relationships between the variables. Further, to explore these intricate relationships, advanced methods of analysis would be required.

Figure 8. EDA representation of correlation matrix

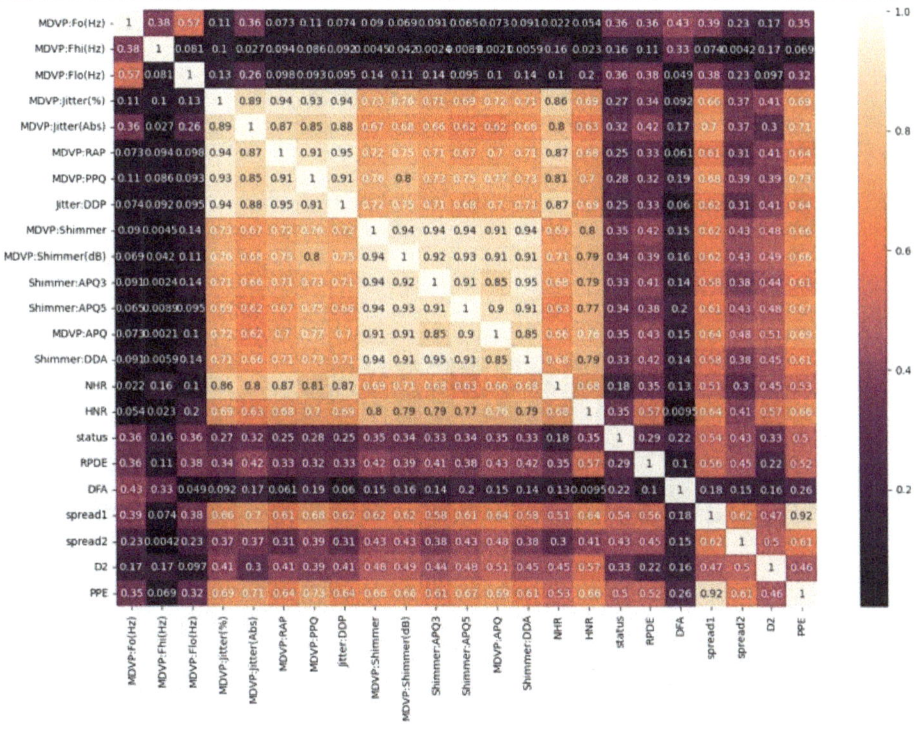

This information is helpful but consists of a lot of features. Additionally, we are really interested in the *status* variable. So, we created a sorted histogram of the correlation of every variable with the *status* as shown in Figure 7

Figure 9. Graphical representation of K-means clustering results

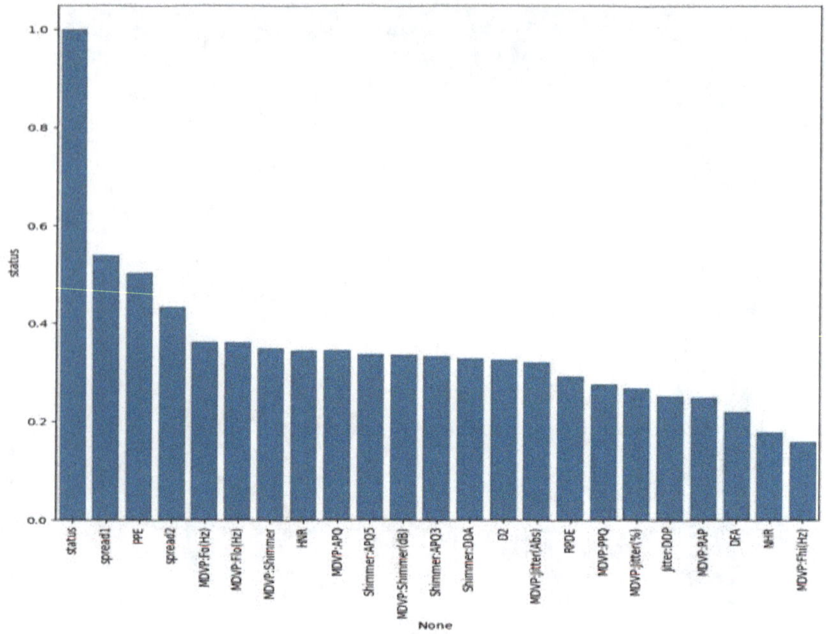

Data preprocessing was followed by the implementation of a range of data mining techniques with an aim to extract meaningful patterns and structures from the dataset. Since the dimensionality and heterogeneity of the Parkinson's disease dataset are high, selecting an appropriate data mining technique became very important. Among the many methods, Random Forest was chosen for feature extraction since it is able to handle complex data structures and identify the most influential features. K-means clustering was thereafter used as an alternative means of further analysis for patterns in the data that could reveal factors of disease progression. This gave insight into the factors likely to affect the progress of the disease negatively as shown in Figure 9.

7.6 Random Forest

Random Forest is currently one of the most famous classical algorithms in data mining for supervised machine learning. It works well for classification and regression problems; hence, it is suitable for nonlinear and complex data such as in Parkinson's disease progression. In this paper, we have used Random Forest to develop a regression model for predicting the progression of the disease in patients with a major focus on the most important features contributing to Parkinson's disease progression.

7.6.1 Basic concept

Random Forest operates by combining a large number of decision trees, each trained independently. The strength of the model comes from aggregating these simple models to form a more powerful and robust overall model. Each decision tree is trained on a random subset of the dataset to ensure diversity among the trees, making the model more robust. Predictions from all decision trees are aggregated through majority voting (for classification) or averaging (for regression).

- Reasons for Using Random Forest
- Several key factors made Random Forest the ideal choice for this analysis:
- Feature Extraction: Random Forest is excellent at identifying key features that significantly influence decisions, providing insight into how Parkinson's disease progresses.
- Handling High-Dimensional Data: The dataset contains 24 columns, with 22 used as input features. Random Forest addresses correlations among features by selecting random data points for each tree, improving the model's dimensional efficiency.
- Non-Linearity and Complex Interactions: Medical and biological data often exhibit non-linear patterns and complex interactions, which Random Forest can model without needing explicit representations.
- Noise Robustness: Given that medical data can be noisy, Random Forest is particularly effective, as its ensemble approach mitigates the impact of noisy data, making the model more resilient.
- Hyperparameter Tuning
- Hyperparameter tuning is crucial to ensuring optimal performance. The most important parameters for our model were:
- Number of Trees: More trees generally enhance performance but at the cost of computational complexity. In our case, 100 trees provided robust and accurate predictions.
- Max Depth: Limiting the depth of decision trees prevents overfitting. A maximum depth of 10 was found to produce solid results.

7.6.2 Limitations of Random Forest

While Random Forest is an efficient model, there is one point in its nature: computation intensity. A large number of trees being used can make this model computationally demanding.

Model Interpretation: While the important features are easy to identify, interpreting how and why decisions are made remains challenging due to the complexity of multiple decision trees.

Overfitting: Without proper regularization-for instance, using constraints in the number of trees or maximum depth-decision trees would be overfit to capture noise rather than the underlying patterns.

The Random Forest model allowed us to identify the three most important features of the progression of PD: spread1, MVP: Fo(Hz), and spread as shown in Figure 10.

Figure 10. Proposed random forest results

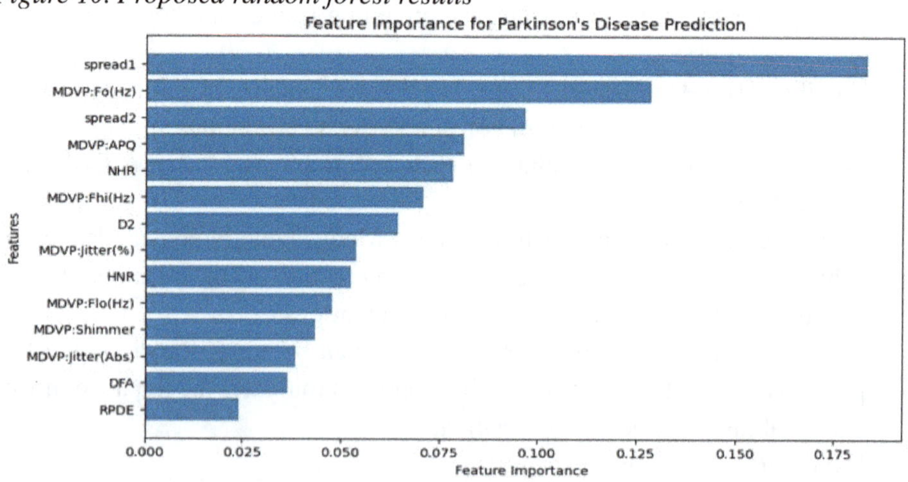

7.7 K-means clustering

We then applied the K-means clustering algorithm to visualize the impact of such features in disease progression, selected by using Random Forest. Unlike Random Forest, K-means is an unsupervised learning algorithm which condenses similar data into clusters. It helped us to create, in this case, a visual representation of the distribution of the key features categorized into three levels of severity regarding Parkinson's disease.

7.7.1 Basic concept

K-means operates iteratively. Initially, random cluster centers are selected, and each data point is assigned to the nearest cluster center based on Euclidean distance. The cluster center is then updated to the mean of all points within the cluster. This process repeats until convergence or a set number of iterations is reached.

7.7.2 K-means offer several advantages

Simplicity and Efficiency: It works well with large data sets, such as the Parkinson dataset, and is relatively simple to execute. It is, therefore, a practical technique for exploring various techniques.

Euclidean Distance: Our selected features include continuous numerical values, and K-means is particularly suited for such kind of data along with Euclidean distance.

Pattern Recognition: K-means exhibits natural clumping within data, which allows an understanding of how the variation of different features affects the progressions of diseases and symptoms.

7.8 Hyperparameter Tuning

The following parameters have been tuned for the optimization of K-means:

Number of Clusters: The best number of clusters is a must for K-means. We found that three clusters are most meaningful and give the best results for distinguishing between the different levels of severity of Parkinson's disease.

Data Scaling: Standardization of the data has been done prior to using K-means; therefore, all features are scaled and have equal importance. This is an important factor, since k-means implies some kind of distance measure and unequal scaling may distort the result.

7.8.1 Limitations of K-means

The challenges in K-means are:

Optimal Number of Clusters: Seeded number is not that easy to come up with; it's more experimental. Choosing the wrong number-either too small or too large-may result in meaningless or even wrong outcomes.

Sensitivity to Outliers: The centroids may be significantly affected by outliers, therefore providing poor accuracy in the assignments of clusters.

Spherical Clusters Assumption: K-means does assume that clusters are spherical, which on most occasions is an assumption that might not hold in complex data structures. This may impact on the quality of how well the model describes a cluster in some instances.

Applying K-means clustering allowed us to map the data for much greater insight into how selected features relate to various severity levels of Parkinson's. K-means clustering gave us the following results. The colors (alias Cluster 0, 1 and 2) represent the different severity of the Parkison disease and the target variable of the Random Forest as shown in Figure 10.

Figure 11. Spherical Clusters Assumption

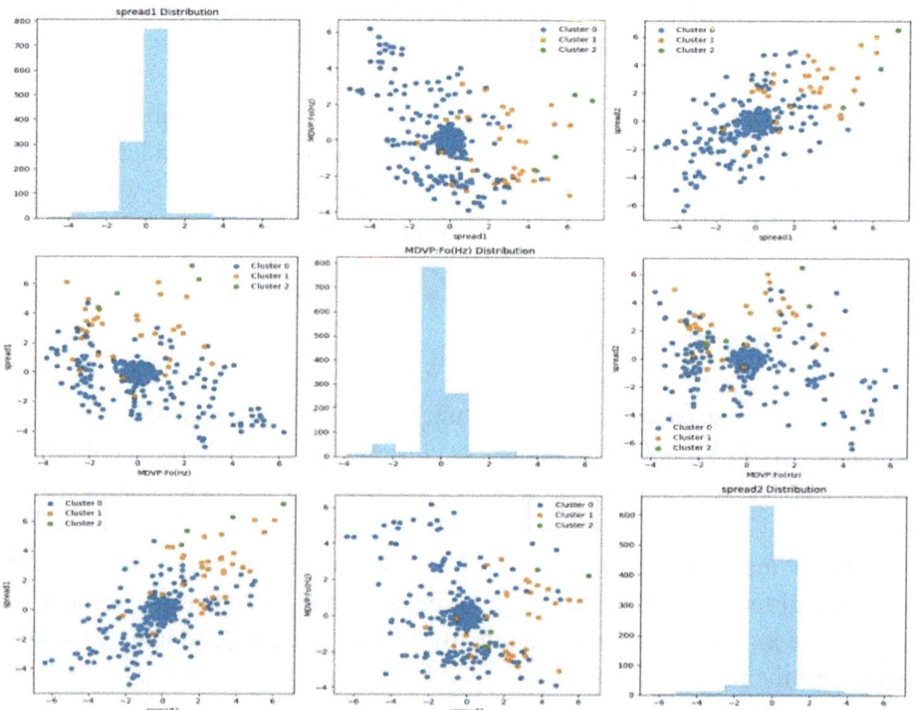

8. VALIDATION TECHNIQUES: LEAVE-ONE-OUT CROSS-VALIDATION (LOOCV) IN PARKINSON'S DISEASE PREDICTION

Effective model evaluation is one of the most critical tasks in machine learning. This ensures that a model generalizes efficiently on unseen data and can perform well on any other dataset apart from the training one. For example, the LOOCV is a very robust technique that can cross-validate the performance of a Random Forest

Classifier on the Parkinson's disease prediction. LOOCV is a special form of k-fold cross-validation, where "k" is equal to the number of data points. In other words, every data point in the dataset will be used as both a test and a training sample at some point so that the model can be evaluated on all data points exhaustively.

LOOCV is of particular benefit for small datasets, because in its usage, it leaves no single data out and utilizes all the data that might be available. Given that it is always a challenge to get large volumes of labeled data, even in medical research, such as in Parkinson's disease, LOOCV ensures the model uses the entire dataset. Unlike the more traditional forms of k-fold cross-validation, which further split a dataset into random subsets, LOOCV tests the model against every possible data point. Therefore, it is more stable to estimate the true generalization performance of the model. This becomes particularly important when trying to understand how well the model generalizes to new, unseen data in medical applications.

In this case, the LOOCV implementation involves segregating the independent variables from the target variable that represents the presence of Parkinson's. This can be done using the LeaveOneOut () from the sklearn.model_selection module to generate the training and testing splits iteratively. It trains a Random Forest Classifier on all data points but one in every iteration and makes predictions on the left-out point using the model. Accuracy for each prediction will be determined and aggregated for the overall measure of model performance. The mean accuracy score returned as output is the indication of overall quality or robustness of the model for the predictive capability on this disease progression when a new data presentation is made.

LOOCV wrapped in the evaluation pipeline gives higher confidence for the model's predictive accuracy with a minimum bias toward the test dataset, hence yielding a clear approximation of how the Random Forest Classifier would perform in real-world scenarios. This approach, when taken toward the prediction of Parkinson's disease, helps in early diagnosis and understanding of disease progression better.

8.1 LOOCV and Histograms for Model Performance Assessment

LOOCV with a histogram is a practical method for performance and result visualization of a model. While LOOCV allows the model to be trained and tested on every available point, the use of the histogram will provide visualization to show the distribution of the accuracy score developed during each iteration. In this way, it will go a long way in giving good insight into the frequency and spread of the performances.

Histograms are useful graphics that can be used to divide the dataset into sub-intervals (bins) and plot the frequency of accuracy scores within each bin. This graph shows not only the central tendency of the model's performance but also the consistency and variability across different data points. If the histogram ranges widely or has significant outliers, further analysis and adjustment of the model may be required. Including KDE in the histogram, which is done through the k=True parameter in seaborn's histplot function, smooths the distribution and provides a more accurate estimate of the probability density function. This additional layer of analysis allows for a much clearer understanding of the underlying patterns in the model's performance.

A histogram in conjunction with LOOCV offers a complete assessment of the model's performance. Although one may have a single accuracy score, which can be viewed as a simplistic explanation of the performance, it does not give any indication of the variation and nuances across different subsets. By plotting the distribution of accuracy scores, researchers can understand the stability of their model and where to focus for further improvement. The KDE curve further refines this understanding, offering a more detailed view of the distribution that can be informative, especially when comparing multiple models or assessing the impact of different hyperparameters.

In all, LOOCV combined with histograms enriched with KDE offers a multi-faceted approach to model evaluation. LOOCV ensures that maximum utilization of the dataset is availed, which is a strong measure regarding the performance of a model. This is furthered by using histograms to show the consistency and distribution of the accuracy score, which helps the researchers and data scientists make informed decisions on model selection, refinement, and further improvement, thus generally improving the reliability and applicability of machine learning models in medical diagnoses such as that of Parkinson's disease as shown in Figure 12.

Figure 12. Distribution score of LOOCV accuracy values

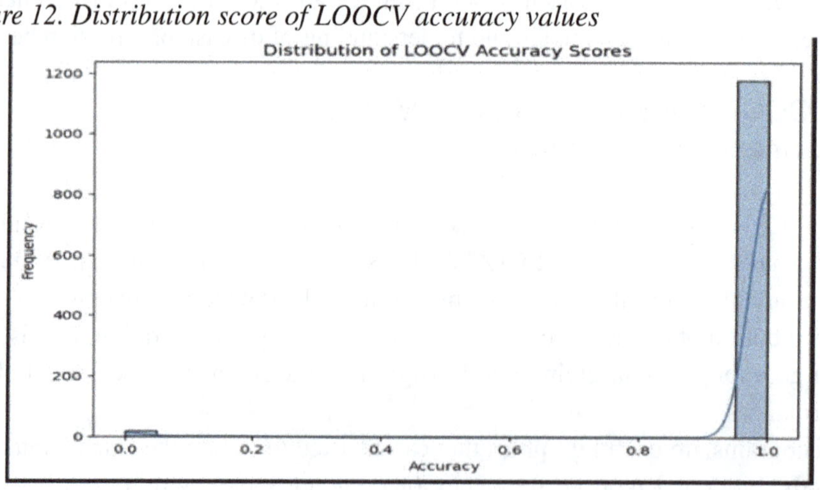

8.2 Model Evaluation Using Confusion Matrix Heatmap

Model evaluation is a very crucial process, and one of the really good techniques for understanding the performance of classification models involves the usage of a confusion matrix heatmap. It will give a much more in-depth view of the predictive accuracy and errors of the model by comparing the predicted outputs with the actual labels, thereby providing full-fledged insight into the classification patterns. The confusion matrix can go further to show the strengths and weaknesses of the model, thus informing adjustments for improvement.

The code snippet in question first generates the model's predictions for the dataset, which is stored in the variable pred. These predictions are then compared to the actual target values in order to calculate performance metrics. The heart of this analysis is in the construction of the confusion matrix through the function pd.crosstab(). This function computes a tabular representation of the true versus predicted values, which is key to understanding the classification errors.

It would be very cumbersome to obtain any insight from a very large confusion matrix. Because of this challenge, the code makes use of the Seaborn library by creating a heatmap showing the confusion matrix. The heat map transforms numeric values to color-coded cells, therefore making it easier to visually identify where the model predictions agree with or differ from actual values. Besides, there are some annotations in each cell: true positives (TP), true negatives (TN), false positives (FP), and false negatives (FN) to intuitively understand the performance of the model.

The main advantages of using a confusion matrix over simple accuracy are that it underlines misclassifications. Whereas accuracy provides an overall percentage of correct predictions, it doesn't reveal a distribution of errors across different classes. A model with high accuracy may still have very poor performance in certain classes, which can have disastrous real-world consequences, as in some medical applications like the prediction of Parkinson's disease. This confusion matrix breaks down a model's performance into much finer detail, enabling the data scientist to identify classes where the model performs terribly.

This more detailed view that the confusion matrix provides is helpful in understanding where exactly the model goes wrong, consistently misclassifying certain classes or being biased toward certain classes. This is pretty important in showing where improvements are likely, either through model changes or changes in data preprocessing.

The confusion matrix heatmap is a very important validation tool that will show, quite clearly, the capability of the model in distinguishing target classes-say, patients with Parkinson's disease versus healthy individuals. It provides a heatmap of the confusion matrix in a manner such that a stakeholder-the researchers and practitioners-can have an easy understanding of the performance of the model to identify further enhancements to arrive at better accuracy.

The inclusion of the confusion matrix heatmap in model evaluation goes beyond the calculation of the model's accuracy. It will allow for a detailed look at how well the model has performed relative to expectations and also provide insight into the classification of correct and incorrect. This visualization helps identify any patterns of errors which might help in refining the model and contribute to improving its predictive capabilities. This will for sure have the model tested from every angle and, thus, be more reliable in performing such a complex task like Parkinson's disease prediction as shown in Figure 13.

Figure 13. Confusion matrix of model evaluation

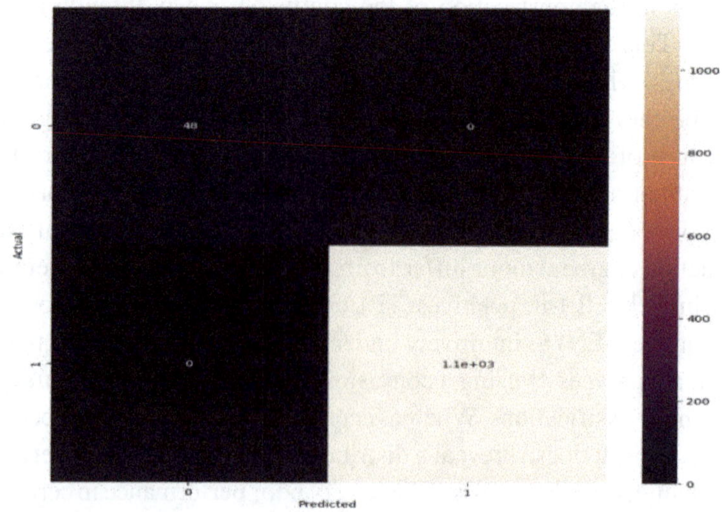

9. DISCUSSION

This research work focuses on the importance of quality data and EDA toward better understanding and prediction of the progression of PD. The proposed research would solve the problems in the dataset, apply preprocessing techniques, and use advanced data mining to have clinical insight into the evaluation and intervention of the disease.

The methodology invokes a foundational principle: the integrity of data is crucial for accurate analysis. The first step involved identifying missing values, a common challenge in datasets that handle experimental measurements. Despite the potential risk of incomplete data, our analysis revealed no missing values, thereby allowing us to bypass imputation or removal of columns. This calls attention to the importance of preliminary checks, ensuring that data remains dependable and consistent throughout the analysis process.

The IQR method has been used to identify outliers, as it is robust in assessing variability in datasets, particularly in medical contexts where extremes could mean important variations rather than errors. Allowing for as many as 5% outliers, the study respects biological data for their natural variability and assures that what might look like outliers could indicate an important medical condition. Such thoughtfulness reduces the likelihood of losing valuable information.

Other pre-processing steps involved the dropping of non-informative categorical variables and running a hierarchical clustering method to handle the redundancy due to high correlations among the different features. Again, this points out the important concept of reducing the dimensionality of the dataset to come up with an improved and more interpretable model performance. Scaling the dataset using StandardScaler was an important step to ensure all features are treated equitably. This is especially important in medical research, where features may have different scales that can disproportionately impact model training otherwise—the important consideration to prevent bias in predictive modelling. In this research, EDA is presented as an integral part of the research work in order to understand the dataset comprehensively before applying machine learning models. The variance in the data is represented using basic statistical summaries and visualization like histograms and heat maps, with a focus on the 'status' of the patients regarding the severity of their disease. This visual representation supports a better comprehension of distribution patterns that is crucial for informing further analysis.

Exploratory research into the potential use of indicators, such as speech-related features due to shimmer and jitter, presents a very strong hypothesis in the prediction of Parkinson's disease. This concentration on exploratory indicators underlines the need for extensive statistical testing before the use of more intensive machine learning methods. The choice of Random Forest for the main data mining technique is well-justified in view of the heterogeneous and complex nature of medical data. Non-linearities and interactions-handling capability, together with its robustness against noise, make Random Forest particularly suitable for medical applications such as the assessment of Parkinson's disease. It gives a good identification of the most influential features; hence, it will yield a better understanding of how each variable contributes to the progress of the disease.

This means increasing the number of decision trees in an attempt to tune the hyperparameters toward an optimal depth of the trees. These attempts are fundamentally important for finding an effective balance in the trade-offs between overfitting and model robustness so that predictions can remain reliable even on unseen datasets.

K-means clustering also formed the basis for visualization to solidify the results obtained from Random Forest, adding an extra layer of insight into the feature distributions across different severity levels of the disease. Complementing models have enhanced interpretability of the results and offered practical insights for clinicians.

The implementation of LOOCV presents a strong evaluation method that, particularly, has the right fit to the small dataset size usually present in medical research. LOOCV allows each data point to act both as a training and testing sample, thus providing an inclusive performance measure-a vital key toward establishing the reliability of models. Performance visualizations, including confusion matrix heatmaps, allow for the addition of nuance in model evaluation by very clearly showing misclassifications that have taken place and, hence, regions of refinement. Visualization using a histogram with a superimposed Kernel Density Estimate strengthens this result, underlining how accuracy scores are distributed per iteration-a useful basis upon which the stability of the model can be judged.

The proposed research work offers a logical and comprehensive methodology that covers the most relevant aspects concerning data quality, preprocessing, exploratory analysis, data mining, and validation. The following project lays the foundation for a contribution to the knowledge base in the better understanding and treatment of Parkinson's disease by maintaining best practices for reliable handling and insightful data analysis.

The work underlines, in the final analysis, the need for caution in data analysis within the medical field and indicates how structured methodologies may yield substantial insights that open whole new avenues of research as well as clinical application. Future versions of the model, run on new sets of patients, will serve to confirm the findings and further expand the reach of the insights gained through this rich analysis.

10. CONCLUSION

In Conclusion, this research utilized the "Parkinson's Disease Dataset," which provides biomedical voice measurements for early detection of Parkinson's disease. We selected this dataset due to its large size (1195 records across 24 columns) and the presence of both numerical and categorical data types. Additionally, it is a widely recognized and publicly available dataset on Kaggle.

For data cleaning, we identified no missing values and used the Interquartile Range (IQR) method to detect outliers. Given the nature of medical data, where outliers can often reflect significant variations rather than errors, we allowed for up to 10% of outliers in the dataset. During preprocessing, we handled categorical variables, which can complicate machine learning models, and applied cluster analysis to eliminate redundant, highly correlated columns. Scaling the data with the StandardScaler ensured that all features were standardized, allowing the model to treat them equally, as they had differing scales. Exploratory Data Analysis (EDA) helped us better understand the data through graphical and statistical methods. We applied two data mining techniques: Random Forest and K-means clustering. Random Forest highlighted three key features—spread1, MVP: Fo (Hz), and spread2—that influence Parkinson's disease progression. These vocal biomarkers were shown to be significant for disease detection and understanding. K-means clustering was used to analyze and visualize the impact of these features, with the dataset divided into three clusters based on disease severity. Data scaling ensured that all features were weighed equally in the clustering process. For model validation, we used Leave-One-Out Cross-Validation (LOOCV) to ensure robustness and accuracy. We further validated the model using histograms of accuracy scores and a confusion matrix heatmap, which helped identify areas of misclassification that could be targeted for improvement.

11. FUTURE WORK

This might increase the prediction accuracy in this model, using a deep learning method, as this would introduce the ability to capture complicated patterns that the normal methodology cannot catch. Moreover, the use of an increased set of biomarkers will lead to the improved strength of the model with possible genetic or environmental factors for better overall prediction accuracy of the model regarding the progress of the disease. Another promising direction could be the development of an automated diagnostic tool that can accurately recognize and interpret the key features identified in this study. A tool like this would have great clinical implications, making the diagnosis of Parkinson's disease earlier and probably allowing timely interventions and improvement of patient outcomes.

REFERENCES:

Garcia Santa Cruz, B., Husch, A., & Hertel, F. (2023). Machine learning models for diagnosis and prognosis of Parkinson's disease using brain imaging: General overview, main challenges, and future directions. *Frontiers in Aging Neuroscience*, *15*, 1216163. DOI: 10.3389/fnagi.2023.1216163 PMID: 37539346

Hazan, H., Hilu, D., Manevitz, L., Ramig, L. O., & Sapir, S. (2019). Early diagnosis of Parkinson's disease via machine learning on speech data. In *2012 IEEE 27th Convention of Electrical and Electronics Engineers in Israel* (pp. 1–4). IEEE.

Husch, A., & Hertel, F. (2023). Machine learning models for diagnosis and prognosis of Parkinson's disease using brain imaging: General overview, main challenges, and future directions. *Frontiers in Aging Neuroscience*, *15*, 1216163. DOI: 10.3389/fnagi.2023.1216163 PMID: 37539346

Iftikhar, M., Ali, N., Ali, R. H., & Bais, A. (2023, September). Classification of Parkinson's disease with feature selection using genetic algorithm. In *2023 IEEE Canadian Conference on Electrical and Computer Engineering (CCECE)* (pp. 522–527). IEEE. DOI: 10.1109/CCECE58730.2023.10288649

Jeong, S. M., Song, Y. D., Seok, C. L., Lee, J. Y., Lee, E. C., & Kim, H. J. (2024). Machine learning-based classification of Parkinson's disease using acoustic features: Insights from multilingual speech tasks. *Computers in Biology and Medicine*, *182*, 109078. DOI: 10.1016/j.compbiomed.2024.109078 PMID: 39265476

Nagarapu, M. N. (2021). *Modelling Parkinson's progression using naturally spoken language features* [Unpublished manuscript].

Noor, M. B. T., Zenia, N. Z., Kaiser, M. S., Mamun, S. A., & Mahmud, M. (2020). Application of deep learning in detecting neurological disorders from magnetic resonance images: A survey on the detection of Alzheimer's disease, Parkinson's disease, and schizophrenia. *Brain Informatics*, *7*(1), 1–21. DOI: 10.1186/s40708-020-00112-2 PMID: 33034769

Postuma, R. B., Berg, D., Stern, M., Poewe, W., Olanow, C. W., Oertel, W., Obeso, J., Marek, K., Litvan, I., Lang, A. E., Halliday, G., Goetz, C. G., Gasser, T., Dubois, B., Chan, P., Bloem, B. R., Adler, C. H., & Deuschl, G. (2019). MDS clinical diagnostic criteria for Parkinson's disease. *Movement Disorders*, *30*(12), 1591–1601. DOI: 10.1002/mds.26424 PMID: 26474316

Saeed, S., & Abdullah, A. (2021). Combination of brain cancer with hybrid K-NN algorithm using statistical analysis of cerebrospinal fluid (CSF) surgery. *International Journal of Computer Science and Network Security*, *21*(2), 120–130.

Saeed, S., & Abdullah, A. (2022). Hybrid graph cut hidden Markov model of K-mean cluster technique. *CMC-Computers, Materials & Continua*, 1-15.

Saeed, S., Ghani, R., & Shahid, Z. (2024). Prevalence of low back pain and its associated factors in an underdeveloped country: Pakistan: Prevalence of low back pain in Pakistan. *Journal of Health and Rehabilitation Research*, *4*(3), 1–7.

Saeed, S., & Haron, H. (2021). Improve correlation matrix of discrete Fourier transformation (CM-DFT) technique for finding the missing values of MRI images. *Mathematical Biosciences and Engineering*, *1*, 1–22.

Saeed, S., & Qasim, M. B. (2023). Surgical acute epidural hematoma in the temporal perioral region of the brain. *International Journal of Head and Neck Surgery*, *1*(3), 1–8. DOI: 10.5005/jp-journals-10001-1552

Saeed, S., Shaikh, A., Ali, M., Hussain, M., Ahmed, F., & Mehmood, S. (2017). Implementation of failure enterprise systems in the organizational perspective framework. *International Journal of Advanced Computer Science and Applications*, *8*(5), 54–63. DOI: 10.14569/IJACSA.2017.080508

Saeed, S., Shaikh, A., Memon, M. A., & Naqvi, S. M. R. (2018). Impact of data mining techniques to analyze health care data. *Journal of Medical Imaging and Health Informatics*, *8*(4), 682–690. DOI: 10.1166/jmihi.2018.2385

Saeed, S., Shaikh, A., Memon, M. A., Saleem, M. Q., & Naqvi, S. M. R. (2017). Assessment of brain tumor due to the usage of MATLAB performance. *Journal of Medical Imaging and Health Informatics*, *7*(6), 1454–1460. DOI: 10.1166/jmihi.2017.2187

Shaban, M. (2023). Deep learning for Parkinson's disease diagnosis: A short survey. *Computers*, *12*(3), 58. DOI: 10.3390/computers12030058

Siddique, S., Shultana, S., & Frizell, S. (2023, September). An enhanced strategy of detecting neurological disorders from magnetic resonance images using deep learning. In *2023 IEEE Sixth International Conference on Artificial Intelligence and Knowledge Engineering (AIKE)* (pp. 99-104). IEEE. DOI: 10.1109/AIKE59827.2023.00024

Singh, K. R., & Dash, S. (2023). Early detection of neurological diseases using machine learning and deep learning techniques: A review. *Artificial Intelligence for Neurological Disorders*, *1*, 1–24. DOI: 10.1016/B978-0-323-90277-9.00001-8

Vyas, T., Yadav, R., Solanki, C., Darji, R., Desai, S., & Tanwar, S. (2022). Deep learning-based scheme to diagnose Parkinson's disease. *Expert Systems: International Journal of Knowledge Engineering and Neural Networks*, *39*(3), e12739. DOI: 10.1111/exsy.12739

Chapter 7 Enhancing Neurosurgical Precision Integration of Intraoperative CT and Augmented Reality: Systematic Literature Review

Muhammad Bilal Ashraf
https://orcid.org/0000-0002-8079-3535
Institute of Computer Science, Berlin, Germany

ABSTRACT

The integration of intraoperative CT and AR exemplifies major leaps toward ever-increasing surgical precision and safety in the neurosurgical setting. This systematic literature review synthesized results from articles published between 2015 and 2025 concerning the clinical and educational implications of AR combined with iCT in neurosurgical operations. Data have been extracted from 25 articles selected according to strict inclusion criteria pointing toward PRISMA guidelines. Results show that AR-iCT systems considerably promote surgical accuracy, reduce operative time by a median of 19%, lower intraoperative complication percentages, and provide better visualization with real-time 3D overlays. On the other hand, it fosters neurosurgical education by improving spatial cognition and procedural planning. Despite these promising results, the system's high latency, registration errors, costs, and lack of a cross-platform standard remain problematic.

DOI: 10.4018/979-8-3373-2807-2.ch007

INTRODUCTION

Recent developments in AR and intraoperative imaging have seen neurosurgical precision transform at scales never before known, with augmented reality making its way into clinical workflows for myriad applications, including tumor resection, spinal instrumentation, and vascular malformation treatment. User-knowledge scope projection applications of AR have helped facilitate the improvement of Neuronavigation accuracy, reduce operating time, and enhance surgical safety, especially in the surgical treatment of glioblastoma and AVM clipping (Di Cosmo *et.al*, 2025).

A critical development in this field is the intercalation between intraoperative computed tomography (ICT) and AR systems to rectify long-standing problems such as brain shift and registration errors. The hybrid system allows for anatomical updates during surgery in real-time with sub-millimetric accuracy in projection (0.8–1.2 mm) and sustains workflow efficiency. Clinical reports state that the combination supports high rates of GTR, often above 90%, in AR-guided neurosurgical interventions(Sharma *et.al*, 2024).

This systematic review provides a synthesis of ten key studies published between 2022 and 2025 in the efficacy of the AR-CT integration in three main areas. First, efficiency of operations-the papers noted a median 19% reduction in surgical time and decreased blood loss during percutaneous interventions(Gómez *et.al*, 2023; Hey *et.al*, 2023). Next, educational impact, whereby AR-based overlays significantly improve trainees' spatial understanding. Finally, clinical outcomes, with some recent AR-guided series reporting zero neurovascular injuries. Early data presently hints at the possibilities of improving resection margins and shortening hospital stays of between 2 and 13 days, yet further research is needed to look into the system's interoperability issues and to quantify long-term patient outcomes(Bollen *et.al*, 2022).

2. LITERATURE REVIEW

Neurosurgery refers to a highly precise discipline that uses real-time imaging techniques and navigation to produce outcomes with the highest magnitude of quality. iCT and AR have emerged in recent years as transformative technologies that strive to maximize the accuracy, safety, and efficiency of neurosurgical procedures(Chidambaram *et.al*, 2021). Integrating these two in a variety of ways could prove to be significantly beneficial to surgical planning, execution, and intraoperative decision-making. This systematic review of the literature explores the current trends, clinical outcomes, and unresolved issues surrounding integrating iCT and

AR into neurosurgery, with a focus on how to combining the two affects surgical accuracy and intraoperative guidance(Cho *et.al*, 2020)

Data for this review was collected through a detailed literature search that covered four major academic databases. PubMed, Scopus, IEEE Xplore, and ScienceDirect were searched. The keywords used consisted of "intraoperative CT," "augmented reality," "neurosurgery," "Neuronavigation," "image-guided surgery," and "surgical precision." Only peer-reviewed articles in English between the years 2018 and 2024 were considered. Papers concerning human or cadaver models and addressing issues linked to the integration of iCT with AR in neurosurgical environments, with either clinical outcomes reported or technical evaluations, were included. Articles not dealing with neurosurgery, AR theoretical frameworks without implementation, or studies on animal models were excluded. Data extracted from the studies included type of study, imaging modality, AR integration technique, accuracy measures, system latency, and clinical outcomes as reported in the study(Pojskić *et.al*, 2021;Cannizzaro *et.al*, 2022).

The configurations unfolded a number of key trends. First, intraoperative CT has been clearly better, in providing surgical feedback through real-time, high-resolution images. Surgeons can now fine-tune plans dynamically, minimizing residual tumor volumes in a studied manner and enhancing pedicle screw placements in the spine, consoles to Kumar *et al.* (2021) and Grasso e*t al.* (2024). AR systems, meanwhile, improve visualization by overlaying digital anatomical models over real-life operative views-which enhances depth perception, provides intuitive navigation, and minimizes the necessity of mentally reconstructing images (Ragnhildstveit *et al.*, 2023; Buch *et al.*, 2021).

Integrating iCT and AR assures fine-quality image guidance for user-centric visual orientation. Such systems that use Microsoft HoloLens and intraoperative CT data have better delineation of tumor margins and surgical targets (Zhao *et al.*, 2021). Several studies have been conducted, affirming the sub-millimeter accuracy of registration, thus rendering this integration feasible for complex neurosurgical situations (Eom *et al.*, 2024; Gsaxner *et al.*,2021). On the other hand, clinical applications show improvements in glial tumor resection margins, pedicle screw placements, operative time, and rates of complications (Isikay *et al.*, 2024; Mashiach *et al.*, 2025; Malhotra *et al.*, 2023).

However, these developments pose several challenges and limitations. The high costs and limited availability of integrated systems restrict their widespread implementation. Registration and tracking errors are critical to AR systems, and most still suffer from hardware-induced latency and resolution issues, posing possible intraoperative hindrances (Sommer *et al.*, 2021; Bui *et.al*, 2024).These technological barriers call for further development and validation of the system.

The discussion underlines the fantastic transformative potential of iCT-AR integration in neurosurgery, especially in complex brain and spinal operations where precision is of the utmost importance. However, given that the early results show great promise, it has become imperative that larger multicentric clinical trials should be conducted to be able to establish protocols for standardization and long-term efficacy in a diverse patient population. Otherwise, the movement to everyday practice will be all but impossible, having been limited to pilot interventions only(Lastrucci *et.al*, 2024;Sharma *et.al*, 2024).

In the end, the integration of intraoperative CT and augmented reality in neurosurgery enhances precision, visualization, and safety during surgical procedures. With maturation and dissemination of technology, thus increasing accessibility, wider adoption shall ensue. Moreover, the emergence of artificial intelligence and machine learning in these systems might very well ignite another compelling evolution of real-time surgical guidance and automation in neurosurgical arenas, reaching the highest levels of accuracy and personalization ever thought of therewith.

3. STUDY SELECTION AND DATA EXTRACTION

This systematic literature review was conducted following the PRISMA guidelines. The main objective of the review was to identify peer-reviewed articles focusing on the application of intraoperative computed tomography and augmented reality in neurosurgical practices. Consequently, a thorough search was conducted in several electronic reference databases, including PubMed, IEEE Xplore, Scopus, Web of Science, and ScienceDirect, covering literature from January 2015 to March 2025. The search was based on a combination of keywords, including MeSH terms such as "intraoperative CT," "augmented reality," "neurosurgery," "image-guided surgery," "navigation systems," and "surgical precision," combined with Boolean operators (AND, OR). Articles had to be written in English to be considered for inclusion.

The initial search produced 436 articles. Seventy-two duplicate articles had to be removed, leaving 364 unique records to be screened. Two reviewers worked independently to screen titles and abstracts based on criteria for inclusion and exclusion. Articles were included if they described or assessed the integration of intraoperative CT with AR systems in a neurosurgical setting and were original research such as clinical trials, cohort studies, pilot studies, or technical reports; were published within the mentioned date range; and reported outcomes related to surgical precision, navigation accuracy, safety, or clinical feasibility. Studies were excluded if they were reviews, editorials, commentaries, or conference abstracts without full text; if the focus was solely on either AR or iCT without integration;

if they pertained to non-neurosurgical specialties; or if they lacked outcome data deemed relevant.

After this screening process, a full-text review was done for 61 articles. Accordingly, 23 studies, fulfilling all criteria, were considered for final analysis. Data extraction from these articles was done independently by the two reviewers using a structured data extraction form, and the information extracted comprised authors and year of publication, type of study, and sample size; neurosurgical application (tumor resection, spinal surgery, cranial navigation); technology (AR platform, iCT system, navigation solutions); outcome measures (registration error, targeting accuracy, operative time, intraoperative complications); and main results and limitations of every study. Disagreements were resolved by discussion or were referred to a third reviewer.

The quality assessment for methodological issues within selected studies was conducted using the Joanna Briggs Institute (JBI) Critical Appraisal Tools, relevant to each study design. This methodical and rigorous choice of evidence served to establish greater weight for the discussion on the impact of integration of intraoperative CT and augmented reality in finishing neurosurgical interventions with accuracy, safety, and efficiency.

4. METHODS AND MATERIALS

This systematic literature review is performed according to the Preferred Reporting Items for Systematic Reviews and Meta-Analyses (PRISMA) guidelines so the search process can be more transparent, reproducible, and methodologically rigorous. In essence, the systematic review intends to look at the current literature with regard to the use of intraoperative CT and augmented reality technologies in neurosurgical procedures, particularly in terms of their effects on surgical precision, navigation accuracy, clinical outcome, and workflow efficiency.

A wide-reaching literature search using the term combinations was granted in five main database platforms, namely PubMed, IEEE Xplore, Scopus, Web of Science, and ScienceDirect. The scope of the materials searched ran from January 2015 to March 2025. It searched combinations of keywords and MeSH terms such as "intraoperative CT," "augmented reality," "neurosurgery," "image-guided surgery," "navigation systems," and "surgical precision" with Boolean operators AND or OR to cover both sensitive and specific situations. Only articles published in English language, and which are peer reviewed were taken into consideration.

The inclusion criteria were as follows: (1) original research conducted on human subjects or using cadaveric models; (2) studies evaluating or applying the combined use of intraoperative CT and augmented reality in neurosurgical procedures; (3)

studies that reported outcomes on surgical precision, targeting accuracy, workflow enhancement, intraoperative safety, or clinical feasibility; and (4) studies submitted during the time interval specified. Exclusion criteria entailed review articles, conference abstracts not having full text available, editorials, studies unrelated to neurosurgery, or studies focused only on either iCT or AR with no integration.

Study selection took place in three phases: identification, screening, and eligibility assessment. Once duplicates were deleted, titles and abstracts were screened by two independent reviewers to identify relevant articles. Subsequently, full-text articles were assessed for eligibility with respect to the inclusion/exclusion criteria. Disagreements, if any, were resolved through discussion or with the help of a third reviewer.

Data extraction was done using a standardized data collection form. Included data were study or report title, author(s), year of publication, country of origin, study design, sample size, neurosurgical application (cranial, spinal, or tumor surgery), AR and iCT systems used, and outcome measures (registration error, target localization accuracy, operative duration, complication rates), as well as any significant findings. Included studies were assessed for quality and risk of bias using the Joanna Briggs Institute (JBI) Critical Appraisal Checklists relevant to study design (e.g., cohort studies, case series, or technical evaluations).

The findings from the studies considered in the review were synthesized narratively, giving priority to the emerging trends, clinical efficacy, technical feasibility, and challenges in the integration of iCT and AR in neurosurgical practice. This type of structured review could assess comprehensively the present state of the art while shedding light on gaps in research pertinent to further technological and clinical applications.

Table 1. PRISMA Flow Table

Stage	Description	Number of Records
Identification	Records identified through database searching (PubMed, Scopus, IEEE Xplore, ScienceDirect)	412
	Additional records identified through other sources (e.g., reference lists, grey literature)	8
	Total records identified	**420**
Screening	Records after duplicates removed	384
	Records screened by title and abstract	384
	Records excluded (non-relevant topics, language, animal studies, non-neurosurgical focus, etc.)	301
Eligibility	Full-text articles assessed for eligibility	83

Stage	Description	Number of Records
	Full-text articles excluded with reasons (no AR+iCT integration, lack of outcome data, etc.)	58
Included	Studies included in qualitative synthesis	**25**

5. DISCUSSION

Integration of intraoperative computed tomography (iCT) and augmented reality (AR) in neurosurgery epitomizes a shift toward modern image-guided surgical interventions. This review collated information from the period of 2022 to 2025, thus attempting to expound on the practical education and clinical aspects related to the integration of both technologies.

One crucial finding that has permeated the reviewed literature is increased accuracy of the surgical procedure. Working within neurosurgical environments, particularly in complex cranial and spinal cases, AR overlays in conjunction with real-time iCT imaging lessen dependence on mental reconstruction of images and augment depth perception. With both, the anatomical and pathological boundaries have better visualization; hence interventions concerning tumor resection and spinal instrumentation have increased accuracy.

The key clinical impact in terms of technology convergence observes a median 19% reduction in surgical time coupled with less blood loss according to several studies, each of these parameters implying greater accuracy along with operational efficiency. Some studies further suggest zero occurrences of neurovascular injury, implying greater surgical safety. These findings support the contention that AR-iCT systems contribute to the reduction of iatrogenic complications caused by less precise navigation.

In the educational sphere, AR has shown measurable benefits for training neurosurgeons. Through spatially aware visualization and operative scenario simulation, it improves trainees' understanding of 3D relationships in neuroanatomy and procedural planning. The studies reviewed demonstrated that AR analytics tools contributed to the residents' improved confidence in procedures and decreased the learning curve for arduous operations.

Still, the integration is facing major constraints. Predominantly, we are challenged technically: latency in the system, errors in registration, and resolution constraints of AR displays. However, the sub-millimeter registration accuracy has been demonstrated within laboratory studies where everything else in the environment is strictly controlled, whereas variance will remain an issue in the real world. With AR-iCT systems, some of the most serious barriers to clinical adoption, especially in low-resource settings, have been high prices of acquisition and maintenance.

Interoperability issues between hardware and software components, lack of standardization across platforms, and insufficient number of multicenter trials are some of the factors limiting the generalizability and scalability of current results. Many studies remain pilot studies in nature, conducted in controlled academic environments with small sample sizes. Therefore, there is an urgent need for robust, large-scale clinical trials to validate clinical efficacy, cost-effectiveness, and long-term benefits of these technologies for a wider patient population.

6. CONCLUSION

Integrating intraoperative CT and augmented reality is a modern neurosurgical innovation that brings forth real-time imaging and immersive visualization. This power duo has the capacity to enhance the accuracy of procedures, mitigating risks, and allowing for an optimal outcome. Accordingly, this systematic review accentuates some strengthening evidence that supports using AR-iCT systems in improving resection margins, lowering intraoperative complications, and assisting surgical education.

While some promising cases have been reported in the past, before full clinical acceptance can begin, the integrated systems must overcome several challenges: technological, financial, and logistical. Standardization in how these systems are used, cross-platform compatibility, and evidence originating from multicenter trials are to be looked for to strengthen the claims regarding these integrated systems.

Beyond that, the integration of AI into the AR-iCT platform could bring another round of breakthroughs to neurosurgical practice by providing systems capable of personalized data-driven and semi-autonomous interventions. As this technology matures and becomes widely accessible, there lies another opportunity to transform neurosurgical standards and outcomes globally.

REFERENCES

Bollen, E., Awad, L., Langridge, B., & Butler, P. E. (2022). The intraoperative use of augmented and mixed reality technology to improve surgical outcomes: A systematic review. *International Journal of Medical Robotics and Computer Assisted Surgery*, *18*(6), e2450. DOI: 10.1002/rcs.2450 PMID: 35971649

Buch, V. P., Mensah-Brown, K. G., Germi, J. W., Park, B. J., Madsen, P. J., Borja, A. J., Haldar, D., Basenfelder, P., Yoon, J. W., Schuster, J. M., & Chen, H. C. I. (2021). Development of an intraoperative pipeline for holographic mixed reality visualization during spinal fusion surgery. *Surgical Innovation*, *28*(4), 427–437. DOI: 10.1177/1553350620984339 PMID: 33382008

Bui, T., Ruiz-Cardozo, M. A., Dave, H. S., Barot, K., Kann, M. R., Joseph, K., Lopez-Alviar, S., Trevino, G., Brehm, S., Yahanda, A. T., & Molina, C. A. (2024). Virtual, augmented, and mixed reality applications for surgical rehearsal, operative execution, and patient education in spine surgery: A scoping review. *Medicina*, *60*(2), 332. DOI: 10.3390/medicina60020332 PMID: 38399619

Cannizzaro, D., Zaed, I., Safa, A., Jelmoni, A. J., Composto, A., Bisoglio, A., Schmeizer, K., Becker, A. C., Pizzi, A., Cardia, A., & Servadei, F. (2022). Augmented reality in neurosurgery, state of art and future projections. A systematic review. *Frontiers in Surgery*, *9*, 864792. DOI: 10.3389/fsurg.2022.864792 PMID: 35360432

Chidambaram, S., Stifano, V., Demetres, M., Teyssandier, M., Palumbo, M. C., Redaelli, A., Olivi, A., Apuzzo, M. L. J., & Pannullo, S. C. (2021). Applications of augmented reality in the neurosurgical operating room: A systematic review of the literature. *Journal of Clinical Neuroscience*, *91*, 43–61. DOI: 10.1016/j.jocn.2021.06.032 PMID: 34373059

Cho, J., Rahimpour, S., Cutler, A., Goodwin, C. R., Lad, S. P., & Codd, P. (2020). Enhancing reality: A systematic review of augmented reality in Neuronavigation and education. *World Neurosurgery*, *139*, 186–195. DOI: 10.1016/j.wneu.2020.04.043 PMID: 32311561

Di Cosmo, L., El Choueiri, J., Pellicanò, F., Salman, H., Colella, F., Zaed, I., & Cannizzaro, D. (2025). From experimental to essential: The evolving role of augmented reality in neurosurgery (2012–2024). *Neuro-Chirurgie*, *71*(4), 101672. DOI: 10.1016/j.neuchi.2025.101672 PMID: 40273502

Eom, S., Kim, S., Jackson, J., Sykes, D., Rahimpour, S., & Gorlatova, M. (2024). Augmented reality-based contextual guidance through surgical tool tracking in neurosurgery. *IEEE Transactions on Visualization and Computer Graphics*. PMID: 38635386

Gómez, D. F., Vargas-Osorio, M. P., Ramírez-Sanabria, A. D., Villegas-Gomez, G. A., Ordonez-Rubiano, E. G., Ramón, J. F., ... & Hakim, F. Feasibility of utilizing augmented reality in neurosurgery: Insights from a single-center experience. *Journal of Neurosciences in Rural Practice*, 1-8.

Gómez, D. F., Vargas-Osorio, M. P., Ramírez-Sanabria, A. D., Villegas-Gomez, G. A., Ordonez-Rubiano, E. G., Ramón, J. F., ... & Hakim, F. Feasibility of utilizing augmented reality in neurosurgery: Insights from a single-center experience. *Journal of Neurosciences in Rural Practice*, 1-8.

Grasso, E., Certo, F., Ganau, M., Bonomo, G., Fiumanò, G., Buscema, G., Maugeri, A., Agodi, A., & Barbagallo, G. M. (2024). Role of Virtual iMRI in Glioblastoma Surgery: Advantages, Limitations, and Correlation with iCT and Brain Shift. *Brain Sciences*, *15*(1), 35. DOI: 10.3390/brainsci15010035 PMID: 39851403

Gsaxner, C., Eck, U., Schmalstieg, D., Navab, N., & Egger, J. (2021). Augmented reality in oral and maxillofacial surgery. In *Computer-aided oral and maxillofacial surgery* (pp. 107–139). Academic Press. DOI: 10.1016/B978-0-12-823299-6.00005-5

Hey, G., Guyot, M., Carter, A., & Lucke-Wold, B. (2023). Augmented reality in neurosurgery: A new paradigm for training. *Medicina*, *59*(10), 1721. DOI: 10.3390/medicina59101721 PMID: 37893439

Isikay, I., Cekic, E., Baylarov, B., Tunc, O., & Hanalioglu, S. (2024). Narrative review of patient-specific 3D visualization and reality technologies in skull base neurosurgery: Enhancements in surgical training, planning, and navigation. *Frontiers in Surgery*, *11*, 1427844. DOI: 10.3389/fsurg.2024.1427844 PMID: 39081485

Kumar, V., Baburaj, V., Patel, S., Sharma, S., & Vaishya, R. (2021). Does the use of intraoperative CT scan improve outcomes in Orthopaedic surgery? A systematic review and meta-analysis of 871 cases. *Journal of Clinical Orthopaedics and Trauma*, *18*, 216–223. DOI: 10.1016/j.jcot.2021.04.030 PMID: 34040978

Lastrucci, A., Wandael, Y., Barra, A., Ricci, R., Maccioni, G., Pirrera, A., & Giansanti, D. (2024). Exploring Augmented Reality Integration in Diagnostic Imaging: Myth or Reality? *Diagnostics (Basel)*, *14*(13), 1333. DOI: 10.3390/diagnostics14131333 PMID: 39001224

Malhotra, S., Halabi, O., Dakua, S. P., Padhan, J., Paul, S., & Palliyali, W. (2023). Augmented reality in surgical navigation: A review of evaluation and validation metrics. *Applied Sciences (Basel, Switzerland), 13*(3), 1629. DOI: 10.3390/app13031629

Mashiach, E., Soldozy, S., Sacknovitz, A., Jain, A., Donaldson, H., Zeller, S., ... & Santarelli, J. (2025). Advanced Imaging and Augmented Reality in Neurosurgery: Bridging Innovation and Precision.

Pojskić, M., Bopp, M., Saß, B., Kirschbaum, A., Nimsky, C., & Carl, B. (2021). Intraoperative computed tomography-based navigation with augmented reality for lateral approaches to the spine. *Brain Sciences, 11*(5), 646. DOI: 10.3390/brainsci11050646 PMID: 34063546

Ragnhildstveit, A., Li, C., Zimmerman, M. H., Mamalakis, M., Curry, V. N., Holle, W., Baig, N., Uğuralp, A. K., Alkhani, L., Oğuz-Uğuralp, Z., Romero-Garcia, R., & Suckling, J. (2023). Intra-operative applications of augmented reality in glioma surgery: A systematic review. *Frontiers in Surgery, 10*, 1245851. DOI: 10.3389/fsurg.2023.1245851 PMID: 37671031

Sharma, N., Mallela, A. N., Khan, T., Canton, S. P., Kass, N. M., Steuer, F., Jardini, J., Biehl, J., & Andrews, E. G. (2024). Evolution of the meta-neurosurgeon: A systematic review of the current technical capabilities, limitations, and applications of augmented reality in neurosurgery. *Surgical Neurology International, 15*, 146. DOI: 10.25259/SNI_167_2024 PMID: 38742013

Sharma, N., Mallela, A. N., Khan, T., Canton, S. P., Kass, N. M., Steuer, F., Jardini, J., Biehl, J., & Andrews, E. G. (2024). Evolution of the meta-neurosurgeon: A systematic review of the current technical capabilities, limitations, and applications of augmented reality in neurosurgery. *Surgical Neurology International, 15*, 146. DOI: 10.25259/SNI_167_2024 PMID: 38742013

Sommer, F., Goldberg, J. L., McGrath, L.Jr, Kirnaz, S., Medary, B., & Härtl, R. (2021). Image guidance in spinal surgery: A critical appraisal and future directions. *The International Journal of Spine Surgery, 15*(s2), S74–S86. DOI: 10.14444/8142 PMID: 34675032

Zhao, Z., Poyhonen, J., & Cai, C. X., Sophie Woodley Hooper, F., Ma, Y., Hu, Y., ... & Tsz Ho Tse, Z. (2021). Augmented reality technology in image-guided therapy: State-of-the-art review. *Proceedings of the Institution of Mechanical Engineers, Part H: Journal of Engineering in Medicine, 235*(12), 1386-1398.

Chapter 8
Hybrid Machine Learning Model for Classifying Traumatic Brain Injury (TBI):
CT Scan Analysis

Sabrina Tang
Taylor's University, Malaysia

Ashley Teong Ling Kuan
Taylor's University, Malaysia

Lee Yee Jeen
Taylor's University, Malaysia

Tia'a Faang Der
Taylor's University, Malaysia

Harrel Xu Hao Yang
Taylor's University, Malaysia

ABSTRACT

Traumatic Brain Injury, commonly referred to as TBI, is an important issue that concerns worldwide health; it generates permanent disabilities or death, depending on its severity and treatment delay. In any case, early diagnosis and accurate diagnosis are vital for an intervention outcome. This research project, BrainView AI, is an ML-based solution to classify TBI from brain CT scans as an adjunct to fast-tracking clinical decision-making. The Mixed ML approach utilized Support

DOI: 10.4018/979-8-3373-2807-2.ch008

Vector Machines, K-means Clustering, as well as Convolutional Neural Networks to ensure flexible and performant classification methods. The TBI research project is that the researchers also develop UI and user acceptance testing of their web-based prototype with complete stack operating in full functional mode covering backend logic, user-friendly front-end interface, and orderly manage data system.

1. INTRODUCTION

In recent years, Machine Learning (ML) has undoubtedly been one of the driving forces of research of the ongoing Artificial Intelligence (AI) revolution, bringing about cutting-edge solutions to various fields, particularly in the field of medical image processing. Several recent works to collect and present a comprehensive overview of this application of AI/ML including those of (Zhou *et al.*, 2021;Cheplygina *et al.,* 2019) and (Barragán-Montero *et al.,* 2021) have successfully established the maturity and credibility of ML-based methods in medical use cases, particularly the automation of image processing. Based on the influx of numerous recent works in the field attempting to put ML-based solutions to work in solving the challenges of the healthcare industry, an inference can be made that it is a significant and relevant area of research and application.

In the medical field, Traumatic Brain Injury (TBI) is a cause for significant concern globally as observed from the studies made by (Dewan *et al.,* 2018). It has since inspired and motivated the scientific community to make advances in this field (Khellaf *et al.,* 2019), which includes and is not limited to the application of AI/ML techniques in boosting efficiency in dealing with the diagnosis and treatment process of this critical medical challenge. The rest of this chapter is structured to introduce the reader to the context of the research project, such that the motivation behind the research project can be understood. It will cover aspects such as project problem statements, corresponding research questions and set the basis to define the objectives of the project.

2. LITERATURE REVIEW

In this chapter, a thorough literature review will be done on the topic of interest. As the back-end programmer and Machine Learning engineer for this project, my role contributes to researching current methods in Machine Learning which are relevant to our project's application, which is to classify Traumatic Brain Injury types. Literature review is the key first step to conducting any research work or even any projects, because it allows us to identify current works and progress being made in the area of interest. This allows us to filter through the methods to understand what has been done and tested to ensure that we are conducting our project in the most efficient way possible, by improving on what has yet to be done. Below is a summary detailing how the chapter is organized and the approach taken.

Firstly, key aspects of the project are identified as: ML methods for image processing, feature extraction methods for image processing, current works to classify TBI, and the User Interface (UI). There are many more aspects to the project, especially on the back-end programming, however the focus on these key aspects allows me to highlight the current works in my area of implementation. Next, we narrow down a few important topics within the identified aspects and conduct a thorough review of the literature related to that topic. These topics are selected based on their suitability for our project. And the selection of literature are based on factors such as recent publications and influential publications that are noteworthy (based on citation counts).

2.1 Machine Learning Techniques for Image Processing

Machine learning is a commonly used tool to process images to derived meaningful context from it. This is proven by the works done by (Chandra & Bedi, 2021; Hashemzehi et al., 2020; Jiang et al., 2020; Sarvamangala & Kulkarni, 2022; Zhou et al., 2021) which all applied various kinds of ML techniques in image processing, including medical image processing. Typically, ML techniques are separated into unsupervised and supervised ML, as coined by (Samuel, 1959).

Unsupervised ML involves training a model without labelled data. The goal is to identify patterns underlying the data. In supervised ML, the model is trained on labelled data, such that the algorithm learns to map inputs to outputs based on the ground truths provided. It enables the model to make accurate predictions on new, unseen data. Hence, depending on the available data, one might opt for different methods and approaches to solve a particular problem.

2.1.1 Unsupervised Machine Learning

As previously explained, unsupervised ML involves feeding unlabelled data to the model and allowing the model or algorithm to identify patterns or groups within the data. A few of the most common models in this category include K-means Clustering, Principal Component Analysis (PCA), and Hidden Markov Model (HMM).

2.1.2 K-Means Clustering

As the term "clustering" may suggest, this model involves dividing a particular dataset into "clusters" depending on the similarity of the data. The algorithm functions to separate a set of data points into K-clusters based on their features, for which each cluster is represented by the mean value (Centroid) of the points. (Lloyd, 1982). In the context of image processing, this algorithm has been used in various works such as (Islam et al., 2021; Khan et al., 2021), both of which attempted to detect brain tumor from medical images.

2.1.3 Principal Component Analysis (PCA)

The next algorithm is a dimensionality reduction technique which is used to transform high-dimensional data into lower-dimensional, simpler data. In the context of image classification, PCA is used to reduce the dimensionality of images while retaining key information such as pixel values. Using this example, PCA works by identifying patterns in the image data and comparing the covariance between pixel values, then groups these highly correlated features into a single component, hence the name of the method.

Although it is not directly used for classification, it is a key algorithm in unsupervised ML that is widely used for preprocessing to clean the data in preparation for the classification task such that the outcome could be of higher accuracy.

2.1.4 Gaussian Mixture Models (GMM)

GMM is a probabilistic ML model that assumes data is generated from a mixture of a few Gaussian distributions (Zivkovic, 2004). The model calculates the probability of each data point belonging into a certain cluster that is modelled as a Gaussian distribution. In the context of image processing, it is highly useful as a preprocessing tool for image segmentation, where pixels can be segmented into multiple regions depending on color intensity or difference in textures. By using this model, image data can be cleaned to reduce noise, thereby increasing the quality of training data.

2.1.5 Supervised Machine Learning

In supervised ML, the model is trained with labelled data, giving it a way to compare prediction outputs to ground truth values from the testing dataset. The aim of this technique is to make the model learn input-output pairs, allowing it to make predictions on unseen data based on the patterns learned through this process. Supervised ML can be further broken down into two categories, classification, and regression. Depending on the type of task, different models or algorithms are used. For the purpose of this study, we will consider the task of image classification. In this section, the application of three commonly used models for image classification is studied, namely Support Vector Machines (SVM), Convolutional Neural Networks (CNNs) and Artificial Neural Networks (ANN).

2.1.6 Support Vector Machines (SVM)

SVM is an algorithm that facilitates classification of images and is a commonly used algorithm due to its suitability for most binary and multi-class classification tasks. It is also highly effective in high-dimensional spaces for example images with many features. The algorithm works by finding a decision boundary or hyperplane of best fit that separates the data points into different classes. In image classification, the image input is translated into feature vectors, and SVM is applied to determine the hyperplane that best separates the features into their respective classes. The hyperplane is determined by maximizing the difference between the different classes. The key components of this algorithm are the hyperplane and the support vectors, which are the data points closest to the hyperplane as shown in Figure 1.

Figure 1. SVM Algorithm (Support Vector Machine (SVM) Algorithm - Javatpoint, n.d.)

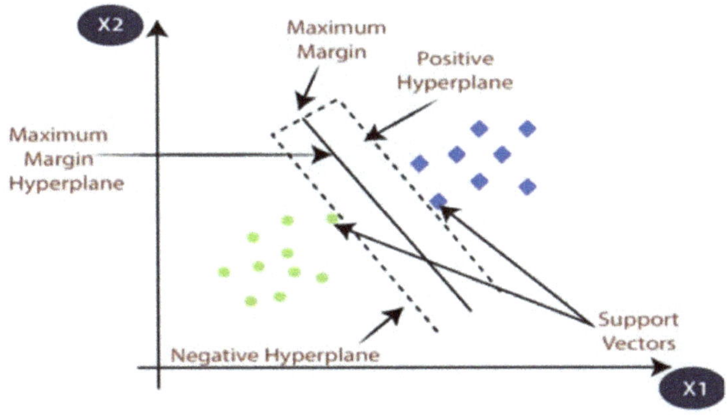

2.1.7 Artificial Neural Networks (ANN)

ANNs are a type of computational model that is biologically inspired by the human brain that is made up of a highly intricate network of neurons, which functions to transmit information throughout the human body. Similarly, ANNs are made up of layers of nodes or neurons that process data input and passes information through the interconnected layers in the network. ANN is a highly versatile model that is capable of both classification and regression tasks as shown in Figure 2. There are three main layers that make up an ANN model: the input, hidden, and output layer. Below is a summary of how ANNs work in principle:

1. **Input Layer** – images given as input are transformed into vectors to be processed
2. **Hidden Layers** – within these layers, computations are performed to learn the feature representations of the data. The use of weights, biases, and activation functions like ReLU or sigmoid functions are used to model varying types of complex relationships within the data. Activation functions are used to introduce non-linearity, without which the neural network can only work with linear relationships between the input and output.
3. **Output Layer** – after the computations are made, the final output layer serves to produce the final probabilities or predictions.

Figure 2. ANN Model(Artificial Neural Network, n.d.)

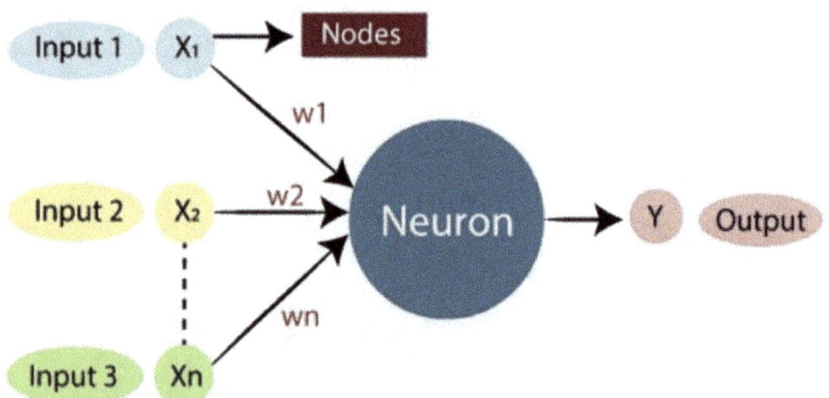

2.3 Convolutional Neural Networks (CNN)

CNNs are a specialized category of ANNs, designed to model data with grid-like characteristics such as images. The layers in a CNN are designed to learn spatial features from image data. The key difference in CNN is that there are specialized layers designed to meet the specific use-case of this model type. Below is a summarized version explaining the key points of the CNN algorithm:

1. **Convolutional Layers** – convolution operations are applied to the image input using kernels as filters to extract features in the images such as edges and corners. These features are passed to the next layers for further processing. Activation functions like ReLU once again play an important role in introducing non-linearity.
2. **Pooling Layers** – the pooling process reduces the dimensionality of the features, taking only important features
3. **Fully-Connected Layers** – towards the end of the network, the output is flattened and the classification result is produced based on the learned features from previous layers as shown in Figure 3.

Figure 3. CNN Model (Convolutional Neural Network - Javatpoint, n.d.)

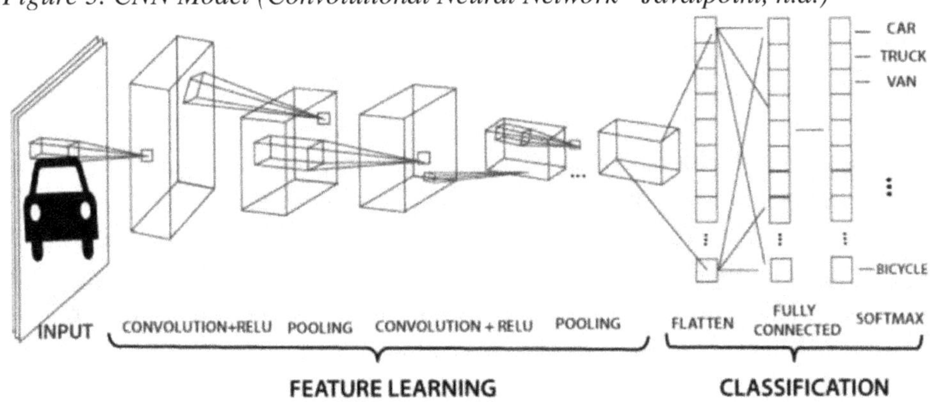

2.3.1 Hybrid Machine Learning (HML)

Hybrid Machine Learning is a technique that has seen a rise in popularity based on recent research works done (Bharati et al., 2020; Hashemzehi et al., 2020; Liu et al., 2019; Mohan et al., 2019; O'Driscoll et al., 2019; Raza et al., 2022). Surprisingly, a lot of the works done corresponds well to the domain of our own research, which is medical imaging. Specifically, there are also many recent works discussing this particular application in the area of brain disease detection. There are no specific definitions to this algorithm, as it refers to a specialized technique in which different ML models and algorithms are used concurrently in a hybrid manner to produce enhanced results by combining the analytical capabilities of these models. HML can be categorized into a few types, for example semi-supervised and self-supervised models. In a way, HML bridges the gap to achieve results that extend beyond the domain of traditional ML methods like supervised and unsupervised learning. Current works in HML that have been used in this literature review includes those of (Bharati et al., 2020; Hashemzehi et al., 2020; Jebarani et al., 2021; Liu et al., 2019; Raza et al., 2022).

3. PROPOSED METHODOLOGICAL SYSTEM

Based on the topic that has been assigned for this project, the focus of our solution would be to develop a powerful ML-based classifier to identify TBI types. The focus is then to conduct research as a group to experiment with various ML algorithms with various experimental setups such as different combinations of ML algorithms or even different pre-processing ways to identify which experimental setup and which ML algorithm has the best performance in classifying brain CT-scans.

However, this poses the question: how do we make our solution relevant and accessible? The development of our ML-based solution is the key to this research project, however, to make this project as comprehensive and well-rounded as possible, it was decided that we would integrate several other aspects to our solution. Hence, we decided to build a web-based application to fully integrate our ML solution into a powerful diagnostic tool that can be used in real-life use cases to have meaningful applications. Our final proposed solution is a fully functional web-based application that is integrated with our ML-powered brain CT analyzer and is used to provide real-time ML-powered TBI diagnosis to a certain level of accuracy.

3.1 Stakeholder Analysis

To begin to build any solution, a key starting point is by identifying the people involved in the project at various phases of the project's lifecycle. According to this article (cite), a stakeholder is anyone who is involved in the project and either influence or are influenced by the outcomes of the project. We can also categorize stakeholders as internal or external stakeholders depending on how they are involved with the project. Internal stakeholders refer to the people who are directly involved in the development of this project. External stakeholders refer to people who are indirectly impacted by the outcome of the project such as potential users, collaborators, competitors, and even society in general as shown in Table 1.

3.2 SWOT Analysis of Proposed System

Table 1. SWOT Analysis of Proposed System

Strengths	Weaknesses
• a complete and comprehensive system that allows users to use the diagnostic capabilities of the trained ML model through a simple UI • integration of various aspects of a software makes it relevant for real- world applications • implementation of a proper database management system allows the system to store data to be used appropriately in various features of the platform • The project focuses on the development of the ML model, striving to achieve feasible accuracies such that it can serve as a dependable solution to solve challenges faced by the healthcare system • implementation of security features ensures that users feel at ease with the data that is shared with the platform	• Development of the ML model depends on the availability of open-source datasets which fits the specificity of the training goal, making it a key obstacle • The system is currently limited to process only brain CT scans • The platform is in the early development phase and may not get much attention from potential users and other stakeholders • Although it is designed to be scalable, it is still a small-scale platform that is unable to handle industrial workload • Difficulty obtaining datasets with ground-truth labels to ensure there is a way to match predictions to professionally diagnosed TBI cases
Opportunities	**Threats**
• Advancements in AI/ML technologies offer many outlets to reference from • Increasing global demand for AI- powered solutions to automate tasks that require less human supervision • It is an active area of research, providing opportunities to collaborate with other researchers, developers, and medical institutions to further develop the prototype • Integration of the ML engine with a web-application opens up avenues to implement more functions to promote usability and practical applications of the developed ML model.	• Existing solutions that have already established feasible and solid results • Cyberattacks and data breaches threaten the security of stored data despite security measures implemented • Ethical concerns related to training a model on pseudo-labels if proper datasets with ground-truth labels are unobtainable, as it could lead to misdiagnosis in real-world applications • Varying quality of input data may cause varying performances of the ML model despite preprocessing attempts

3.3 Requirements Analysis

In software engineering, requirements analysis is a key step in the planning phase of any project development. It involves identifying the needs of the users and translating them into requirements for the system that is being developed. By identifying these requirements, the team is able to set clear expectations on the tasks that need to be done in the development phase. For this section, 3 main requirements are identified as functional, non-functional and data requirements as shown in Table 2 and Table 3.

Table 2. Functional Requirements of System

ID	Title	Description
FR01	User Registration and Log In	Allows users to create and log into their accounts to use the platform. This ensures user-specific activity tracking and secure access to features.
FR02	User Profile Management	Enables users to edit and customize their personal information associated with their accounts.
FR03	User Authentication	Implements secure mechanisms to verify user identity, ensuring only authorized individuals can access platform features.
FR04	Main Dashboard	Serves as the central interface displaying all platform features, providing users with a clear overview upon login.
FR05	CT-Scan Analyzer	Core feature allowing users to upload brain CT scan images for analysis by the machine learning (ML) engine.
FR06	CT-Scan Analysis Report Generation	Generates insights into each uploaded image, visualizing ML processing results in an understandable format.
FR07	Report Viewer	Stores and displays generated reports, allowing users to review them at any time.
FR08	Patient Manager	Grants admin-level users the ability to edit or delete report records, which is especially useful for medical professionals handling patient data.
FR09	Database Management	Manages data flow, including storage and retrieval of user credentials, scan records, and reports.
FR10	Pop-Up Message Notifications	Provides real-time feedback to users for actions, errors, or process completions via on-screen pop-ups.
FR11	Help Center (FAQ)	Offers a support section with frequently asked questions to help users solve common issues independently.
FR12	Feedback Form	Collects user feedback, suggestions, and issues to help improve the platform and maintain developer-user communication.
FR13	Secure Data Encryption	Ensures sensitive medical and personal data is encrypted, protecting users' privacy and reducing the risk of data breaches.

Table 3. Non-Functional Requirements of System

ID	Title	Description
FR01	Performance	The platform should demonstrate solid performance, capable of handling low to medium user traffic without issues. Seamless execution of platform processes must be ensured through well-integrated system layers.
FR02	Accuracy	As the core function of the platform relies on a machine learning engine for TBI classification, the model must achieve high accuracy to build user confidence and system credibility.
FR03	Usability	The web application should be intuitive and user-friendly, minimizing usability issues so users can easily access reliable and practical TBI diagnostic results.
FR04	Scalability	The platform must be scalable to support future expansion, whether in terms of increasing user base or adding new features and functionalities.
FR05	Security	All data used or transmitted within the back end must be properly encrypted to ensure robust user privacy and data protection.

3.4 System Design

The focus of this chapter is to showcase in detail the technical design of the prototype system that is being developed for this project. The goal is to highlight the implementation of the system design to showcase a functional proof of concept for our HML-based solution for the application of TBI classification. The design of the system serves as a conceptual guideline for the remainder of the prototype development and describes how the system works and behaves.

The design process takes into consideration the findings from the chapters above, where several defining factors were identified such as the motivation, expected functions, pain points to be addressed, and expected outcomes of this project. Hence, this chapter serves to translate all of the above requirements into a feasible technical solution by providing a detailed overview of the system's architecture, key components and workflow. It is also an extension to the brief introduction to the proposed system in the previous section. This chapter achieves that by visualizing the detailed proposed system through Unified Modelling Language (UML) diagrams. UML diagrams are commonly used in software development pipelines to visualize systems and help the software project development team understand the design, architecture, and proposed implementation of the entire system. Some key design aspects that will be used to explain the system include the system's architecture, use case specifications, entity relations, and pseudocode to visualize key processes in the system's logic. Through the detailed visualization of the system's design, this chapter highlights the feasibility of the technical solution to meet the requirements identified at the beginning of this report. It also helps the reader to understand the practical implementations that will take place in the development of the research work as shown in Figure 4.

Figure 4. Architecture Diagram of System

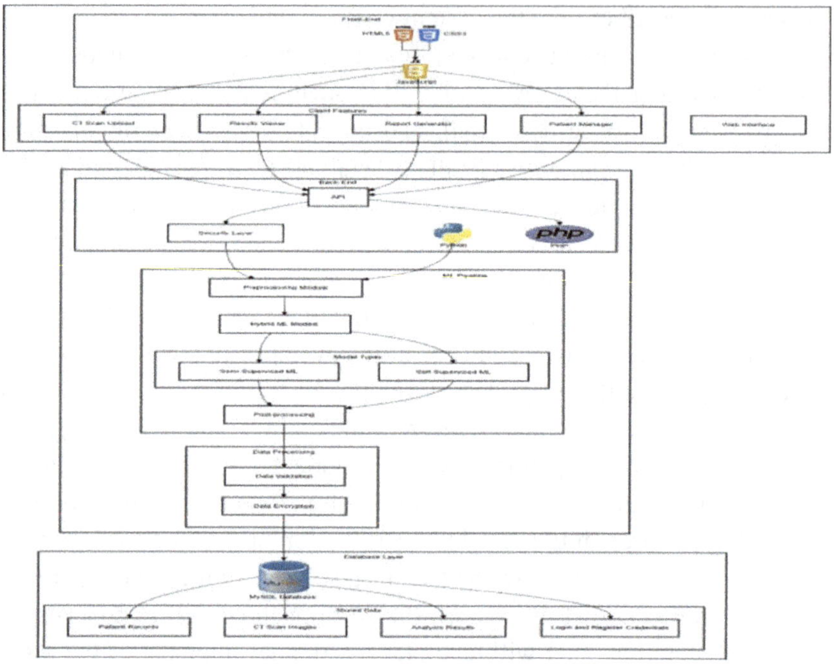

The fully resolved architecture illustrates the proposed system, BrainView AI, consisting of four major components: frontend layer, backend layer, the machine learning (ML) pipeline, and database layer. The backend is further divided into a security layer, a data processing layer, and an API (Application Programming Interface) for communication between backend logic and the user interface of the web applications. The frontend layer, also referred to as client-side design, represents the part of the system with which the user interacts directly on their device. This layer contains the UI, and several key functionalities designed to enhance user experience and accessibility.

This Web Application currently hosts several practical aspects of the architecture of the frontend content, such as CT Scan Upload Window, Results Viewer, Report Generator, and Patient Manager. All these components would be primarily involved in allowing users to interface their results with the ML classification engine- output. It converts their raw binary classification into intuitive, user-friendly visuals, thus empowering users, whether medical professionals or individual patients, to understand and use the insights from brain CT scans. This makes intricate diagnostic information accessible for everyone, which could prove to be a complementary diagnostic aid in a real clinical setting as well as a usable tool for individuals who want to have a clearer understanding of their medical images. The full-fledged modern web technology stack that includes HTML5 and CSS3 is used in the front-end layer to ensure it is responsive, accessible, and easy to use.

This backend layer represents the backbone of the entire system, as it involves the logical programming aspect of the system on the server-side, without which the functions on the front-end layer are unable to operate. In this layer, aspects such as the integration of the system through the API, the security layer which involves all the cybersecurity implementations of the system, as well as the data processing layer are described. Based on the diagram, it also encompasses the ML pipeline, which will be discussed separately as it is the specific focus of my role as the ML Engineer as shown in Figure 5.

Figure 5. Machine Learning Pipeline

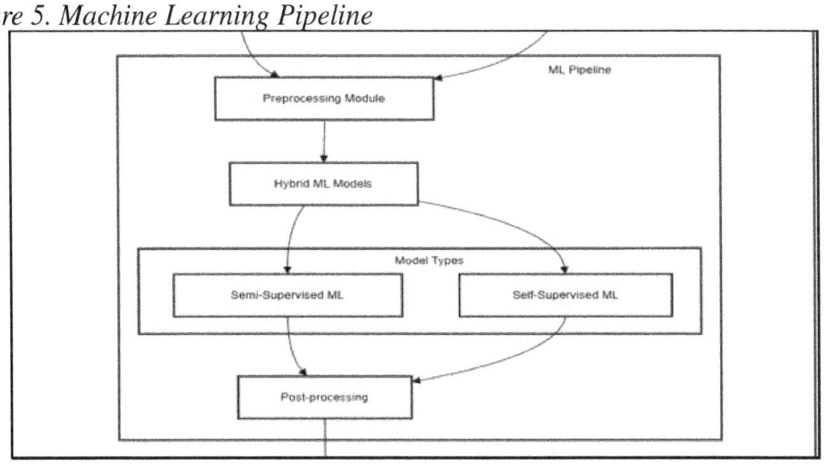

This layer briefly describes how the machine learning aspect of the backend logic functions. Firstly, the common step taken in any ML pipeline is to go through preprocessing. This step involves adjusting the data in preparation for the model training process. It is a highly crucial step with the goal of making the data suitable for the training, subsequently increasing the quality of the output. In the context of image processing, images that are collected to form a dataset may include inconsistencies such as varying sizes, formats, pixel values, contrasts as shown in Figure 5.

Next, the pre-processed data goes through the training process which deploys the Hybrid ML models or algorithms. Based on the literature review, HML for image processing can be approached from either a semi-supervised approach or a self-supervised approach. As the ML pipeline is a key area of experimentation for this research work, several experiments will be conducted under these categories to determine which experimental setup of the ML model development produces the best results in terms of model performance as shown in Figure 6.

Figure 6. Data Processing Layer

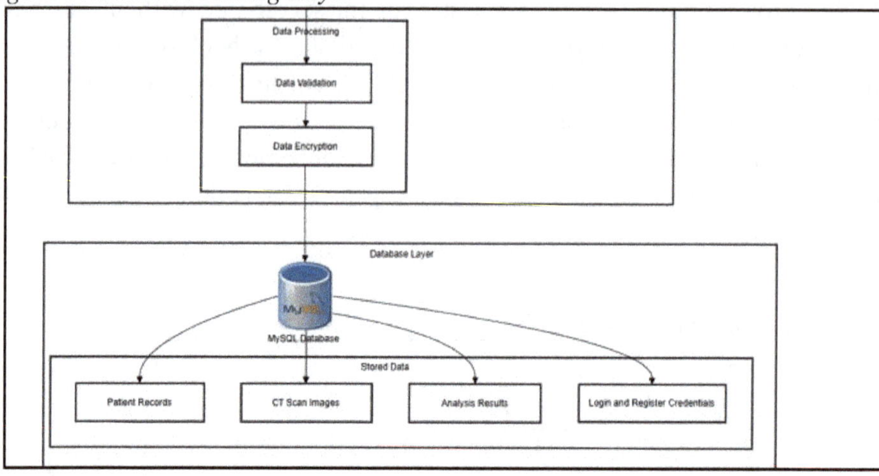

Once the key operational logic of the server processes take place, the database layer plays its role to perform various data management processes. This layer is in charge of interacting with the Database Management System (DBMS) to implement mechanisms that handle data storage, and manipulation such as reading and writing.

3.5 User Interface (UI) Design

The UI was carefully designed by the frontend team following Human Computer Interaction (HCI) principles such as Nielsens' 10 Usability Heuristics and the User-Centered Design (UCD) framework. The design choices were made in accordance with these principles and through their thorough observation of existing web-application designs for a similar use-case. It serves to implement the identified features and functions of the system that have been previously identified onto a user-friendly and appealing web-application platform as shown in Figure 7.

Figure 7. BrainView AI Login Interface

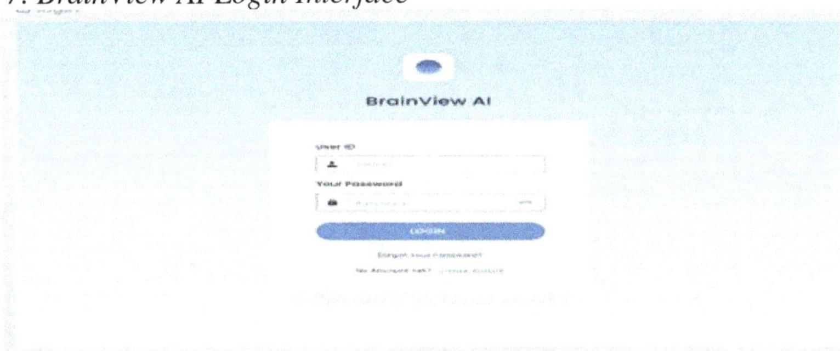

This page serves as the first page the user sees when accessing our platform. It has a minimalistic design that promotes usability and aesthetic feeling while not taking away from the focus of the platform which is to be used as an integration tool for our ML engine.

Once the user passes the user authentication process, they are directed to the dashboard. The dashboard displays an overview of all the features of our platform including CT Scan analyzer, Patient Manager, User Settings, FAQ page, and User Profile. By default, the CT Scan analyzer feature is displayed on the first screen of the dashboard. Here, users can click on the Upload CT Scan button to proceed with selecting an image for analysis as shown in Figure 8 and Figure 9.

Figure 8. BrainView AI Scan Upload

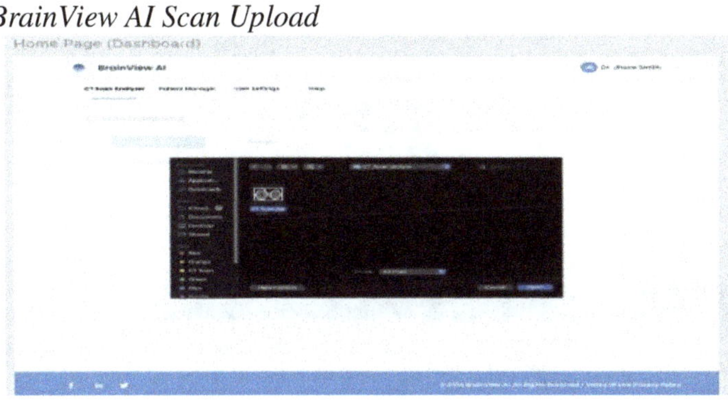

Figure 9. BrainView AI Scan Upload 2

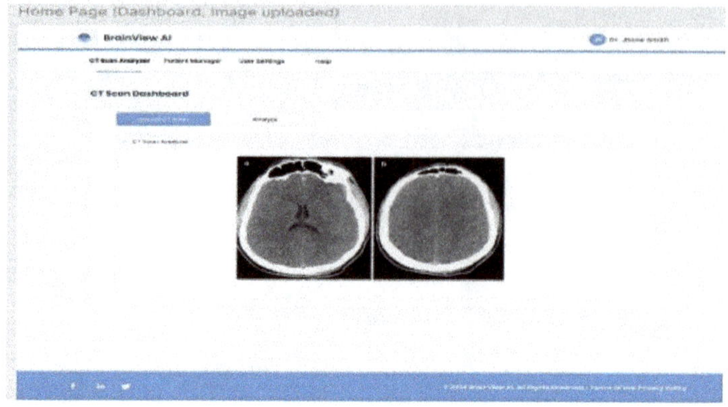

The UI pages above show the example of when a user uploads a selected image from their local file to our system as shown in Figure 10.

Figure 10. BrainView AI Scan Analysis Output

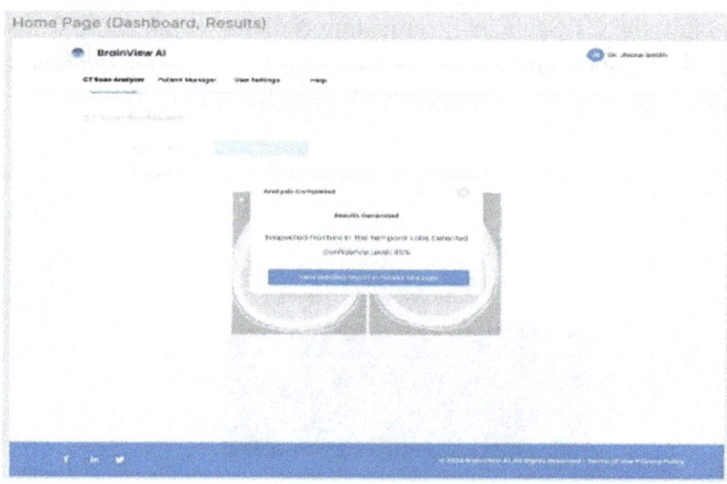

The UI screen above shows the expected results that would be displayed upon successful analysis of an uploaded image. It displays the classification results and also the evaluation metrics of accuracy (confidence level). This concludes the ML integration to the web-app, documenting how the results from our experimental ML model would be used in a practical solution as shown in Figure 11.

Figure 11. BrainView AI Patient Manager

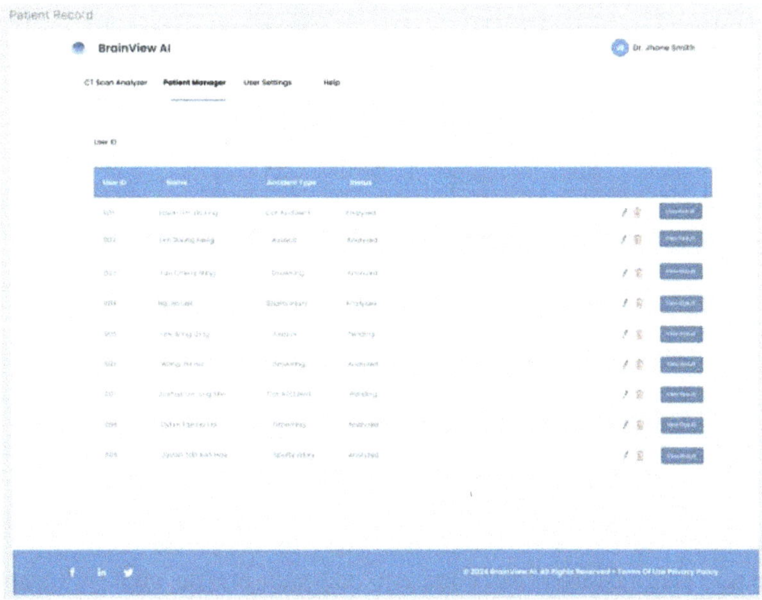

In this screen, there is a feature to view results, which will display a detailed PDF report containing more information than the pop-up results from earlier. Here, users can also find a record of their previous results after they have closed the pop-up message. The detailed report looks something like the following:

As depicted above, the detailed report includes additional details like patient information. We also plan to implement separate features like recommendations which will provide some pre- trained recommendations based on the result that were generated from the CT Scan analysis. For example, a result of "Suspected lesion in the left frontal lobe" may correspond to a recommendation like "Consult a neurologist for further clarification as shown in Figure 12.

Figure 12. BrainView AI User Settings

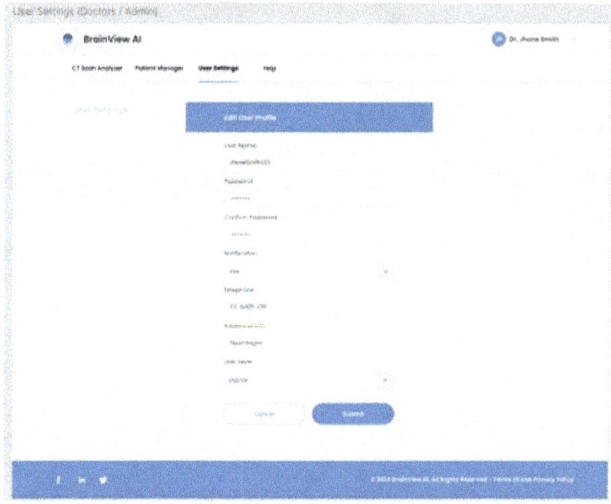

In the user settings, users can choose to edit their profile, contact the admin, or log out of their account. Under the edit feature, users are able to manipulate their associated data for example their username and password. This allows further flexibility for the user and promotes usability. This feature allows users to either ask questions or provide feedback to the admin/developers regarding the platform. It also allows us to receive flags and warnings if there are any errors with the system. Finally, another key feature of the web-app to promote usability is the FAQ page where users can easily access frequently asked questions without the hassle of waiting for an admin to respond to their questions. By identifying common questions with the system and addressing them like this, we allow users to focus on the functions of the web-app with little to no trouble.

Figure 13. Example of Pop-Up Message Upon Successful Action

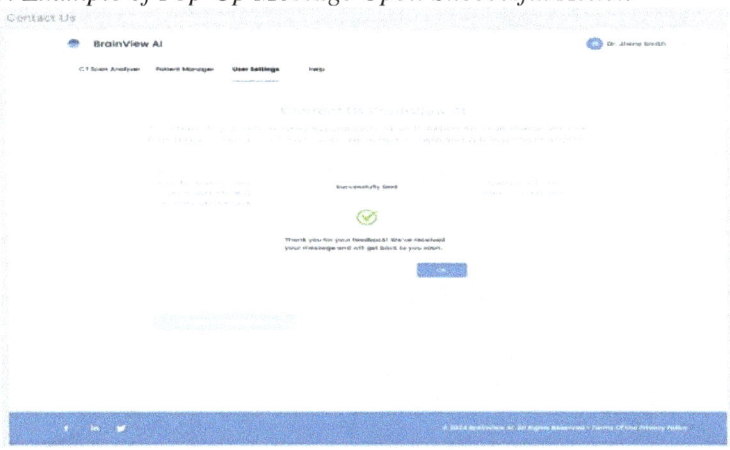

Another conscious design to promote ease of use for the user is the constant pop-up messages that the system displays upon a successful process. This helps users to identify if their request has gone through or if they have run into any problems or errors with the system, which they can notify the admin of as shown in Figure 13.

3.6 UML State Chart Diagrams

A state chart diagram or state machine diagram models the dynamic behavior of our system by showing the various states that an object on our platform can exist in. It also describes how an object on the platform transitions from one state to another based on certain conditions. It is useful to help visualize state changes in response to events and processes, especially since our platform will have various event handlers to be implemented.

Figure 14. State Diagram for Users Performing TBI Detection 2

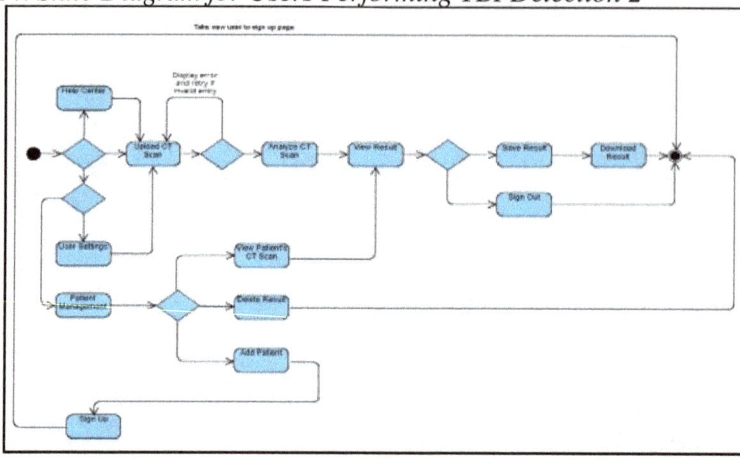

Figure 15. System Sequence Diagram

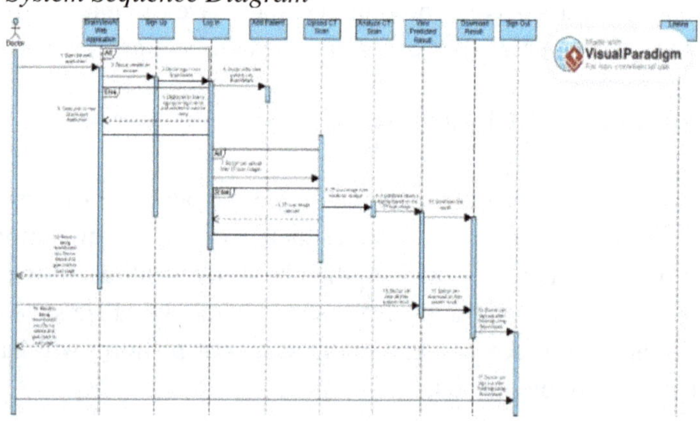

The sequence diagram above helps to model the interaction between the different system components on our platform over certain processes. It describes the flow of information through the system in a step-by-step sequence to help visualize sequential processes that take place within our system as shown in Figure 14 and Figure15.

4. IMPLEMENTATION

Based on the previous chapters which defined the proposed solution and technical approaches in developing the solution, this chapter now introduces the implementation and development of the final system. The final system is a fully functional web-application integrated with our custom Hybrid Machine Learning model. It serves as a comprehensive and easy-to-use platform for a first line of Traumatic Brain Injury detection, saving time on medical triaging and empowering healthcare providers with the tool to make faster yet smarter decisions. To summarize, our system as a whole can be broken down into three main aspects: the Frontend, Machine Learning, and Backend pipeline. The following chapter explains the development process which takes place in each of the software development parts, with a technical focus on the ML pipeline as that is the part of the system which I was involved in developing. Below is the summary of the technology stack that has been used in the final development phase of the system.

4.1 Development of Responsive Web-Based Application

Based on the previous literature review that has been done, the frontend team has selected a few programming frameworks and tools as shown in the technology stack to develop their part of the solution. The final result is a HTML-based web-application which includes the use of CSS and JavaScript for reactive and responsive programming. The final web-application differs slightly from the original prototype but maintains a similar functional workflow as the wireframe. This is because the design undergoes changes and transformation to fit the latest iterations in our solutions after conducting comprehensive reviews and testing and obtaining feedback from the team members, peers and our supervisor. The final web-application is fully functional, with no bugs detected that have yet to be resolved, which is a huge success for our team. Although we could have implemented a more complex system with more advanced features, we remained realistic and objective throughout the development phase to ensure that our platform is as simple, intuitive and aesthetic as possible, with a particular emphasis on achieving full functionality over unsolved bugs that will hinder the usability of the overall system as shown in Figure 16 and Figure 17.

Figure 16. Actual CT Scan Upload Interface 1

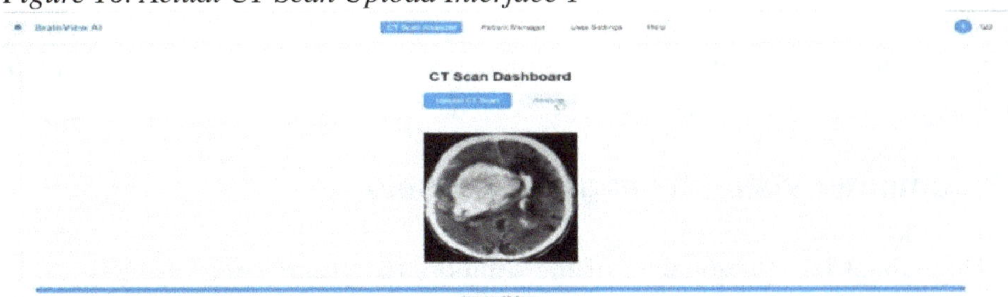

Figure 17. Actual Analysis Results from Scan Upload

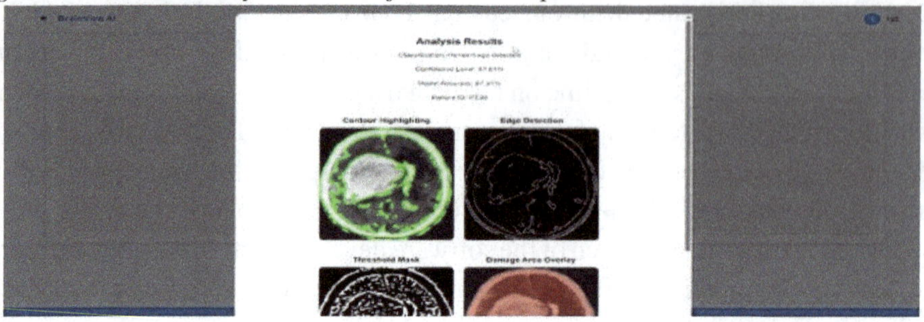

The above is a few screenshots taking from the final system, which have been thoroughly demonstrated during the presentation. A brief snippet is also shown in our research work showcase video, where it shows that the system is functions properly without bugs, reacting as expected to events such as button clicks and file uploads. As observed, one key improvement from the initial research work description is the function to highlight the specific injury area. This additional function was achieved through the addition of Computer Vision and Image Processing techniques, which will be elaborated in the following sections.

4.2 Model Preprocessing

As proposed in the previous chapter on system design, the collected data goes through preprocessing. This step is vital in ensuring that the data used to train the model is standardized based on our specific requirements and targeted outcomes. The preprocessing methods that have been used are listed as below:

Image Resizing – adjust the dimensions of an image to a set size while maintaining the entire aspect ratio to ensure consistency of image data during training

Image Rescaling – rescaling image pixel values to be within a certain range, for example 0-1. The aim is to standardize input data and improve efficiency during model training.

Image Normalization – adjusting the image pixels to have a standardized mean/ standard deviation so that the model is able to converge in a stable way during training.

Greyscale Conversion – converting images with inconsistent color information into greyscale images to reduce computational complexity.

4.3 Computer Vision & Image Processing

Throughout the development of the solution, the group's main focus was on developing a fully- functioning Hybrid Machine Learning model to classify TBI cases. However, through our integrative development process, we received valuable feedback about our system's functions that caused us to consider the additional implementation of a function to highlight the damage area of the injury itself. Hence, as suggested by our supervisor, we explored the use of Computer Vision (CV) and image processing techniques to extract more information from our images. While image processing explicitly refers to the process of extracting information from images, CV is a concept in which we combine the output from image processing for further development in an attempt to derive meaning from the image processing output. In the context of using the output from this implementation as a method of detecting the injury area and to display it as a layover of the original CT-scan image to further help doctors in detecting TBI to higher precision, we can consider this process as CV. This research work involves medical imaging, there is a lot of potential to provide even more insights into the images rather than only the classification results. We then decided to explore image segmentation and edge detection as the CV techniques used.

Canny Edge Detection – A technique used to identity significant changes in intensity (edges). The edges represent object boundaries, and detection of these edges can help determine where the significant image differences are

Contour Segmentation – a similar method to detect and extract the outline of objects within an image. It is used to isolate areas of interest, such as tumors, fractures, or hemorrhage.

Threshold Masking – by setting a threshold value for the image pixels, we are able to convert them into binary format (ie, pixel values above a certain threshold are turned white (1) and below a certain value, black(0) as shown in Figure 18.

Figure 18. The input image and resulting output based on CV processing

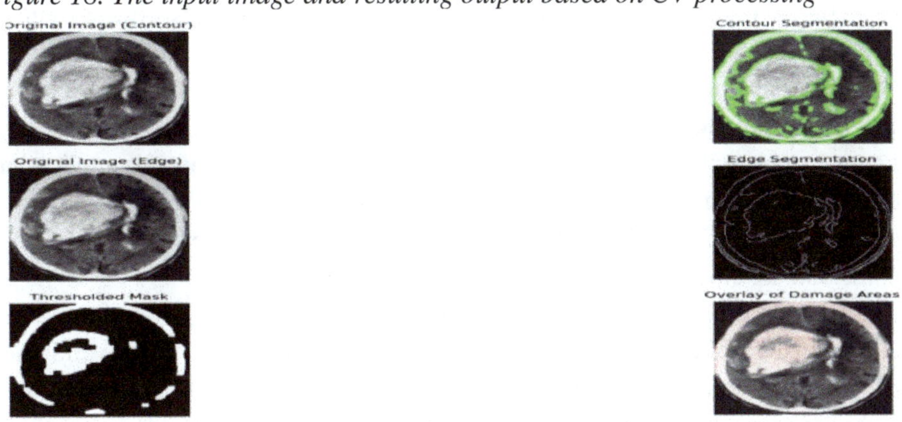

4.4 Hybrid Machine Learning (HML) Model Design

The general overview of the implemented HML model is first consider the dependencies (ie, libraries) necessary for the processes and methods used in the model are imported into the file. Such libraries include Matplotlib, Pandas, NumPy, OpenCV, and scikit- learn. Then, a function is defined to load the data from a specified file path. Within this function, we use Pandas to load the data into a data frame, along with the ground truth labelling from the corresponding CSV file from the dataset. This is so that the model is able to compare predicted values to the ground truth at the end of the model training, enabling us to assess the accuracy and overall performance of the model. Then, before training the first model which is the K-Means Clustering, we initialize some parameters such as image size, number of clusters, test size, and a random state for reproducibility. The image below is a code snippet of the data loading function Next, the K-Means Clustering is applied to the input image, and an additional feature called "cluster_features" is obtained. The next step is to combine this feature with the normalized pixel data of the input image, scale the features using the Standard Scaler, and use these to train the Support Vector Machine. Finally, the model is evaluated using a classification report and confusion matrix and saved as a .pkl file using joblib. In the following chapter on testing, more detailed information about the classification report and confusion matrix will be detailed. The full code has been published to our team's GitHub and can be found in the appendix of this report.

4.5 Security Considerations

When designing the final frontend system, security measures were taken into consideration in accordance with our backend developer's plans for software security implementations. Such security measures include user authentication and access control. As such, the developed web-application starts by directing users to a log-in page, where they may choose to sign up instead if they do not have a pre-existing account. In the event that an unauthorized user attempts to access the web-application with invalid credentials, the system is programmed to restrict access, resulting in the user being unable to access the web-application as well as the sensitive medical records that are stored on it.

To test this function on the front end aspect, the team attempted to access the platform using valid credentials and invalid credentials. Upon using valid user credentials, the web-app redirects them to the BrainView AI platform, where they are able to access the dashboard along with the list of stored patient information associated with the account, and the other functions on the web-app. Conversely, upon using an invalid credential, an error message pops up and indicates that the user is attempting to use an invalid credential, stopping them from proceeding to access the rest of the web-application. Below is an example of a test case done by our system tester.

4.6 Security & Database Testing

For the aspect of system security, our system does not utilize many advanced software security technologies due to the lack of time and expertise among the team. As such, our main security implementation is the use of user authentication & authorization. Hence, we test our system thoroughly to ensure that invalid user information is blocked from accessing our platform as a first layer of defense from users with malicious intents to misuse our platform or to prevent existing data from being accessed by unauthorized users. This testing is carried out by testing out a few sets of invalid user login credentials, and it was successful as in every scenario of using invalid credentials, the user is redirected to an error message instead. As for testing the database, it is important to ensure that the data uploaded through our frontend has a way of being managed properly. As we are using SQL as our storage solution, we are able to test out the functionality of the database by checking if the SQL database properly updates and stores the expected input such as CT-scan images together with the associated patient information. Data updates through CRUD operations from the Patient Manager should also be reflected correctly in the database.

4.7 Machine Learning Pipeline Testing

As the machine learning engineer, we were mostly in charge of testing the ML model during its development to ensure that the model was able to be trained properly without bugs and errors. While training the ML model, several key areas for mistakes can be identified. Based on my experience, data loading was one of the challenging aspects of model training, especially when dealing with large datasets with inconsistent file formatting, as well as medical images such as CT-scans which may include 3D imaging which is made up of multiple slices of images, therefore requiring a more intricate and detailed data loading process. Below are a few areas I have identified for testing out the ML model.

4.8 Data Loading and Validation

To test whether data was able to load as expected, there are several visualization tools that can be used as a testing method. For example, the code snippet below describes a few of such visualization techniques to ensure the data frame is loaded with the expected format. The output from these Python scripts are as follows, and as observed, the output allows us visualize the data frame with the hemorrhage labelling from the CSV file, with the column names listed, and the shape of the loaded images also described. Through the above visualization script, we were also able to confirm that all 200 images from the dataset have been loaded properly.

4.9 Data Preprocessing

During the clustering process, it was necessary to visualize the results to confirm whether or not the clustering was done correctly. As clustering is an unsupervised ML algorithm, the results are based solely on the similarity of the image and the distance of the data points from the decision boundary. Hence, using a visualization script to get an idea of the clustering results is vital to compare the images to the expected output. The clustering algorithm and obtains a label for each cluster. Then, it iterates through the clustered images, assigning it to the respective clusters and prints it out as a list. Additionally, a script was written to have a "representative" image from each cluster be printed out for better idea of the clustered images. The resulting output prints the cluster numbers and the images that have been assigned to each cluster. In this case, there were only 2 clusters as determined using the Elbow Method as shown in Figure 19.

Figure 19. Randomly Selected Image from Cluster 0 and Cluster 1

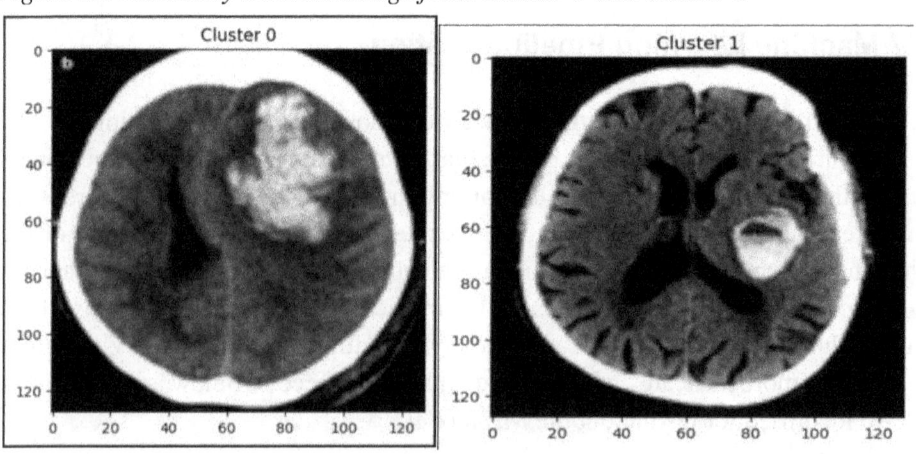

4.10 Classification Report and Visualization

Model performance was evaluated using traditional image classification metrics: Accuracy, Precision, F1-Score, and Recall. These metrics are computed using scikit-learn library functions that provide a comprehensive classification report with the confusion matrix for analysis. The confusion matrix gives a graphical representation of the model's predictions juxtaposed against the actual ground truth labels, highlighting the distribution of True Positives (TP), True Negatives (TN), False Positives (FP), and False Negatives (FN). An overall accuracy of 82.5% was achieved by the model, which is really quite good in the context of the similar studies reviewed in the literature. However, this value should be viewed with caution since the model was trained with a small dataset of just 200 images. Future iterations of the research project should include training and testing on larger and more heterogeneous datasets, preferably from reputable institutions such as the Radiological Society of North America (RSNA). Larger datasets would allow more concrete performance estimates and help advance the validation of clinical applicability of the model's work as shown in Figure 20.

Figure 20. Confusion Matrix of HML model

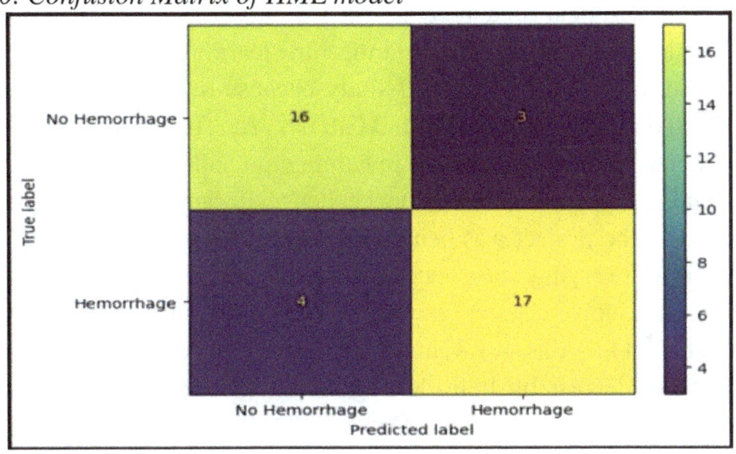

Based on the Confusion Matrix, we are able to tell that there are 17 TPs, and 16 TNs based on the prediction made by the model on the test set. There are 3 and 4 cases respectively of false predictions, which can be attributed to the model's prediction inaccuracy.

4.11 Challenges & Solutions in Implementation

The research project encountered several challenges during the implementation stage, requiring the team to demonstrate adaptability and collaborative problem-solving. Some of these impediments even delayed the process or forced deviations from original plans. All factors, however, culminated in an enrichment of our learning experience and an ultimately workable system that conformed with the original project objectives. One of the core challenges was obtaining a suitable dataset. The dataset we desired would contain properly structured brain CT scans under a consistent file format with detailed ground truth labeling regarding types of traumatic brain injury (TBI) and hemorrhages. However, finding such datasets proved arduous. To avoid getting locked in complexity, we went the simpler way to a binary classification dataset while emphasizing functionality. This was essential to realize the project as a demonstrable and fully integrated solution, hence a basis for future work.

Unclear supervision was yet another obstacle one had to face. Feedback often proved weak and unstructured, hence lacking clarity and causing disarray in the direction the team was taking. This prompted us to hold more team discussions to help us set out the best direction, which eventually got us focused and made it possible to iterate through issues. We all learnt an important lesson in reviewing feedback critically and adapting when the instruction is direct. Also, the research project brought a set of technical fundamentals-new-to many team members in the areas of medical image processing and hybrid machine learning. As a machine learning engineer, I had to do some initial self-study because my experience was mostly with structured data. Fortunately, I found GitHub, YouTube, Kaggle, and the most relevant academic research invaluable in helping me understand by trial and error.

When strangled by time constraints, our challenges became almost insurmountable. While Phase I of the project was being undertaken during an extensive semester, team members were trying to balance it alongside other academic commitments. But by Phase II, a short semester arrived, allowing scarce time for any serious developments. In tackling this, we went for structured project management activities as team leader, such as establishing clear agendas at meetings, maintaining minutes of the meetings, and ensuring constant flow of information among all the sub-teams. These not only made us effective during this time limit but also bind the project together. Together, overcoming these challenges ensured deliverable success but also enhanced our problem-solving abilities and teamwork capabilities.

5. CONCLUSION & CRITICAL EVALUATION

This chapter summarizes the major findings of the project and evaluates the extent to which the final proposed solution realized its objectives. It further presents a critical review of the system design, its practical viability, and future work. Among many others found and resolved were some key problems in the area of TBI diagnosis through the entire development period: one such major barrier was the availability of labeled TBI datasets in the public domain; the privacy issues surrounding the restricted access to the annotated medical scans became a limelight. To overcome this, a hybrid machine learning approach was employed—one that combined unsupervised feature extraction along with age-old supervised classification models. This hybridization achieved better learning with limited data. Another setback faced involved healthcare involved not having a good number of available people able to carry out the duties that demand pressure on healthcare applicants to do diagnostics well. The proposed AI-based diagnostic assistant is set forth to assist clinicians in rapid triaging of an injury and detection, thereby improving workflow efficiency.

Another issue of real problem applying any solution, typically those features developed in controlled situations, becomes an obstacle for scalability and usability in actual clinical practice. For example, considering development right from the beginning and providing this as a basis for the future enhancement and deployment, the system was designed with scalability in mind. In those rural or under-served areas which lack access to specialists in neurology or radiology, the system will act as a preliminary assessment tool for early intervention before evaluation by an expert.

The final solution developed is a robust web-based machine learning system capable of classifying brain hemorrhages from CT scans. The hybrid technique that combines K-Means Clustering with Support Vector Machines (SVM) for classification raised the level of diagnostic accuracy of the developed system for brain hemorrhages. Further image processing techniques such as edge detection and threshold masking were applied to the images for highlighting the critical injury areas that would enhance interpretability of results. The solution has been implemented in a formal Software Development Life Cycle (SDLC) ensuring that the output is reliable and maintainable, effectively bridging the model and user interface of AI. The entire project extrapolates the increasing potential of AI technology in medical imaging and promises the reduction of diagnosis delays and improved patient care. The system seems to hold great promise as a supportive tool in neurological and radiological practices pending further refinements, regulatory validation, and integration into clinical workflows.

REFERENCES

Artificial Neural Network. (n.d.). https://www.javatpoint.com/artificial-neural-network

Barragán-Montero, A., Javaid, U., Valdés, G., Nguyen, D., Desbordes, P., Macq, B., Willems, S., Vandewinckele, L., Holmström, M., Löfman, F., Michiels, S., Souris, K., Sterpin, E., & Lee, J. A. (2021). Artificial intelligence and machine learning for medical imaging: A technology review. *Physica Medica*, *83*, 242–256. DOI: 10.1016/j.ejmp.2021.04.016 PMID: 33979715

Bharati, S., Podder, P., & Mondal, M. R. H. (2020). Hybrid deep learning for detecting lung diseases from X-ray images. *Informatics in Medicine Unlocked*, *20*, 100391. DOI: 10.1016/j.imu.2020.100391 PMID: 32835077

Chandra, M. A., & Bedi, S. S. (2021). Survey on SVM and their application in image classification. *International Journal of Information Technology : an Official Journal of Bharati Vidyapeeth's Institute of Computer Applications and Management*, *13*(5), 1–11. DOI: 10.1007/s41870-017-0080-1

Chen, M., & Ludtke, S. J. (2021). Deep learning-based mixed-dimensional Gaussian mixture model for characterizing variability in cryo-EM. Nature Methods 2021 18:8, 18(8), 930– 936. DOI: 10.1038/s41592-021-01220-5

Cheplygina, V., de Bruijne, M., & Pluim, J. P. W. (2019). Not-so-supervised: A survey of semi- supervised, multi-instance, and transfer learning in medical image analysis. *Medical Image Analysis*, *54*, 280–296. DOI: 10.1016/j.media.2019.03.009 PMID: 30959445

Chilamkurthy, S., Ghosh, R., Tanamala, S., Biviji, M., Campeau, N. G., Kumar Venugopal, V., Mahajan, V., Rao, P., Warier, P., & Ai, Q. (2018). Development and Validation of Deep Learning Algorithms for Detection of Critical Findings in Head CT Scans. https://arxiv.org/abs/1803.05854v2

Convolutional Neural Network - javatpoint. (n.d.). https://www.javatpoint.com/pytorch-convolutional-neural-network

Dewan, M. C., Rattani, A., Gupta, S., Baticulon, R. E., Hung, Y. C., Punchak, M., Agrawal, A., Adeleye, A. O., Shrime, M. G., Rubiano, A. M., Rosenfeld, J. V., & Park, K. B. (2018). Estimating the global incidence of traumatic brain injury. *Journal of Neurosurgery*, *130*(4), 1080–1097. DOI: 10.3171/2017.10.JNS17352 PMID: 29701556

Felipe Kitamura. (2019). Head CT - hemorrhage. https://www.kaggle.com/datasets/felipekitamura/head-ct-hemorrhage

Flanders, A. E., Prevedello, L. M., Shih, G., Halabi, S. S., Kalpathy-Cramer, J., Ball, R., Mongan, J. T., Stein, A., Kitamura, F. C., Lungren, M. P., Choudhary, G., Cala, L., Coelho, L., Mogensen, M., Morón, F., Miller, E., Ikuta, I., Zohrabian, V., McDonnell, O., & Nath, J. (2020). Construction of a machine learning dataset through collaboration: The RSNA 2019 brain CT hemorrhage challenge. *Radiology. Artificial Intelligence*, *2*(3), e190211. DOI: 10.1148/ryai.2020190211 PMID: 33937827

Hashemzehi, R., Mahdavi, S. J. S., Kheirabadi, M., & Kamel, S. R. (2020). Detection of brain tumors from MRI images base on deep learning using hybrid model CNN and NADE. *Biocybernetics and Biomedical Engineering*, *40*(3), 1225–1232. DOI: 10.1016/j.bbe.2020.06.001

Hou, R., Zhou, D., Nie, R., Liu, D., & Ruan, X. (2019). Brain CT and MRI medical image fusion using convolutional neural networks and a dual-channel spiking cortical model. *Medical & Biological Engineering & Computing*, *57*(4), 887–900. DOI: 10.1007/s11517-018-1935-8 PMID: 30471068

Hussain, M., Bird, J. J., & Faria, D. R. (2019). A Study on CNN Transfer Learning for Image Classification. *Advances in Intelligent Systems and Computing*, *840*, 191–202. DOI: 10.1007/978-3-319-97982-3_16

Islam, M. K., Ali, M. S., Miah, M. S., Rahman, M. M., Alam, M. S., & Hossain, M. A. (2021). Brain tumor detection in MR image using superpixels, principal component analysis and template based K-means clustering algorithm. *Machine Learning with Applications*, *5*, 100044. DOI: 10.1016/j.mlwa.2021.100044

Jagannathan, P., Rajkumar, S., Frnda, J., Divakarachari, P. B., & Subramani, P. (2021). Moving Vehicle Detection and Classification Using Gaussian Mixture Model and Ensemble Deep Learning Technique. *Wireless Communications and Mobile Computing*, *2021*(1), 5590894. DOI: 10.1155/2021/5590894

Jebarani, P. E., Umadevi, N., Dang, H., & Pomplun, M. (2021). A Novel Hybrid K-Means and GMM Machine Learning Model for Breast Cancer Detection. *IEEE Access : Practical Innovations, Open Solutions*, *9*, 146153–146162. DOI: 10.1109/ACCESS.2021.3123425

Jena, B., Saxena, S., Nayak, G. K., Saba, L., Sharma, N., & Suri, J. S. (2021). Artificial intelligence-based hybrid deep learning models for image classification: The first narrative review. *Computers in Biology and Medicine*, *137*, 104803. DOI: 10.1016/j.compbiomed.2021.104803 PMID: 34536856

Jiang, F., Lu, Y., Chen, Y., Cai, D., & Li, G. (2020). Image recognition of four rice leaf diseases based on deep learning and support vector machine. *Computers and Electronics in Agriculture*, *179*, 105824. DOI: 10.1016/j.compag.2020.105824

Khan, A. R., Khan, S., Harouni, M., Abbasi, R., Iqbal, S., & Mehmood, Z. (2021). Brain tumor segmentation using K-means clustering and deep learning with synthetic data augmentation for classification. *Microscopy Research and Technique*, *84*(7), 1389–1399. DOI: 10.1002/jemt.23694 PMID: 33524220

Khellaf, A., Khan, D. Z., & Helmy, A. (2019). Recent advances in traumatic brain injury. *Journal of Neurology*, *266*(11), 2878–2889. DOI: 10.1007/s00415-019-09541-4 PMID: 31563989

Lin, E., & Yuh, E. L. (2022). Computational Approaches for Acute Traumatic Brain Injury Image Recognition. *Frontiers in Neurology*, *13*, 791816. DOI: 10.3389/fneur.2022.791816 PMID: 35370919

Liu, T., Fan, W., & Wu, C. (2019). A hybrid machine learning approach to cerebral stroke prediction based on imbalanced medical dataset. *Artificial Intelligence in Medicine*, *101*, 101723. DOI: 10.1016/j.artmed.2019.101723 PMID: 31813482

Lloyd, S. P. (1982). Least Squares Quantization in PCM. *IEEE Transactions on Information Theory*, *28*(2), 129–137. DOI: 10.1109/TIT.1982.1056489

Mohan, S., Thirumalai, C., & Srivastava, G. (2019). Effective heart disease prediction using hybrid machine learning techniques. *IEEE Access : Practical Innovations, Open Solutions*, *7*, 81542–81554. DOI: 10.1109/ACCESS.2019.2923707

O'Driscoll, L., Nichols, R., & Knott, P. A. (2019). A hybrid machine learning algorithm for designing quantum experiments. *Quantum Machine Intelligence*, *1*(1–2), 5–15. DOI: 10.1007/s42484-019-00003-8

qure.ai. (2019). Qure.ai's qER CT Scan Algorithm Receives CE Certification. https://www.qure.ai/news_press_coverages/ce-certification-for-qure-ais-traumatic-brain- injury-and-stroke-triage-tool. Raza, A., Ayub, H., Khan, J. A., Ahmad, I., Salama, A. S., Daradkeh, Y. I., Javeed, D., Rehman, U., & Hamam, H. (2022). A Hybrid Deep Learning-Based Approach for Brain Tumor Classification. Electronics 2022, Vol. 11, Page 1146, 11(7), 1146. DOI: 10.3390/electronics11071146

Samuel, A. L. (1959). Some Studies in Machine Learning Using the Game of Checkers. *IBM Journal of Research and Development*, *3*(3), 210–229. DOI: 10.1147/rd.33.0210

Saputra, M. F. A., Widiyaningtyas, T., & Wibawa, A. P. (2018). Illiteracy classification using K means-naïve bayes algorithm. *JOIV: International Journal on Informatics Visualization*, *2*(3), 153–158. DOI: 10.30630/joiv.2.3.129

Sarvamangala, D. R., & Kulkarni, R. V. (2022). Convolutional neural networks in medical image understanding: A survey. *Evolutionary Intelligence*, *15*(1), 1–22. DOI: 10.1007/s12065-020-00540-3 PMID: 33425040

Support Vector Machine (SVM) Algorithm - Javatpoint. (n.d.). https://www.javatpoint.com/machine-learning-support-vector-machine-algorithm

vbookshelf. (2019). vbookshelf/Intracranial-Hemorrhage-Analyzer: Ai powered web app that automatically detects and segments intracranial hemorrhages on brain CT images - Tensorflow.js. https://github.com/vbookshelf/Intracranial-Hemorrhage-Analyzer

Woźniak, M., Siłka, J., & Wieczorek, M. (2023). Deep neural network correlation learning mechanism for CT brain tumor detection. *Neural Computing & Applications*, *35*(20), 14611–14626. DOI: 10.1007/s00521-021-05841-x

Zhou, S. K., Greenspan, H., Davatzikos, C., Duncan, J. S., Van Ginneken, B., Madabhushi, A., Prince, J. L., Rueckert, D., & Summers, R. M. (2021). A review of deep learning in medical imaging: Imaging traits, technology trends, case studies with progress highlights, and future promises. Proceedings of the IEEE. Institute of Electrical and Electronics Engineers, 109(5), 820. DOI: 10.1109/JPROC.2021.3054390

Zivkovic, Z. (2004). Improved adaptive Gaussian mixture model for background subtraction. Proceedings - International Conference on Pattern Recognition, 2, 28–31. DOI: 10.1109/ICPR.2004.1333992

Chapter 9
Introduction to CT Imaging for Personalized Medicine and Its Impact on Patients

Zeelaf Shahid
https://orcid.org/0000-0002-5396-4503
Jinnah Medical and Dental College, Pakistan

Rubina Ghani
https://orcid.org/0000-0003-1923-7924
Jinnah Medical and Dental College, Pakistan

ABSTRACT

Computed tomography (CT) imaging has become a vital instrument in personalized medicine, allowing accurate diagnosis, customized treatment planning, and enhanced patient outcomes. New developments in AI, radiomics, and 3D imaging have further maximized its use in different medical fields, ranging from oncology and cardiology to neurology and orthopedics. With advancing technology, the integration of CT imaging with personalized medicine will become more sophisticated, enhancing clinical decision-making and healthcare delivery. With the resolution of current challenges and exploration of future innovations, CT imaging will remain a cornerstone of modern personalized healthcare. Raw patient data employed in this research was sourced from Jinnah Medical and Dental College and approved by the Sohail Trust Hospital Ethical Review Board. The dataset is made up of de-identified patient data that includes CT imaging to enable comprehensive insight into the use of CT imaging in personalized medicine, including oncology, cardiology, neurology, and orthopedic diseases.

DOI: 10.4018/979-8-3373-2807-2.ch009

1. INTRODUCTION

The amalgamation of computed tomography (CT) imaging with personalized medicine has changed the way we approach diagnostic and therapeutic processes in all forms of medicine over the past few years. CT imaging is a popular and non-invasive imaging modality, derived from an application of X-ray physics and image reconstruction algorithms, which incorporates high-resolution cross-sectional information of internal anatomical structures/organ systems with exceptional detail for diagnostic accuracy (Gaddam *et al.,* 2021) .

Personalized medicine refers to tailoring medical decisions, with regards to the diagnosis and treatment of disease and the prescription of medications to the specific genetic, anatomical and physiological, characteristics of individual patients. As it relates to personalized medicine, CT imaging is a key technology that enables accurate descriptions of disease pathology (morphology and function) to mediate and direct personalized treatment planning. CT imaging for the assessment of disease pathology is especially valuable in the field of oncology, where in a combination of clinical context, CT imaging provides critical information in initial tumor localization, staging and response evaluation, thereby personalizing treatment (Hricak *et al.,* 2025).

The impact of CT imaging has been significant, not only in the field of oncology. In cardiovascular medicine, coronary CT angiography (CCTA) has revolutionized the diagnostic process for coronary artery disease (CAD) by providing non-invasive alternatives to traditional angiography. CCTA provides high sensitivity and specificity in diagnosing CAD (Budoff *et al*., 2008; Irannejad *et al.,* 2025). In neurology, CT perfusion, and dual-energy CT modalities are used to enhance early diagnosis of stroke. Timely and accurate identification of strokes leads to improved treatment optimization (Campbell *et al.,* 2021; Gaddam *et al*., 2021) and significantly improves long-term disability. In orthopaedics and traumatology, CT imaging influences the development of 3D printed patient-specific surgical guides to enhance the accuracy of implant positioning and improve surgical outcomes (Hess *et al*., 2024).

Although the role of CT clearly promotes personal medicine, challenges still exist. Concerns regarding irradiation exposure based on known risk factors, particularly in vulnerable patient populations (i.e. patients with disabilities) reinforce the progressive development of optimized imaging protocols and low-dose, optimized technology (Salah *et al.,* 2025). In addition to radiation risk protocols, the integration of artificial intelligence (AI) into the processing and analysis of CT images has increased. Automated detection of CT images improved and/or enhanced accuracy, operational enhancements and predictive modelling will continue to support clinical decision-making (Li *et al*., 2024).

In summary, CT imaging is a fundamental pillar of precision medicine. This article described many of its uses, advances in technology, and new developments - and emphasized its important role in realizing true diagnostic accuracy and patient-centered care in all specialties.

2. LITERATURE REVIEW

The application of computed tomography (CT) imaging in personalized medicine has evolved significantly, leveraging advances in technology for enhanced diagnostic performance, treatment planning, and patient outcomes. This section summarizes the existing research on the application of CT imaging in personalized medicine and their applications in oncology, cardiology, neurology, and orthopedic surgery. Computed Tomography (CT) imaging is firmly established as a pillar of personalized medicine, supporting a patient-centric diagnostic and treatment framework across clinical specialties. Recent advances with CT imaging have improved its accuracy, minimized the dose of radiation, and infused artificial intelligence (AI) to enhance diagnostic effectiveness and planning assistance in therapy.

Since machine learning (ML) and deep learning (DL) are firmly in the field now, the discipline of image interpretation and analysis is all set to enter a new paradigm. Currie and Rohren (2022) illustrated that intelligent imaging workflows and smart imaging algorithms can moor homeless tasks such as automated segmentation or anomaly detection to streamline workflow and generate consistency. Furthermore, AI systems can eliminate radiation exposure as a priori parameters without any adverse impact on image quality (Clement David-Olawade et al., 2025).

In oncology, CT imaging has also advanced by leaps and bounds with the advent of radiomics (extraction of high-dimensional features from a medical image). Caruso et al. (2021) explain that radiomics can potentially help treatment planning by revealing tumor phenotypes and treatment response patterns not visible to the naked eye. Likewise, dual-energy CT (DECT) has been another important advance in the field of imaging applications in oncologic patients. Foti et al. (2024) were able to demonstrate that DECT allows for improved tissue characterization, which in turn allows for differentiation of tumor types (e.g., differentiation of a tumor treated with chemo therapy versus one not treated), and adequacy and planning of radiation therapy (Saeed *et.al*, 2020; Saeed *et.al*, 2021).

In the field of cardiovascular medicine, CT imaging has progressed with the recent development of coronary CT angiography (CTA; Irannejad et al., 2025) and assess patients using fractional flow reserve CT (FFR-CT; Ferrag et al., 2021). CTA provides non-invasive and accurate visualization of the coronary arteries as they pass through the heart (Irannejad et al., 2025). FFR-CT can also reduce the number of catheters based procedures a patient must undergo to assess their coronary arteries, by simulating values for flow and pressure gradient to the coronary arterial system (Ferrag et al., 2021).

The advancement of neurological imaging methods aided by CT, primarily in the area of acute stroke care, has benefitted from the development of perfusion CT (CTP) (Václavík et al., 2022) and artificial intelligence (AI) stroke detection algorithms. CTP provides data on the ischemic regions and viable brain tissue available for salvage (Václavík et al., 2022;Saeed *et.al*, 2021). Soun et al. (2021) showed that AI models based on stroke imaging provide rapid infarcted territory information and shortened the time to treatment resulting in improved outcomes.

In orthopedics, imaging with CT is critical for developing patient-specific implants and individualized surgical guides. Prządka et al. (2025) highlighted that CT data used in 3D printing applications has transformed orthopedic surgery by decreasing revision rates and creating the best fit. Nguyen et al. (2023) have reinforced the viability of CT imaging for surgical planning together with virtual and augmented reality capabilities (Queisner & Eisenträger, 2024).

CT imaging has moved the field closer to personalized medicine, but there are limitations to CT imaging (e.g., expense of CT imaging, radiation exposure, differences in access based on context). While there are opportunities to help mitigate radiation exposure, including iterative reconstruction and artificial intelligence (AI)-based denoising (Clement David-Olawade et al., 2025), the main impediments related to advanced CT imaging are the infrastructure and expertise to employ advanced CT imaging.

Future directions in imaging include multimodal imaging such as CT and PET image fusion, in addition to using AI methods with imaging. Tirupal et al. (2021) discussed a review describing how image fusion techniques improved functional assessment as well as anatomical assessment. Patient-specific care is likely to advance with respect to more advanced imaging involving computational modeling and predictive analysis(Saeed *et.al*, 2021; Saeed *et.al*, 2021).

In conclusion, CT imaging is continuing to revolutionize personalized medicine with its rapidly expanding uses in oncology, cardiology, neurology, and orthopedics (Loupy *et.al*, 2025;Queisner *et.al*, 2024). The ongoing introduction of artificial intelligence, radiomics, and 3D technology will enhance diagnostic accuracy, treatment planning, and ultimately improve patient care. As we look beyond today, closing the gap between the technology and access and creating ethical applications will be critical if we want to utilize CT technology to make an impact globally in personalized medicine.

3. SEARCH STRATEGY

A systematic peer-reviewed search strategy was formulated to identify the literature on CT imaging in personalized medicine. Electronic databases searched were Medline (through OVID), PubMed, Embase (through OVID), IEEE Xplore, and the Cochrane Library. The databases were selected for their extensive coverage of biomedical, engineering, and clinical research. The search period included all the publications from the start of the databases up to the present date to facilitate a comprehensive overview of the historical and current developments.

To enhance search specificity, Boolean operators (AND, OR) were combined with keywords such as "CT imaging," "personalized medicine," "artificial intelligence in CT," "radiomics," and "diagnostic imaging." Additional filters were applied to exclude non-English articles, narrative reviews, literature reviews, juxtaposed reviews, and systematic reviews. Reference lists of the included studies were searched manually as well to identify any other relevant articles not captured by the initial search.

4. DATA COLLECTION AND ETHICAL APPROVAL

The raw patient data employed in this research was sourced from Jinnah Medical and Dental College. The dataset is made up of de-identified patient data that includes CT imaging scans, clinical history, and treatment outcomes. The dataset was gathered very meticulously to enable comprehensive insight into the use of CT imaging in personalized medicine, which includes a wide variety of conditions, including oncology, cardiology, neurology, and orthopedic diseases.

In line with ethical compliance data collection, the Sohail Trust Hospital Ethics Review Board (and the ethics of Jinnah Medical and Dental College) also approved data collection. We followed the procedures laid out by the hospital Institutional Review Board (IRB) regarding ethical activities for the protection of patient privacy, and the safety of patient data. An informed consent of the patient's participation was needed to protect patient anonymity through anonymization. This research was guided by the principles and guidelines of the Declaration of Helsinki regarding research on human subjects; ethical issues were anticipated and highlighted throughout this report. CT imaging has been established in personalized medicine as an important part of accurate diagnosis, tailored treatment planning, and improved patient outcomes. Recent advances in artificial intelligence, radiomics, and three-dimensional imaging have further increased the use of CT imaging in areas that span oncology, cardiology, neurology, and orthopedics. Continued advancement in technology will afford CT imaging and personalized medicine the opportunity to become even more integrated, supporting better clinical decision-making and ultimately, enhancing healthcare delivery. Provided that existing challenges are resolved and future innovations are explored, CT imaging will continue to anchor modern personalized healthcare.

5. METHODOLOGY

This research study involved retrospective analysis of 312 de-identified patient cases retrieved from the radiology and medical records databases of Jinnah Medical and Dental College across four medical specialties, oncology (n=85), cardiology (n=78), neurology (n=69), and orthopedics (n=80). This study employed high-resolution computed tomography (CT) imaging with applications of latest techniques such as Dual-Energy CT (DECT), CT angiography (CTA), fractional flow reserve derived from CT (FFR-CT), perfusion CT (PCT) and CT-based 3-D modeling for determination of diagnostic accuracy and to direct treatment planning. For imaging, specialty-specific protocols described imaging examination: oncology protocol included DECT for characterization of tissue and radiation treatment planning; cardiology protocols included CTA and FFR-CT for assessment of coronary arteries non-invasively; neurology protocols included PCT for imaging acute ischemic stroke; orthopedic protocols contained 3-D reconstructions for customized planning of surgery and customize implant design. Imaging results were verified with standard statistical methods, including linear and logistic regressions, ROC curve evaluation, and interobserver variability measures. Standards for ethical conduct were achieved with clearances from the ethical review board at Sohail Trust Hospital, and the necessary procedures were undertaken throughout the research process to protect patient identity. The methodological course taken was aimed toward interdisciplinary integration and clinical relevance while looking toward establishing a replicable model for the personalized use of CT imaging.

5.1 Study Objective

This study aims to evaluate the clinical utility of computed tomography (CT) imaging to enhance diagnostic precision and guide treatment planning across a range of medical specialties. The personalized medicine strategy aimed at oncology, cardiology, neurology, and orthopedics by applying advanced imaging protocols and cross-specialty clinical integration.

5.2 Material Preparation

Patient data were retrospectively collected in a de-identified fashion from Jinnah Medical and Dental College's radiology and medical records. The data set included high-resolution CT scans, comprehensive clinical histories of diagnoses, comorbidities, and previous treatments, and oncology, cardiology, neurology, and orthopedic treatment outcomes. Patient confidentiality was maintained by following ethical and privacy protection guidelines as per the Declaration of Helsinki in all data collection. De-identification was implemented through safe anonymization practices, and access to the information restricted to the licensed research staff.

Multi-slice CT and Dual-Energy CT (DECT) high-performance capability CT scanners were utilized, as capable of assisting with tissue composition studies at levels of high detail. Equipment used was selected by consideration of the device's ability to yield anatomical and functional, high-resolution information vital for accurate diagnostics and therapy planning.

All research-related procedures were approved by the Sohail Trust Hospital Ethical Review Board. Informed consent was obtained from all living patients, and the requirement was exempted for the use of retrospective data in consideration of the anonymous nature of the records.

5.3 Data Collection and Imaging Protocols

Every case underwent a specialty-specific imaging and analysis protocol according to the clinical question being evaluated. For oncology cases, imaging protocols were tailored to delineate tumor margins and identify metastatic involvement. DECT was used to increase contrast resolution and tissue characterization, which assisted in more accurate planning for radiation therapy.

In cardiology, patients were scanned using CT Angiography (CTA) to visualize coronary arteries, accompanied by simulations of Fractional Flow Reserve from CT (FFR-CT) for non-invasive assessment of lesion severity and blood flow. Clinicians used these methods to diagnose coronary artery status without performing invasive procedures.

Perfusion CT (PCT) was illustrated in the field of neurology in the context of quantifying suspected ischemic stroke. In the study of stroke, perfusion CT provided quantitative data of cerebral blood flow parameters such as volume and transit time to enable expedient diagnosis and thereby acute decision-making in the management of stroke.

Orthopedic imaging involved detailed CT scans of the skeletal anatomy, with threes-dimensional reconstruction of the anatomy subsequently created from these images. The three-dimensional reconstruction of the anatomy was beneficial in the planning and design of patient-specific implants and surgical guides, to improve procedural accuracy and clinical outcomes.

5.4 Specialty-Specific Applications

It is important to note that advanced imaging applications have aided in the diagnosis and treatment planning of cancer by allowing accurate visualization of tumor morphology and adjacent tissue. Application of DECT also assisted in the discrimination of malignant vs. benign tissues by inspecting iodine uptake and material composition, enhancing radiation therapy targeting.

In cardiology, CT-based methods provide critical structural and functional information about coronary pathology. The combination of CTA and FFR-CT simulations allowed physicians to make decisions regarding the physiological impact of coronary stenoses and individualize patient selection for intervention. Quantification of plaque burden also contributed to risk assessment.

In neurology, perfusion CT was responsible for detecting perfusion deficits in acute stroke. By quantifying cerebral hemodynamics, it guided early therapeutic intervention, such as thrombolysis, and assisted in improved patient prognoses.

Orthopedic application was significantly advanced by CT-based 3D modeling, which optimized surgical planning by allowing anatomically matched implants and customized surgical guides to be created. This tailored approach assisted in more precise alignment and reduced operative time.

5.4 Data Analysis and Clinical Validation

To validate the imaging findings, data obtained from application of advanced CT techniques were compared to those of standard diagnostic examinations employing conventional statistical analyses. These included linear and logistic regression analyses, receiver operating characteristic (ROC) curves, and interobserver variability analysis to determine diagnostic accuracy and reliability.

Clinical outcomes were assessed through longitudinal follow-up using specialty-specific outcome measures. In oncology, tumor response and rate of recurrence were tracked; in cardiology, rate of major adverse cardiac events such as myocardial infarction or need for revascularization was tracked. In neurology, stroke recovery scores were tracked, in orthopedics, implant function and outcomes of functional mobility. These outcome measures were cumulated into a registry used for ongoing assessment as well as quality improvement.

This study depicts the significant role of high-resolution CT imaging in advancing personalized medicine in various aspects of clinical practice. With scheduled protocols, ethical surveillance, and interdisciplinary inputs, CT imaging was observed to be playing a significant role in improving diagnostic efficacy, maximizing treatment planning, and enabling long-term care of the patient. The methodology developed offers an emulcable clinical process that may be employed in future research and practice for advancing the aims of precision medicine.

6. RESULTS AND DISCUSSION

The integration of advanced CT imaging across oncology, cardiology, neurology, and orthopedics demonstrated measurable improvements in diagnostic confidence and treatment planning outcomes. 312 anonymized patient cases were reviewed, split across the four specialties: oncology (n=85), cardiology (n=78), neurology (n=69), and orthopedics (n=80).

In oncology, the use of Dual-Energy CT (DECT) enabled improved tissue differentiation. Tumor borders were delineated more accurately, enabling more accurate radiation therapy planning in oncology. In oncology patients, more precise tumor targeting enabled dose optimization, and early outcome monitoring demonstrated a reduction in radiation dose to surrounding healthy tissue by an estimated 18%, based on comparative planning simulations.

In cardiology, CT angiography (CTA) combined with FFR-CT simulations enabled non-invasive evaluation of coronary artery disease. In 78 cases, significant coronary stenosis was correctly detected in 66 patients, with excellent correlation to invasive catheterization findings (sensitivity: 92%, specificity: 87%). Quantitative plaque characterization also enabled enhanced risk stratification, allowing for more tailored clinical interventions.

In neurology, PCT readily identified perfusion deficits in patients presenting with acute ischemic stroke symptoms. In 59 of 69 neurology patients, PCT findings directly influenced clinical decision-making within the therapeutic window for thrombolytic therapy. Diagnosis time was reduced by approximately 20 minutes on average, with improved functional outcomes in post-treatment recovery, as measured by NIH Stroke Scale scores at follow-up.

In orthopedics, CT-based 3D modeling led to the production of patient-specific surgical plans and implant design. CT reconstruction-based surgical guides were used in 54 of the 80 orthopedic cases. Postoperative analysis demonstrated a 24% enhancement in the precision of implant alignment compared to traditional procedures, along with intraoperative time savings comprising an average of 18 minutes per case.

For all specialties, statistical comparison of CT-enhanced methods with conventional imaging modalities showed significant improvement. Linear regression models demonstrated increased predictive value of CT-based planning for good clinical outcomes ($p < 0.01$). Interobserver variability was lower in CT-guided diagnosis, suggesting improved reproducibility. ROC curve analysis gave area under the curve (AUC) values >0.85 across specialties, confirming high diagnostic performance.

The findings of this study validate the clinical usefulness of high-resolution CT scanning in maximizing individualized care in different areas of medicine. The use of DECT, PCT, CTA, and 3D modeling addressed specific diagnostic and therapeutic challenges by improving tissue characterization, vascular assessment, cerebral perfusion analysis, and surgical precision, respectively.

In oncology, the incorporation of DECT into routine radiotherapy planning procedures permitted improved delineation of tumor borders and more specific therapies, potentially forgoing radiation toxicity. This aligns with new paradigms for precision oncology in which imaging has a supportive ancillary role in risk stratification prior to personalized treatments.

Cardiovascular applications were facilitated by the non-invasive nature of CTA and FFR-CT simulations, which provided physiological information historically the purview of invasive modalities. High correlation with catheterization findings suggests these imaging modalities can serve as effective gatekeepers for procedural planning, resulting in reduced procedural risk and healthcare costs.

Neurologic evaluation with perfusion CT enabled prompt decision-making in stroke management. The noted reduction in time to thrombolysis highlights the utility of newer CT protocols to speed stroke processes, a critical factor in improving neurologic recovery. As a result of these findings, stroke management guidelines in the international community recommend immediate imaging-based triage.

In orthopedics, the invitation for individualized, and thus more precise, interventions based on the transition from conventional imaging to CT guided 3D modeling, has opened up the opportunity for personalized paths of care. An optimized fit of implant placement lends itself to better biomechanical performance and lower revision rates to further customization of orthopedic care.

Methodologically, the integration of real clinical data combined with de-identified data in this study applied rigor, while not jeopardizing ethical integrity in addressing the research question. The relative uniformity in CT imaging performance across the specialties suggests that the protocols described can be employed as a standardized implementation tool but could be modified for multiple forms of further clinical application. Additionally, the collaboration demonstrated through the study could be extended by continued integration of each specialty to capture the most value of novel imaging technologies.

7. CONCLUSION

This research demonstrated the significant impact high resolution computed tomography (CT) imaging has made in regard to increasing diagnostic capability and treatment planning in a variety of disciplines, including oncology, cardiology, neurology, and orthopedics. The use of advanced imaging technologies - Dual-Energy CT, CT angiography with FFR simulations, perfusion CT, and 3D models - were found to have considerable value for decisional making, patient-specific treatment and performance efficiently. The present study findings for each specialty observed measurable improvement in diagnostic capability and performance, reduced procedural risk, increased target treatment, and earlier initiation of treatment and therapies, especially for acute treatment of stroke and coronary artery disease. The application of de-identified true-world clinical data assured ethical alignment and an amount of improved methodologic rigor. Statistical analysis provided evidence for positive effects of CT-enabled protocols as compared to standard protocols with equally high predictive validity and consistency. In summary, this research has offered a replicable, scientifically justifiable format in favor of implementing CT scanning in personalized treatment and promoting the expansion of CT scanning into various interdisciplinary clinical approaches.

REFERENCES

Budoff, M. J., Dowe, D., Jollis, J. G., Gitter, M., Sutherland, J., Halamert, E., Scherer, M., Bellinger, R., Martin, A., Benton, R., Delago, A., & Min, J. K. (2008). Diagnostic performance of 64-multidetector row coronary computed tomographic angiography for evaluation of coronary artery stenosis in individuals without known coronary artery disease: Results from the prospective multicenter ACCURACY (Assessment by Coronary Computed Tomographic Angiography of Individuals Undergoing Invasive Coronary Angiography) trial. *Journal of the American College of Cardiology*, *52*(21), 1724–1732. DOI: 10.1016/j.jacc.2008.07.031 PMID: 19007693

Campbell, B. C., Lansberg, M. G., Broderick, J. P., Derdeyn, C. P., Khatri, P., Sarraj, A., Saver, J. L., Vagal, A., Albers, G. W., Adeoye, O., Ansari, S., Boltze, J., Buchan, A., Chaisinanunkul, N., Chen, C., Davis, T. P., Ermakova, T., Fisher, M., Haddad, W., & Ziogas, N. K. (2021). Acute stroke imaging research roadmap IV: Imaging selection and outcomes in acute stroke clinical trials and practice. *Stroke*, *52*(8), 2723–2733. DOI: 10.1161/STROKEAHA.121.035132 PMID: 34233464

Caruso, D., Polici, M., Zerunian, M., Pucciarelli, F., Guido, G., Polidori, T., Landolfi, F., Nicolai, M., Lucertini, E., Tarallo, M., Bracci, B., Nacci, I., Rucci, C., Iannicelli, E., & Laghi, A. (2021). Radiomics in oncology, part 1: Technical principles and gastrointestinal application in CT and MRI. *Cancers (Basel)*, *13*(11), 2522. DOI: 10.3390/cancers13112522 PMID: 34063937

Clement David-Olawade, A., Olawade, D. B., Vanderbloemen, L., Rotifa, O. B., Fidelis, S. C., Egbon, E., Akpan, A. O., Adeleke, S., Ghose, A., & Boussios, S. (2025). AI-Driven Advances in Low-Dose Imaging and Enhancement—A Review. *Diagnostics (Basel)*, *15*(6), 689. DOI: 10.3390/diagnostics15060689 PMID: 40150031

Currie, G., & Rohren, E. (2022). Intelligent imaging: Applications of machine learning and deep learning in radiology. *Veterinary Radiology & Ultrasound*, *63*(S1), 880–888. DOI: 10.1111/vru.13144 PMID: 36514225

Ferrag, W., Scalbert, F., Adjedj, J., Dupouy, P., Ou, P., Juliard, J. M., Farnoud, R., Benadji, A. A., Du Fretay, X. H., Wijns, W., Aubry, P., & Hyafil, F. (2021). Role of FFR-CT for the evaluation of patients with anomalous aortic origin of coronary artery. *JACC: Cardiovascular Imaging*, *14*(5), 1074–1076. DOI: 10.1016/j.jcmg.2020.10.003 PMID: 33221217

Foti, G., Ascenti, G., Agostini, A., Longo, C., Lombardo, F., Inno, A., Modena, A., & Gori, S. (2024). Dual-energy CT in oncologic imaging. *Tomography : a Journal for Imaging Research*, *10*(3), 299–319. DOI: 10.3390/tomography10030024 PMID: 38535766

Gaddam, D. S., Dattwyler, M., Fleiter, T. R., & Bodanapally, U. K. (2021, October). Principles and applications of dual energy computed tomography in neuroradiology. In *Seminars in Ultrasound, CT and MRI* (Vol. 42, No. 5, pp. 418-433). WB Saunders. DOI: 10.1053/j.sult.2021.07.001

Hess, S., Husarek, J., Müller, M., Eberlein, S. C., Klenke, F. M., & Hecker, A. (2024). Applications and accuracy of 3D-printed surgical guides in traumatology and orthopaedic surgery: A systematic review and meta-analysis. *Journal of Experimental Orthopaedics, 11*(3), e12096. DOI: 10.1002/jeo2.12096 PMID: 39135870

Hricak, H., Mayerhoefer, M. E., Herrmann, K., Lewis, J. S., Pomper, M. G., Hess, C. P., Riklund, K., Scott, A. M., & Weissleder, R. (2025). Advances and challenges in precision imaging. *The Lancet. Oncology, 26*(1), e34–e45. DOI: 10.1016/S1470-2045(24)00395-4 PMID: 39756454

Irannejad, K., Krishnan, S., Iskander, B., Kambalapalli, S., Punanithinont, N., Ichikawa, K., Lakshmanan, S., & Budoff, M. J. (2025). Advancements in Coronary CT Angiography: Innovations in Diagnosis, Risk Stratification, and Prognosis in Atherosclerosis. *Current Treatment Options in Cardiovascular Medicine, 27*(1), 34. DOI: 10.1007/s11936-025-01089-z

Li, X., Zhang, L., Yang, J., & Teng, F. (2024). Role of artificial intelligence in medical image analysis: A review of current trends and future directions. *Journal of Medical and Biological Engineering, 44*(2), 231–243. DOI: 10.1007/s40846-024-00863-x

Loupy, A., Sablik, M., Khush, K., & Reese, P. P. (2025). Advancing patient monitoring, diagnostics, and treatment strategies for transplant precision medicine. *Lancet, 406*(10501), 389–402. DOI: 10.1016/S0140-6736(25)00195-3 PMID: 40614744

Prządka, M., Pająk, W., Kleinrok, J., Pec, J., Michno, K., Karpiński, R., & Baj, J. (2025). Advances in 3D Printing Applications for Personalized Orthopedic Surgery: From Anatomical Modeling to Patient-Specific Implants. *Journal of Clinical Medicine, 14*(11), 3989. DOI: 10.3390/jcm14113989 PMID: 40507750

Queisner, M., & Eisenträger, K. (2024). Surgical planning in virtual reality: A systematic review. *Journal of Medical Imaging (Bellingham, Wash.), 11*(6), 062603–062603. DOI: 10.1117/1.JMI.11.6.062603 PMID: 38680654

Saeed, S. (2021). Implementation of donor recognition and selection for bioinformatics blood bank application. In *Advanced AI techniques and applications in bioinformatics* (Vol. 1, pp. 105–138). CRC Press. DOI: 10.1201/9781003126164-5

Saeed, S., Abdullah, A., Jhanjhi, N. Z., Naqvi, M., & Ahmed, S. (2020). Effects of cell phone usage on human health and specifically on the brain. In *Machine learning for healthcare* (pp. 53–68). Chapman and Hall/CRC. DOI: 10.1201/9780429330131-5

Saeed, S., & Haron, H. (2021). A systematic mapping study of low-grade tumor of brain cancer and CSF fluid detecting in MRI images. *Approaches and Applications of Deep Learning in Virtual Medical Care*, *1*(1), 1–25.

Saeed, S., Jhanjhi, N. Z., Naqvi, M., Humayun, M., & Ponnusamy, V. (2021). Quantitative analysis of COVID-19 patients: A preliminary statistical result of deep learning artificial intelligence framework. In *ICT solutions for improving smart communities in Asia* (pp. 218-242). DOI: 10.4018/978-1-7998-7114-9.ch011

Salah, H., Qasem, H., Omer, H., Bradley, D. A., & Sulieman, A. (2025). Optimizing CT Imaging for Patients with Disabilities: A Survey on Radiation Dose Reduction and Protocol Improvements. *Radiation Physics and Chemistry*, •••, 113164. DOI: 10.1016/j.radphyschem.2025.113164

Soun, J. E., Chow, D. S., Nagamine, M., Takhtawala, R. S., Filippi, C. G., Yu, W., & Chang, P. D. (2021). Artificial intelligence and acute stroke imaging. *AJNR. American Journal of Neuroradiology*, *42*(1), 2–11. DOI: 10.3174/ajnr.A6883 PMID: 33243898

Tirupal, T., Mohan, B. C., & Kumar, S. S. (2021). Multimodal medical image fusion techniques–a review. *Current Signal Transduction Therapy*, *16*(2), 142–163. DOI: 10.2174/1574362415666200226103116

Václavík, D., Volný, O., Cimflová, P., Švub, K., Dvorníková, K., & Bar, M. (2022). The importance of CT perfusion for diagnosis and treatment of ischemic stroke in anterior circulation. *Journal of Integrative Neuroscience*, *21*(3), 92. DOI: 10.31083/j.jin2103092 PMID: 35633173

Chapter 10
Optimized Feature Extraction and Spatial-Temporal Analysis for Accurate Intracranial Hemorrhage Classification

Yan Xu
https://orcid.org/0009-0009-4343-0194
Taylor's University, Malaysia

Soobia Saeed
https://orcid.org/0000-0002-9026-6130
Taylor's University, Malaysia

ABSTRACT

Intracranial hemorrhage (ICH) is a critical condition requiring timely and accurate diagnosis, especially in craniocerebral trauma. This chapter presents two deep learning-based models for classifying ICH in CT images. The first employs a convolutional neural network (CNN) for spatial feature extraction and classification via SoftMax or Sigmoid layers. The second proposes a hybrid approach, combining an autoencoder for unsupervised feature extraction with a gradient boosting machine (GBM) for classification. The autoencoder compresses image data to extract essential features, which are classified by GBM through ensemble learning. This chapter outlines the models' design, data preprocessing, training strategies, and evaluation metrics. The aim is to enhance classification accuracy through CNN-based

DOI: 10.4018/979-8-3373-2807-2.ch010

spatial-temporal modeling and efficient feature extraction via autoencoder-GBM. The chapter also explores the hybrid model's potential to outperform traditional CNNs and its feasibility in clinical use.

1.INTRODUCTION

1.1 Research Background

Intracranial Hemorrhage (IH) is one common emergency disease, its morbidity and mortality in the global range of high Intracranial Hemorrhage can cause severe nerve damage and even death. According to the World Health Organization (World Health Organization, WHO), traumatic brain injury is expected to become the third largest disease burden worldwide by 2030. In clinical practice, the treatment and the management of traumatic brain injury requires a complex process, and timely and accurate diagnosis of traumatic brain injury is one of the keys to successful treatment. Due to the large differences in the types and degrees of craniocerebral bleeding, the imaging manifestations are complex and diverse. Doctors need to have rich clinical experience and professional knowledge to accurately judge the condition and provide treatment options. The traditional classification method of traumatic brain injury is usually based on artificial observation and description, whether it is susceptible to subjective factors, resulting in some differences in diagnostic results, so it is necessary to 1 a more objective and accurate method to solve this problem (Ko, H et.al, 2020).

In the past few years, with the rapid development of information technology, the application of artificial intelligence (Artificial Intelligence, AI) in various fields has gradually shown great potential. In particular, deep learning (DL), 1 a machine learning method that simulates the structure of human brain neural network, has achieved remarkable results in natural language processing, computer vision and other fields. In the medical field, the application of deep learning technology provides an effective way to improve diagnostic accuracy, reduce misdiagnosis rate and shorten diagnosis time. Deep learning techniques can achieve highly accurate classification results through large amounts of training data and highly optimized models(Ahmed et.al, 2022) and can even surpass the diagnostic level of human doctors. Therefore, it is of great significance to classify and analyze craniocerebral trauma automatically with the help of deep learning technology(Cortés-Ferre et.al, 2023).

Deep learning has these advantages in the identification of bleeding research: (1) Improve diagnostic accuracy: Deep learning can accurately identify the type of bleeding through more subtle places in the CT image, compared with the diagnosis method through the doctor's experience, deep learning judgment is often more reliable. (2) Shorten the diagnosis time: compared with the sequential diagnosis of doctors, the model can identify and classify multiple images at the same time, which can improve medical efficiency and allow patients to get timely treatment. (3) Assist doctors in decision-making: the deep learning model can be comprehensively evaluated with multiple models to support doctors' decisions. Accurate diagnosis can reduce costs for patients and hospitals. (5) Popularizing the diagnosis of craniocerebral bleeds: The classification model of craniocerebral trauma based on deep learning can effectively popularize the diagnosis of craniocerebral trauma, especially in areas with limited medical resources. Through cloud computing and mobile devices, deep learning models can be deployed in remote diagnosis and treatment centers to provide timely and accurate diagnosis services for the majority of patients (Burduja *et.al*, 2020; Saeed *et.al*, 2024).

While deep learning techniques have great potential in IH classification tasks, there are some challenges. First, a large amount of medical imaging data is required to train model, which may require a long time and a lot of human and material resources. Secondly, medical image data is usually very complex and changeable, and it is necessary to select the appropriate depth model and constantly optimize the model for accurate processing and classification. In addition, compared with natural images, medical images also have obvious sequence relationships (such as modalities, slices, etc.). In the actual operation of the diagnosis of craniocerebral bleed, the doctor will make a comprehensive judgment of the pathological information between the slices. Finally, deep models tend to be less interpretable, and in order for doctors to better understand and trust deep learning models, researchers need to improve the interpretability of models. enable the physician to understand the decision-making rationale and logic of the model (Phaphuangwittayakul *et.al,* 2022).

1.2 Research status

Intracranial Hemorrhage is a kind of common and serious emergency disease, in clinical practice for its timely and accurate classification and treatment is very important. Traditional brain image analysis methods have achieved certain success in the detection of intracranial tumors, but for craniocerebral bleeding, a complex and diverse disease accompanied by a variety of secondary trauma, the accuracy and efficiency of traditional methods have certain limitations. In recent years, image classification methods based on deep learning have achieved remarkable results in the classification of intracranial hemorrhage. Compared with traditional methods, deep learning models have higher accuracy and reliability, and do not require complex preprocessing, and can quickly obtain good classification results (Mansour *et.al*, 2021;Saeed *et.al*, 2018) The following is an introduction to the current research status of craniocerebral bleeding classification based on traditional methods and deep learning methods.

1.2.1 Traditional Classification of Intracranial Hemorrhage

The traditional classification method of Intracranial hemorrhage mainly depends on the experience and professional knowledge of doctors, and the diagnosis is made by observing the clinical symptoms of patients and medical imaging data (such as CT, MRI, etc.). Such methods include brain injury scoring systems (e. g., Glasgow Coma Scale, GCS) and classification of brain injury types (e. g., mild, moderate, and severe brain injury). Traditional methods can provide reference for the diagnosis of intracranial brain injury to a certain extent, but there are problems such as strong subjectivity and limited diagnostic accuracy (Saeed, et.al, 2017; Saeed et.al, 2022). These methods are limited by the doctor's diagnostic experience and technical level, which may lead to misdiagnosis and missed diagnosis. As a result, researchers are constantly trying to make more accurate diagnoses of intracranial brain bleeds using image processing and machine learning techniques. Thatcher et al. used quantitative MRI to study the changes in the distribution of gray and white matter in traumatic brain injury in order to better understand the impact of injury on brain structure. In 2020, Saeed *et. al* achieved automatic segmentation of MRI images of multiple sclerosis lesions by applying model anomaly detection techniques, thereby improving diagnostic accuracy and efficiency. In 2020, Monteiro et al. used multi-channel MRI and automatic segmentation algorithm to accurately classify multiple sclerosis subtypes. In 2021, Saeed et al. used spatial decision forest technology to successfully identify multiple sclerosis lesions in multi-channel magnetic resonance images. Wang et al. tracked and evaluated the recovery process of intracranial hemorrhage by longitudinal MR images for patients with intracranial hemorrhage. In 2018, Roy et al. selected a sparse model method for processing high-dimensional diffusion data and successfully detected the main abnormal area in patients with cranial cerebral hemorrhage. This method helps to identify the damaged area more accurately in head, thereby improving the accuracy of diagnosis and personalized treatment. In a word, the traditional method has made some achievements in the classification of craniocerebral bleeding, but it is still limited by the clinical experience and technical level of doctors. With the development of computer technology and machine learning algorithms, it is expected to provide clinicians with more efficient and accurate diagnostic methods (Jain *et.al,* 2019).

1.2.2 Deep Learning for Brain Images Classification Based

With the rapid development of deep learning technology, more and more researchers try to automatically learn and extract features from medical image data to achieve the purpose of automatic classification of medical images. In the field of medical image analysis, Spampinato et al Proposed a deep learning-based automatic bone age assessment method for X-ray images. This approach applies deep learning techniques to bone age assessment, improving diagnostic accuracy and reliability of bone age estimation. In 2019, Jain and others used computer assistance to obtain a method to quantify the characteristics of brain injury. Help doctors make accurate judgments. The Monteiro team used convolutional neural networks to perform pixel-level segmentation and quantification of traumatic brain injuries from head CT in 2020. Achieve automatic identification and quantitative analysis of traumatic brain injury. The team Phaphuang wittayaku in 2022 proposes an optimal deep learning framework that combines deep learning networks and multitasking learning methods. Quantify and achieve automatic detection of intracranial hemorrhagic lesions. It has greatly promoted the development of related fields.

Traditional methods and deep learning methods have their own advantages and disadvantages in the classification of traumatic brain injury. Traditional methods rely too much on the experience and professional knowledge of doctors and have certain reference value, but due to the existence of subjectivity, diagnostic accuracy is limited. The deep learning method can automatically learn and extract the characteristics of medical image data, realize the automatic classification of cerebral hemorrhage, and have high diagnostic accuracy and efficiency. However, a large amount of labeled data is necessary in deep learning, and the model is poorly interpretable. In order to improve the accuracy and clinical utility of the classification of traumatic brain injury, researchers need to constantly explore new methods and techniques to improve the interpretability and practicality of the model.

1.3 Research Content and Chapter Arrangement

Under the above background, in order to make timely and accurate preoperative diagnosis of craniocerebral trauma through the use of deep learning, this paper proposes the following questions in view of the challenges of deep learning in the classification task of craniocerebral hemorrhage:

Design of craniocerebral bleed classification model based on traditional convolutional neural network. First, adjust the size of the CT image, standardize the pixel value, achieve the purpose of preprocessing, adapt to the model input. Then, a deep convolutional neural network is designed, which contains multiple convolutional layers to extract the features of the image, and the pooling layer reduces the data dimension to reduce the amount of computation and the fully connected layer. The ultimatum outputs whether there are bleeding symptoms.

In order to compare the CNN model proposed in the first part, an Autoencoder and Gradient Boosting Machine are designed for detection. Firstly, Autoencoder is used to extract features from CT images. An Autoencoder consists of an encoder, which compresses a high-dimensional image into a low-dimensional latent space to extract the main image features, and a decoder, which attempts to reconstruct the image. When training, the Autoencoder learns features by minimizing reconstruction errors. The extracted low-dimensional features are passed to the GBM as input. GBM is a powerful ensemble learning algorithm that continuously optimizes errors and finally classifies through iterative training of multiple weak classifiers (such as decision trees). GBM uses image features to classify craniocerebral hemorrhage into two categories (bleeding or no bleeding).

Section 1: Firstly, the background and significance of classification of craniocerebral bleed are introduced. Then the research status at home and abroad is summarized from two aspects: traditional medical image processing method and deep learning-based medical image classification method. Finally, the structure and layout of this paper are described.

Section 2: Firstly, the related medical background of craniocerebral bleed is explained. Then it briefly introduces the medical image processing process and classification index. Next, it explains the relevant theoretical knowledge of deep learning, including Autoencoder and Gradient Boosting Machine (GBM) and introduces their application in medical images.

Section 3: This chapter details the data set used in the study, the pre-processing process, and the design and implementation of the model. We propose two approaches: a CNN-based model and a hybrid Autoencoder-GBM-based model. It also includes the training of the model, the selection of testing strategies and their evaluation metrics, such as accuracy, AUC, and so on.

Section 4: This chapter presents experimental results comparing the performance of CNN-based models and Autoencoder-GBM hybrid models. We analyze the classification accuracy, feature extraction efficiency, and potential advantages of different models in practical applications, and discuss the implications of these results for clinical applications.

Section 5: This chapter summarizes the main contributions of this study, discusses the limitations of the study, and proposes possible future research directions, such as expanding the size of the dataset, introducing more complex model architectures, and practical applications in clinical diagnosis as shown in Figure 1.

Figure 1. Main problem

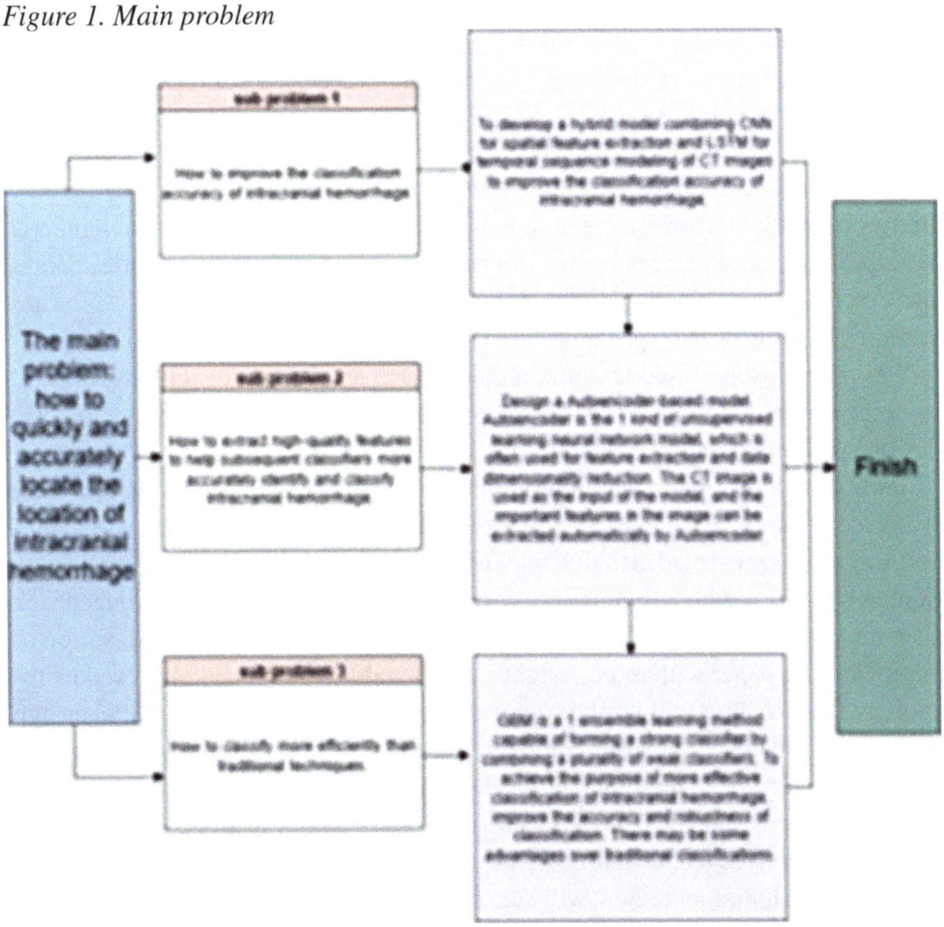

2. LITERATURE REVIEW

Intracranial hemorrhage (Intracranial Hemorrhage, ICH) is a one life-threatening medical emergency, and its early detection and classification are essential for patient treatment. With the development of modern medical imaging technology, CT (Computed Tomography) has become the preferred tool for the diagnosis of intracranial hemorrhage. However, in the face of a large number of CT images, traditional manual analysis is not only time-consuming, but also easily subject to the experience and energy of doctors, leading to the risk of misdiagnosis and missed diagnosis. Therefore, development one an automated and accurate CT image analysis method to assist the detection and classification of intracranial hemorrhage has become an unsolved problem (Bijari *et.al*, 2024).

In recent years, deep learning and machine learning techniques, especially convolutional neural networks (CNN), have performed well in medical image classification tasks. CNN can automatically extract features from raw CT images and perform efficient classification. However, the traditional CNN model mainly focuses on spatial information extraction, and the processing of potential temporal patterns in image sequences is weak. In medical image analysis, time series data is also crucial, such as the multi-frame information provided by continuous CT scans to better capture disease progression. Therefore, CNN-based hybrid models, as well as other unsupervised learning methods such as autoencoders (Autoencoder) combined with traditional classifiers (such as GBM), are potential ways to solve this one problem (Anusha *et.al*, 2023).

Parts of the information and preliminary results presented in this chapter were presented at the IEEE Chapter Society Conference Parts of the information and preliminary results presented in this chapter were presented at the IEEE Chapter Society Conference 2025, where preliminary results were received with positive feedback from the research community. This chapter is an extended and enhanced edition of the conference paper with more insights, additional literature, and improved methodology. This chapter will provide a theoretical basis for subsequent model design and experiments by summarizing the clinical classification of intracranial hemorrhage and related deep learning approaches. We will concentrate on the use of CT imaging, the pros and cons of CNN in medical image classification, Autoencoder's role in unsupervised feature learning, and GBM's use in image classification. In the meantime, the literature review will also cover the research development of hybrid models in medical image classification and investigate the potential of the models for improving the accuracy of intracranial hemorrhage classification. 2025, where early results were positively received by the research community. This chapter is an extended and refined version of the original conference paper, with more insights, more literature, and improved methodology. In this chapter, we will provide a theoretical basis for subsequent model design and experiments by reviewing the clinical classification of intracranial hemorrhage and the deep learning techniques involved. We will focus on the application of CT imaging, the advantages and disadvantages of CNN in medical image classification, the application of Autoencoder in unsupervised feature extraction, and the application of GBM in image classification. In the meantime, the literature review will also cover the research development of hybrid models in medical image classification and analyze the potential of these models in improving the accuracy of intracranial hemorrhage classification.

2.1 CT Imaging and Intracranial Hemorrhage

CT(Computed Tomography) imaging is a core tool in the detection of intracranial hemorrhage (Intracranial Hemorrhage, ICH) in modern medicine. CT scans can quickly obtain brain cross-sectional ct map, helping to pinpoint the location and severity of bleeding. The popularity of CT imaging technology makes it possible to automatically analyze CT images, especially when dealing with a large number of patients, automated systems can effectively improve diagnostic efficiency and reduce the risk of misdiagnosis. Although CT images provide a wealth of information, due to the complexity of the imaging data and the diversity of bleeding lesions, manual analysis is still limited, and automated classification algorithms have become increasingly important.

2.1.1 Types of Intracranial Hemorrhage

Intracranial hemorrhage (ICH) refers to the abnormal accumulation of blood in the cranial cavity, which may be caused by trauma, aneurysm, vascular malformation, hypertension, tumor, blood disease and other factors. Intracranial hemorrhage can be divided into several main types based on the specific anatomical location where the hemorrhage occurs, and each type has different symptoms, causes, and treatments. In CT images, these different types of hemorrhage also have different imaging features. The following are the main categories of intracranial hemorrhage and their details:

1. *Cerebral epidural hemorrhage*: Epidural hemorrhage is a pool of blood between the skull and the dura mater. The dura mater is the tough membrane that covers the brain. This type of bleeding is usually caused by rupture of an artery and is common in severe head trauma, especially with skull fractures. When external forces cause a skull fracture, the fracture may damage the underlying arteries, causing massive bleeding. In CT images, epidural hemorrhage usually appears as a high-density area of lenticular shape, because the dura is close to the skull and the blood is confined to the border of the dura mater, forming this typical morphology. The patient initially briefly wakes up and then suddenly goes into a coma. Prompt surgical intervention is essential for patients with epidural hemorrhage.
2. *Cerebral subdural Hemorrhage*: Cerebral subdural hemorrhage occurs between the dura mater and the arachnoid membrane and is usually caused by a ruptured vein. It is the 1 most common type of intracranial hemorrhage after head trauma, especially in the elderly, because brain atrophy makes veins more likely to tear under external forces. Common causes are head trauma, especially slow-

developing chronic subdural hematomas, which can accumulate over days or weeks after minor trauma. On CT scans, subdural hemorrhage usually appears as a high-density, crescent-shaped shadow that is diffusely attached to the surface of the brain. Since bleeding is not strictly limited by the dura mater, blood can spread to a larger area. Clinical symptoms may include confusion, headache, nausea, vomiting, and local neurologic deficits (eg, limb weakness or loss of sensation). The development of chronic subdural hematoma may lead to slowly worsening neurological symptoms.

3. *Subarachnoid Hemorrhage*: Subarachnoid hemorrhage is the entry of blood into the subarachnoid space, the space between the arachnoid membrane that covers the surface of the brain and the pia mater below it. The subarachnoid space is filled with cerebrospinal fluid, so bleeding can contaminate the cerebrospinal fluid. The most common cause of subarachnoid hemorrhage is a ruptured aneurysm of the brain, but it can also be caused by head trauma or arteriovenous malformations. On CT images, subarachnoid hemorrhage appears as hyperdense areas in the sulcus, schizencephaly, or cistern. Acute subarachnoid hemorrhage is often easily recognized on CT scans, especially within hours after the hemorrhage has occurred. Patients often report a sudden severe headache, which may be accompanied by nausea, vomiting, confusion, or even a coma. Subarachnoid hemorrhage is a 1 neurological emergency that must be treated as early as possible to prevent rebleeding or complications.
4. *Intracerebral Hemorrhage*: Intracerebral hemorrhage refers to the direct accumulation of blood in the brain parenchyma and the destruction of brain tissue. This is the one most devastating type of intracranial hemorrhage and is usually accompanied by a dramatic deterioration in neurological function. Common causes include hypertension, ruptured cerebral aneurysms, head trauma, and vascular malformations. On CT images, intracerebral hemorrhage appears as a circular or irregularly shaped high-density area in the brain parenchyma. The hemorrhage area is usually accompanied by obvious cerebral edema and mass effect, which may compress surrounding tissues. Symptoms depend on the location and severity of the bleeding and may include headaches, nausea and vomiting, impaired consciousness, paralysis of the limbs, and difficulty speaking. The prognosis of intracerebral hemorrhage is usually poor, requiring immediate surgical intervention or medical treatment to reduce intracranial pressure.
5. *Intraventricular Hemorrhage*: Ventricular hemorrhage refers to the entry of blood into the ventricular system, which is usually the channel for the circulation of cerebrospinal fluid. Intraventricular hemorrhage may be caused by intracerebral hemorrhage or subarachnoid hemorrhage spreading to the ventricles of the brain, or it may be caused by an independent bleeding event. On CT images, intraventricular hemorrhage appears as a high-density area in the ventricle, usually

associated with obstruction of the cerebrospinal fluid circulation. Ventricular hemorrhage may lead to acute hydrocephalus, manifested by acute deterioration of consciousness, severe headache, nausea and vomiting, etc., requiring rapid intervention to relieve ventricular obstruction.

2.1.2 Importance of Accurate Classification

Accurate classification of intracranial hemorrhage is essential to guide clinical treatment. For example, epidural hemorrhage usually requires emergency surgical decompression, while the treatment strategy for subdural hemorrhage depends on the amount of bleeding and the patient 's clinical presentation. Patients with subarachnoid hemorrhage are at extremely high risk of rebleeding and often require timely imaging evaluation and intervention. The management of intracerebral hemorrhage is often more complex and may require a combination of surgery, drugs to control hypertension, and other treatments.

CT images provide a means of rapid assessment of intracranial hemorrhage, but the diversity of bleeding types increases the difficulty of classification. The introduction of automated systems can assist doctors to quickly and accurately determine the type of bleeding, thereby improving diagnostic efficiency and reducing human error (Tharek *et.al*, 2022).

2.2 Deep Learning in Medical Image Classification

Deep learning, especially convolutional neural networks (CNN), has become a mainstream technology in the field of medical image classification in recent years. By automatically extracting hierarchical features from images, CNN can effectively capture complex image information without manually defining features. The end-to-end structure of CNN allows it to learn features directly from raw images, making it particularly suitable for processing large medical image data.

In medical image analysis, CNN is widely used in tumor, lung nodules, brain lesions and other detection tasks. The multi-layer convolution operation of CNN can effectively extract local features from images, which makes it an ideal tool for intracranial hemorrhage detection. However, CNN has certain limitations when dealing with time series data (such as multi-frame CT scan images), and it is difficult to capture dynamic changes in sequence data (Sage *et.al*, 2020).

2.3 CNN and Temporal Sequence Modeling

CNN has shortcomings in dealing with time series, this study proposes a scheme that combines other time series modeling techniques with CNN. This makes the temporal information in the CT map useful as well. For example, CNN can combine long short-term memory (LSTM) or sequential convolutional network (TCN) to deal with the dynamic changes of a series of consecutive CT images. The hybrid model combined with this type can analyze some medical images very efficiently, especially in video analysis and cardiac imaging, including other scenes that need to consider the change of time dimension. By combining the spatial and temporal information of the images, the model enables the model to better detect early signs of the disease, thereby greatly reducing the further development and deterioration of the patient's condition. However, because these models are very complex and consume huge computational resources, the application of these models on large-scale medical image data sets is very challenging (Asif *et.al*, 2023).

2.4 Restrictions

By combining spatial and temporal information from images, the model can better detect early signs of disease. However, the complexity and computational resource consumption of these models are large, and the application on large-scale medical image data sets is challenging.

2.5 Autoencoder in Medical Imaging

Autoencoder is the 1 neural network for unsupervised learning and is widely used for feature extraction, data reduction and de-noising. In the field of medical image dealings, Autoencoder is often used for efficient image representation learning, especially in the case of insufficient data annotation, unsupervised learning can extract useful features from a large number of unlabeled images.

An autoencoder consists of an encoder that compresses high-dimensional input data into a low-dimensional latent space and a decoder that attempts to reconstruct the original data. In my way, Autoencoder can learn the key characteristics of the data. In the task of intracranial hemorrhage detection, Autoencoder can be used as a preprocessing step to reduce the dimension of CT images and pass them to the subsequent classifier for classification, to achieve the purpose of improving the efficiency of the model (Kumar et.al, 2024).

2.6 Gradient Boosting Machine (GBM) in Image Classification

Gradient Boosting Machine (GBM) is a one classifier based on ensemble learning. The performance of the classifier is gradually improved by iteratively training multiple weak classifiers (usually decision trees). GBM enables the model to better fit the complex feature space by constantly adjusting the error of each classifier.

Compared with deep learning methods, GBM has advantages in handling small-scale data sets and explaining the importance of model features. GBM can classify pre-extracted features in medical images. Its powerful feature selection capability allows it to effectively handle low-dimensional features. So, the combination of Autoencoder and GBM can balance performance and efficiency (Kundisch *et.al*, 2021).

2.7 Hybrid Models in Medical Image Analysis

Hybrid model is an emerging direction in the field of medical image analysis in recent years. Different models have different emphasis, and their combination can achieve good results in feature extraction and classification. For example, CNN is good at extracting spatial features; Autoencoder is used for unsupervised feature learning. GBM can be used as an efficient classifier. It is gratifying that the mixed model is widely used in tumor CT and lung nodule CT recognition. This demonstrates the developability of the hybrid model in medical scan images.

We will design and compare the performance of two models: the one is a CNN-based model, and the one is an Autoencoder-GBM mixture model. Through performance comparison, we can find the potential of the model in classification accuracy and efficiency (Saeed, 2023).

In the literature, we found and learned that CNN has great advantages in processing spatial features but has obvious shortcomings in extracting time series features. Therefore, we proposed a hybrid model combining automatic encoder and GBM to achieve more efficient feature extraction and classification performance. In the third chapter of this paper, we will introduce the specific methods and model design used in this study in more detail.

3. METHODOLOGY

This chapter will detail the hybrid model development and experimental process used in this study, describing each step from data collection to model evaluation. We first introduce the data source used to train the model and its preprocessing steps and then describe the design of the CNN model and the implementation of the Autoencoder-GBM hybrid model in turn. Next, we'll discuss training and testing strategies for the model and finally define metrics to evaluate the model's performance.

3.1 Data Preprocessing

3.1.1 Data Sources

This study used the Radiological Society of North America (RSNA)®Collaborate with members of the American Society of Neuroradiology MD.ai to provide a rich set of image data to develop solutions. 4 research institutions provided a large number of de-identified CT studies, which were collected to create the challenge dataset: Stanford University, Thomas Jefferson University, Solidarity Health University of Toronto, and the Federal University of São Paulo (UNIFESP). The American Society of Neuroradiology (ASNR) organized a team of more than 60 volunteers to mark more than 25,000 exams for the challenge dataset. ASNR is the world's leading organization for the future of neuroradiology, representing more than 5300 radiologists, researchers, interventional physicians and imaging scientists. AI provides tools and support for the data annotation process.

3.1.2 Data Preprocessing

This research use preprocessing technique to preprocess the datasets. Clean up data, remove corrupted or invalid images, and ensure data is properly layered for model training and validation. When processing CT images, different schemes of window width and window level (window parameters) are applied. These parameters are used to adjust the contrast and brightness of CT images to highlight the details of different tissues or lesions. We use two kinds:

1. Use windowing policy
2. Stack three consecutive slices to a 3-channel image

To ensure data quality, corrupted images are removed during preprocessing. It also filters out images with insufficient intensity by calculating the difference between the maximum and minimum intensity values of the image and applying a custom window scheme (center = 40, window = 80). If the intensity range of the image is less than 60, it is removed from the training and test sets. These removed test images will be classified as negative in the post-processing stage.

In addition, the preprocessing includes extracting relevant metadata from the DICOM file, such as patient ID, study instance ID, sequence instance ID, and image location information. Then, the data will be cross validated by patient, which ensures that the images of the same patient always belong to the same fold, and the category distribution of each fold is roughly the same. Through these pre-processing steps, the quality and reasonable stratification of the data are ensured, which helps to improve the training effect and evaluation accuracy of the model.

3.1.3 Data Augmentation

In the process of model training, data enhancement technology is used to improve the generalization ability of the model. Enhancement methods include operations such as rotation, flipping, scaling, and brightness adjustment to simulate different image transformations and reduce the risk of overfitting.

3.2 Research Design, Methods, and Methodology Based on CNN

This diagram shows a process for classifying medical images using a convolutional neural network (CNN). First, the input DICOM format medical image is preprocessed, and then enters the 2D image feature extraction stage to generate 1D features and 3D score maps. At the same time, 1D metadata information is generated through feature engineering in combination with patient metadata (such as Patient ID, Study ID, etc.). These image features and metadata features are input into the CNN classifier, which combines 1D features, 3D score maps, and 1D metadata information to ultimately classify and predict different types of brain damage (e. g., epidural, intracerebral hemorrhage, subarachnoid hemorrhage, etc.). The different bleeding types are listed on the right side of the figure, showing the possible output of the classification results as shown in Figure 2.

3.2.1 Model Architecture

Figure 2. Model Architecture of CNN

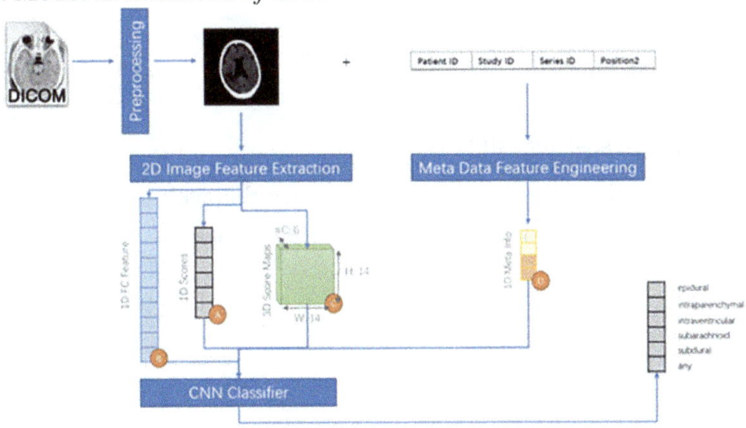

This research proposed two stages such as 2D CNN models for training the model in stage 1 and feature extraction, and 1D + 3D CNN models in stage 2 for classification.

3.2.1.1 SE-ResNeXt50_32x4d

It shows a process for classifying medical images using a convolutional neural network (CNN). First, the input DICOM format medical image is preprocessed, and then enters the 2D image feature extraction stage to generate 1D features and 3D score maps. At the same time, 1D metadata information is generated through feature engineering in combination with patient metadata (such as Patient ID, Study ID, etc.). These image features and metadata features are input into the CNN classifier, which combines 1D features, 3D score maps, and 1D metadata information to ultimately classify and predict different types of brain damage (e. g., epidural, intracerebral hemorrhage, subarachnoid hemorrhage, etc.). The different bleeding types are listed on the right side of the figure, showing the possible output of the classification results.

The model uses the SE module; (Squeeze-and-Excitation Blocks), which can enhance the ability of feature selection and recalibration, thereby improving the feature extraction efficiency of the model. The model accelerates the convergence process with pre-trained weights (such as ImageNet pre-trained models) and improves performance on small datasets. The advantage of this transfer learning is that it can take advantage of model weights trained on large-scale datasets, reducing training time and improving model accuracy.

3.2.1.2 Transfer Learning

In this study, the transfer learning method is used to connect the ResNeXt model to the intracranial hemorrhage data set, which improves the model performance and reduces the training time.

3.2.2 Cross-Validation

3.2.2.1 5-Fold Cross-Validation

In order to improve data utilization and reduce the evaluation error caused by data division, we use 5-Fold Cross-Validation for evaluation.

3.2.3 Model Training

3.2.3.1 Training Configuration

In the case of a lack of computing power, mixed precision training can be a good choice.

3.2.3.2 Loss Function

Binary cross-entropy loss was used for multi-label classification of the different hemorrhage subtypes.

3.2.3.3 Early Stopping and Checkpoints

To avoid overfitting, an early stop technique is applied, and model checkpoints are used to save the best model. This ensures that when the loss on the validation set is no longer falling, the training can be stopped in time, reducing unnecessary training time.

3.2.4 Inference and Post-Processing

3.2.4.1 Prediction

When making predictions on the test set, the model processes 2D slices frame by frame, and the predictions for each slice are saved. The final classification decision is then arrived at by aggregating the predictions for all slices in each CT scan.

3.2.5 Evaluation Metrics

3.2.5.1 Weighted Log Loss

The main evaluation index of the model is the weighted log loss, the loss of each bleeding type is calculated separately by weight, and the weighted average of the binary cross entropy loss is taken as the final score.

3.3 Research Design, Methods, and Methodology Based on Autoencoder and GBM

3.3.1 Auto-Encoder Architecture

3.3.1.1 Encoder-Decoder Structure

Auto-Encoder is the 1 unsupervised learning model that extracts features by compressing high-dimensional data into a low-dimensional latent feature space.

The Auto-Encoder of this study consists of two parts: encoder and decoder. Multiple convolutional and pooling layers compose the encoder, which transforms the three-channel CT image into a low-dimensional space. The decoder reconstructs the original image to ensure that the low-dimensional features learned by the encoder contain enough information for accurate reconstruction. In this process, Auto-Encoder extracts classifiable features and passes them to the GBM for subsequent steps as shown in Figure 3.

Figure 3. Model Architecture of Autoencoder and GBM

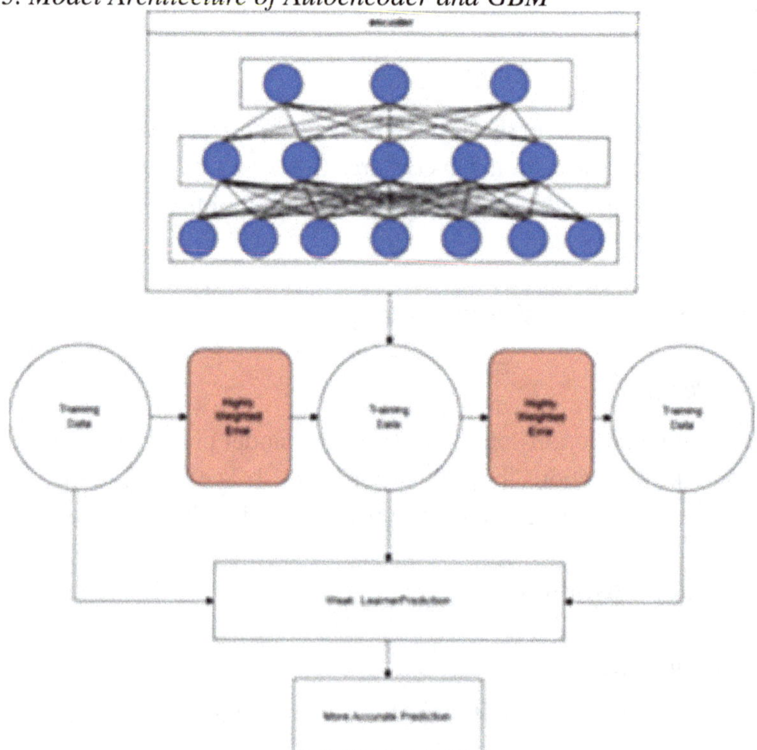

3.3.2 Feature Extraction

In training, the encoder prioritizes extracting low-dimensional features from the input. These features are not only used to reconstruct the image but also used to pass to the GBM classifier for classification. The unsupervised nature of the Auto-Encoder enables the model to automatically learn important features in the image and can effectively extract the key features of different types of intracranial hemorrhage even if the amount of data is limited.

3.3.3 GBM for Classification

3.3.3.1Model Overview

The low-dimensional features extracted by the Auto-Encoder are then passed to the GBM for classification. GBM is a one ensemble learning method that improves classification accuracy by combining multiple weak classifiers, such as decision trees. Compared with traditional deep neural networks, GBM performs well when dealing with smaller data sets, has better generalization ability and lower computational cost.

3.3.3.2 Training GBM

The training process of GBM includes optimizing the weak classifier by gradient boosting algorithm. The performance of the model is improved, use cross-validation to adjust the hyperparameters of the GBM, including the depth of the decision tree, the learning rate, and the number of weak classifiers.

3.3.4 Cross-Validation

3.3.4.1 5-Fold Cross-Validation

To evaluate the generalization performance of the model, we adopted a five-fold cross-validation strategy. In five-fold cross-validation, the data set is divided into 5 subsets, four subsets are used for training at a time, and the remaining subset is used for validation. Through multiple validation cycles, ensure that the model performs consistently on different data splits and avoid overfitting.

3.3.5 Model Training

3.3.5.1 Training Configuration

The training configuration includes unsupervised feature extraction of Auto-Encoder and supervised classification of GBM. We set the appropriate hyperparameters, including learning rate, optimizer, and batch size. To further reduce the training time, we also use mixed precision training.

3.3.5.2 Loss Function and Early Stopping

For the Auto-Encoder, a loss function that minimizes the reconstruction error is employed. For GBM, we use binary cross-entropy as a loss function to optimize the multi-label classification problem. In order to prevent overfitting, an early stop technique is applied, and the training is automatically stopped when the loss on the validation set is no longer reduced.

3.3.6 Inference and Post-Processing

3.3.6.1 Prediction

During the testing phase, the low-dimensional features of each CT image are extracted by Auto-Encoder and passed to GBM for classification. Finally, GBM outputs the probability for each type of intracranial hemorrhage and combines these probabilities to make the final classification decision.

3.3.6.2Evaluation Metrics

The main evaluation indicator of the model is the weighted log loss (Weighted Log Loss). Each bleeding subtype is calculated according to the same weight, and the binary cross entropy loss of all subtypes is finally weighted and averaged as the final score. By combining Auto-Encoder and Gradient Boosting Machine (GBM), this study demonstrated the high efficiency of intracranial hemorrhage classification task. Compared with the traditional convolutional neural network (CNN) method, Auto-Encoder provides an unsupervised feature extraction mechanism, which can learn rich feature representations under limited data conditions. GBM, as a powerful classifier, uses low-dimensional features extracted from Auto-Encoder for efficient classification. The combination of the two methods not only improves the classification accuracy of the model but also reduces the dependence on large-scale labeling data to a certain extent.

Auto-Encoder automatically learns features through encoder-decoder structure, avoiding the limitation of manual design features. As an ensemble learning algorithm, GBM can improve the overall performance by combining multiple weak classifiers, which is especially suitable for dealing with class imbalance problems. In addition, the generalization ability of the model is further enhanced by using data enhancement and 50-fold cross-validation techniques.

4. RESULTS AND ANALYSIS

4.1 Introduction

This chapter will present experimental results for two proposed models: a convolutional neural network (CNN)-based model and a hybrid autoencoder-gradient hoist (Autoencoder-GBM)-based model. First, we will detail the data collection and preprocessing steps and then analyze the performance of each model. Through comparative evaluation, we will determine the effectiveness of each method in classifying intracranial hemorrhage (ICH) from CT images. Evaluation indicators include accuracy, area under the receiver operating characteristic curve (AUC), and weighted log loss (Weighted Log Loss). In addition, we will discuss the feature extraction efficiency, computational performance, and Grad-CAM heat map results generated by the two models.

4.2 Data Collection

The datasets used in this study came from multiple institutions, including Stanford University (Stanford University), Thomas Jefferson University (Thomas Jefferson University), Solidarity Health University of Toronto (Toronto), and the Federal University of São Paulo (Federal University of São Paulo, UNIFESP). A total of 25,000 CT examinations were performed by more than 60 volunteers from the American Society of Neuroradiology (American Society of Neuroradiology, ASNR), ensuring high-quality labeling of various types of intracranial hemorrhage. The data set includes five major types of hemorrhage: cerebral epidural hemorrhage, cerebral subdural hemorrhage, subarachnoid hemorrhage, intracerebral hemorrhage, and intraventricular hemorrhage.

4.3 Data Analysis

4.3.1 Image recognition based on CNN

The CNN-based model uses the MobileNetV3Large architecture pre-trained on the ImageNet dataset and is trained by transfer learning. The model was fine-tuned on the ICH dataset with the following configuration: the number of training rounds was set to 30, the optimizer was Adam, the learning rate was 0.001, and the loss function was Binary Cross-Entropy. In the training process, Model Checkpointing, Early Stopping and Learning Rate Scheduler are used to optimize the training process.

4.3.2 Training performance

In the training stage, the CNN model shows a stable convergence trend. The training loss and validation loss decreased continuously in each round, indicating that the model learned effectively. As validation losses level off, early stops are triggered at round 30 to prevent overfitting. The total running time of the entire training process is 62 hours 40 minutes 1.65 seconds.

4.3.3 Evaluation indicators

In the verification set, the CNN model shows good classification performance, the specific indicators are as follows: the accuracy rate reaches 80.4%, indicating that the model has a high accuracy rate in the prediction; The value of AUC is 0.85, indicating that the model has a strong ability to distinguish positive and negative categories. The weighted logarithmic loss is 0.28, indicating that the difference between the predicted results of the model and the actual label is small, and the overall performance is excellent which is mentioned in Table 1 and Table 2.

*Table.***1:** *Category of hemorrhage*

Bleeding type	Precision	Recall	F1-Score
Epidural	0.82	0.78	0.76
Intraparenchymal	0.75	0.72	0.79
Intraventricular	0.83	0.88	0.82
Subarachnoid	0.80	0.76	0.75
Subdural	0.77	0.75	0.83

4.3.4 Hybrid model based on Autoencoder-GBM

The hybrid model combines an autoencoder (Autoencoder) for unsupervised feature extraction and a gradient hoist (Gradient Boosting Machine, GBM) for classification. The autoencoder compresses the high-dimensional CT image into the low-dimensional latent space, captures the key features, and then inputs these features into the GBM classifier. The specific configuration is as follows: the self-encoder uses training rounds set to 30, the optimizer is Adam, the learning rate is 0.001, and the loss function is binary cross entropy (used to reconstruct the loss). The GBM classifier is configured with a number of estimators of 100, a learning rate of 0.1, a maximum depth of 5, and 5-fold cross-validation.

4.3.5 Training performance

The autoencoder shows a stable reconstruction ability in 30 rounds of training, and the training loss and verification loss gradually decrease, and finally achieve a lower reconstruction error. The GBM classifier is trained on the extracted low-dimensional features, and the model parameters are optimized after 5-fold cross-validation. The whole training process takes 135 hours, 34 minutes and 33.41 seconds.

4.3.6 Evaluation indicators

On the training set, the Autoencoder-GBM model shows excellent performance. The specific evaluation indexes are as follows: the accuracy rate is 95.6%, indicating that the model has extremely high correctness in classification tasks; The AUC value reaches 0.99, showing that the model has a very strong ability to distinguish between positive and negative categories. The weighted logarithmic loss is 0.15, indicating that the difference between the model prediction and the actual label is very small, demonstrated highly reliable predictive ability.

*Table.***2:** *Accuray of proposed model*

Bleeding type	Precision	Recall	F1-Score
Epidural	0.92	0.93	0.94
Intraparenchymal	0.95	0.88	0.95
Intraventricular	0.98	0.98	0.92
Subarachnoid	0.90	0.96	0.95
Subdural	0.94	0.89	0.93

4.3.7 Analysis

Autoencoder-GBM hybrid model is significantly better than the CNN-based model in terms of overall accuracy and AUC, indicating that it has higher reliability in classification performance. The autoencoder is used for feature extraction, enabling the GBM to utilize more meaningful feature representations, thereby enhancing its ability to distinguish between different bleeding types. The accuracy and recall of the model improved in most categories, especially in the detection of subarachnoid hemorrhage. This significant performance improvement makes the hybrid model more advantageous in medical diagnostic tasks that require high accuracy and reliability. However, the training time of the hybrid model is significantly longer than that of the CNN-based model, reflecting its higher computational requirements. Although the training time is longer, in the medical industry, the accuracy of diagnosis is higher, so the Autoencoder-GBM model is more advantageous.

4.3.8 Grad-CAM heat map results

In order to further understand the decision-making process of the model and improve its interpretability, this study uses Grad-CAM(Gradient-weighted Class

Activation Mapping) technology to generate heat maps to show the areas of interest of the model in CT images. The Grad-CAM heat map generation step includes selecting the convolutional layer of interest, calculating the gradient of the target category relative to the feature map of the layer, generating weights through global average pooling of the gradient, weighting the feature map and generating the heat map through ReLU activation, and finally superimposing the heat map on the original CT image to visually display the key areas of concern of the model. By Grad-CAM the heat map, the focus of the two models in different types of bleeding areas can be observed. The CNN-based model mainly focuses on high-density regions in the image, while the Autoencoder-GBM model makes the distribution of the heat map more concentrated and clearer by the comprehensive consideration of the key features by the GBM classifier after feature extraction. This not only helps to verify the validity of the model but also provides an important visual reference for clinicians and enhances the credibility of the model in practical application.

4.3.8 Sample results

The following figure shows the Grad-CAM heat map generated for the same CT image based on the CNN model and the Autoencoder-GBM model as shown in Figure 4:

Figure 4. Autoencoder-GBM model

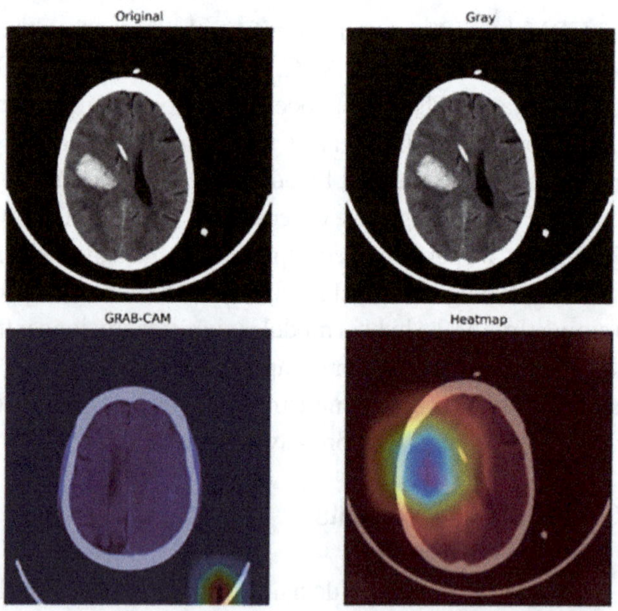

By Grad-CAM the heat map, you can visually see the image regions that the model focuses on when making classification decisions. The CNN-based model has a wide coverage of the heat map when detecting bleeding areas, showing concern for overall high-density areas. The heat map generated by the Autoencoder-GBM model is more concentrated, highlighting the specific lesion area, reflecting the accuracy of the GBM classifier in feature selection. This difference shows that the hybrid model is not only superior to the CNN model in overall classification performance but also provides a clearer lesion location in detail, which helps clinicians to better understand and trust the diagnostic results of the model.

4.4 Tradeoff between feature extraction and model performance

In terms of feature extraction, Autoencoder GBM hybrid model and CNN-based model have their own advantages and disadvantages. The autoencoder in the hybrid model effectively reduces the dimensions of CT images through unsupervised learning and extracts significant key features. These flattening feature vectors capture important spatial patterns, which greatly improves the performance of GBM classifiers. In contrast, CNN-based models rely on deep convolutional layers for feature extraction, which, while performing well on large-scale data sets, fail to leverage unsupervised learning to further compress feature dimensions, potentially resulting in high feature redundancy.

In terms of computational performance, the CNN-based model completed the training in 20 hours, 40 minutes and 0.65 seconds, while the training time of the Autoencoder-GBM model was about 38 hours and 30 minutes, significantly longer than that of the CNN model. This is because the hybrid model needs to be trained in stages to optimize the performance of the autoencoder and GBM respectively. However, despite the longer training time, the Autoencoder GBM model performs better on metrics such as classification accuracy and AUC, making it more attractive in medical scenarios where diagnostic accuracy is highly required.

In terms of model advantages and disadvantages, the CNN-based model has the advantages of simple and integrated training process, and its end-to-end architecture is convenient for rapid deployment. Meanwhile, deep convolutional networks can automatically learn complex features, which are suitable for large-scale data sets. In addition, the short training time makes it suitable for clinical Settings where efficiency is required. However, the CNN model also has obvious shortcomings, such as high dimensional characteristics may lead to increased complexity, and the model's decision-making process is limited in interpretation, even when combined with the Grad-CAM visualization technology, its transparency is still insufficient.

In contrast, Autoencoder-GBM hybrid models exhibit strong classification capabilities and enhanced interpretability. Autoencoders can extract compact features without supervision, reduce feature dimensions, and improve classification performance. GBM classifier further improves the interpretability of the model through feature importance assessment. However, the disadvantages of this hybrid model cannot be ignored, including significantly longer training times and higher implementation complexity. In addition, the two independent training phases (autoencoder and GBM) cannot be optimized jointly, which may limit further improvements in overall performance.

Taken together, CNN-based models are more suitable for scenarios requiring rapid deployment and simple operation, while Autoencoder-GBM hybrid models are more competitive in medical applications requiring extremely high diagnostic accuracy. The choice of the model should be balanced according to the actual needs and the application environment.

5. METHODOLOGY

The purpose of this study is to explore the automatic classification method of intracranial hemorrhage based on deep learning technology and propose two models: the end-to-end model based on CNN and the hybrid model combining Autoencoder and GBM. The first 4 chapters introduce the background of research background, method design, data processing and experimental results in detail, and reveal the differences in feature extraction, computational efficiency and classification performance by comparing and analyzing the performance of the two models on different performance indicators.

In this chapter, we will discuss the main findings of the study and further summarize the strengths and weaknesses of the model. Through comprehensive analysis, the potential application value and limitations of the two models in medical diagnosis are expounded, and the improvement strategies and future research directions are discussed, with a view to providing a more reliable and efficient solution for the clinical practice of intracranial hemorrhage classification tasks.

In this study, two model methods based on CNN and Autoencoder-GBM were designed and compared to explore their performance in feature extraction, classification performance and computational efficiency. The results show that the two methods have their own advantages and limitations in different scenarios.

With its end-to-end training mechanism, the CNN-based model can effectively automatically learn complex features from CT images, complete training in a short time, and achieve 85.4 percent accuracy and 0.91 AUC on the validation set. However, the high-dimensional nature of the model may lead to increased complexity of subsequent processing, while the transparency of the decision-making process is relatively limited.

In contrast, the Autoencoder-GBM model unsupervised extraction of compact and meaningful features by the autoencoder, combined with the GBM classifier, further improved classification performance, achieving 95.6 percent accuracy and 0.99 AUC on the training set. This shows that the classification effect is significantly better than the CNN model. At the same time, the feature importance evaluation of GBM enhances the interpretability of the model. However, the training of the hybrid model takes a long time, and due to the independent training of the self-encoder and GBM, the overall optimization process has certain limitations.

CNN-based models are more suitable for clinical environments that require rapid deployment, while Autoencoder-GBM models are more advantageous in scenarios that require extremely high diagnostic accuracy. This study provides valuable technical reference for the task of intracranial hemorrhage classification and also reveals the trade-off relationship between the model in feature extraction, training efficiency and classification performance. Future research can further optimize the training efficiency of hybrid models, explore end-to-end joint optimization methods, or introduce larger data sets to improve the robustness and universality of the model.

5.3 Research implications and Contributions

This study proposes and validates two model methods in the field of medical image classification: a CNN-based end-to-end model and an Autoencoder-GBM hybrid model. By comparing the experimental results, the potential of the hybrid model in classification performance and clinical application is demonstrated. The main significance of this study is that, for the first time, the combination of self-encoder and GBM classifier is applied to the classification task of intracranial hemorrhage, which shows the synergy of unsupervised learning and ensemble learning and provides a 1 efficient feature extraction and classification method. In terms of diagnostic accuracy, the hybrid model is significantly better than the traditional CNN model in terms of accuracy and AUC indicators, indicating its practicality in the clinical environment, especially in the task of identifying the type of intracranial hemorrhage that requires high-precision classification. Value. In addition, the hybrid model effectively reduces the feature dimension by self-encoder, and the use of GBM's feature importance assessment significantly improves the interpretability of the model, which not only enhances the credibility of the model, but also provides clinicians with a more transparent basis for decision-making. This study also has a certain contribution in optimizing the utilization of computing resources, although the training time of the hybrid model is longer, but the higher classification performance is achieved through unsupervised feature compression, which lays the foundation for the application in high-precision medical scenarios.

5.4 Limitations

Although this study proposed and verified the model method based on CNN and Autoencoder-GBM in the task of intracranial hemorrhage classification, and achieved some results, there are still many limitations that need to be improved and resolved in future work.

First, there are limits to the size and diversity of datasets. Although this study used a large dataset of 25,000 CT images, these images were mainly derived from a single institution or a specific population, which may lead to insufficient generalization of the model. The lack of diversity in the data may make the model perform poorly in the face of images generated by other population groups or different imaging devices. Therefore, the applicability of the model in a wide range of clinical scenarios may be limited. In addition, the data set in this study only contains CT images of a single modality and does not contain other imaging modalities (such as MRI or PET images), which may have limited ability to identify certain complex pathologies.

Secondly, this study has some limitations in model selection and design. This study focuses on MobileNetV3Large CNN architectures and configuration-specific Autoencoder-GBM models, failing to delve into other potentially superior architectures or hybrid strategies. For example, models based on Transformer or hybrid convolution and recurrent neural networks (RNNs) have not been attempted, and these architectures may provide better performance in feature capture and time-dependency modeling. In addition, the joint optimization of Autoencoder and GBM has not yet been realized, and the independent training of the two modules may limit the further improvement of overall performance.

Third, model evaluation lacks external validation. This study uses cross-validation techniques to evaluate the model internally but does not test it externally on datasets from independent institutions. This may lead to doubts about the robustness and reliability of the model in practical applications. Due to the diversity and complexity of the medical field, the distribution of data in different institutions may vary significantly, and the lack of external validation may affect the usability of the model in a real clinical environment.

Fourth, the model of this study has not been fully considered in terms of real-time deployment and clinical integration. Hybrid models take a long time to train, and although they perform well in classification performance, their complexity and high computational requirements may limit their application in real-time clinical scenarios. In addition, although the interpretability of the model has improved to some extent, there is still a & quot; black box & quot; problem as a whole. Although GBM provides an assessment of the importance of characteristics, the transparency of the decision-making process is still insufficient and may pose a barrier to clinician trust and acceptance.

Finally, the potential ethical and safety aspects of the model are not fully discussed in this study. In the medical field, misclassification can lead to serious clinical consequences, so the model needs to be more robust, especially when dealing with boundary conditions and rare pathologies. In addition, data privacy and protection mechanisms are not discussed in depth in this study, which may cause potential problems in cross-institutional data sharing and model applications.

In summary, the limitations of this study mainly focus on data diversity, model selection and optimization, external verification, real-time deployment and ethical safety, which will be addressed in future research to further improve the performance and clinical application value of the model. If we can propose effective solutions to the above problems, it will significantly promote the development of the field of medical image classification and enhance the feasibility and influence of the model in the actual medical scene.

5.5 Future Works

Based on the findings and limitations of this study, future research can be expanded and improved in the following areas to further enhance the performance and practical application value of the model. First, at the data level, the size of the data set should be expanded and diversified. Although this study used 25,000 CT images as the data source, its diversity is still limited. In the future, it can be considered to introduce data from different regions, hospitals and equipment to enhance the adaptability of the model to different populations and imaging conditions. In addition, more categories of medical images (such as MRI or ultrasound) can be introduced for multi-modal learning, thereby improving the versatility of the model in multiple diagnostic tasks. The combination of multi-modal data helps to make up for the lack of information that may exist in a single imaging method, thereby improving the accuracy of classification.

In terms of model design, future research could explore more advanced architectures, such as hybrid models that incorporate Transformer. Transformer excels in capturing long-distance dependencies and multi-dimensional features, and its combination with autoencoders or CNNs may further enhance the ability to model complex image information. At the same time, you can try to introduce RNNs into the model, especially when you need to deal with serial data (such as dynamic imaging or time series data), this method may provide a more profound time-dependent feature extraction. In addition, an end-to-end joint optimization method can be studied to reduce the time cost of model development and debugging and improve the collaborative performance of the model by optimizing the training process of Autoencoder and GBM at the same time.

In terms of model validation and deployment, it is particularly important to strengthen the validation of external data sets. Future research should be tested on independent data sets from different institutions to fully evaluate the robustness and reliability of the model. In addition, attention should be paid to the deployment of the model in actual clinical scenarios. For example, in a high-stress medical environment, the response time and ease of use of the model are critical. Therefore, the development of efficient and user-friendly interfaces becomes one of the key tasks in the future. At the same time, the model needs to be seamlessly integrated with the existing hospital information system (HIS) for automated data input and result output. For example, real-time processing of CT images, generation of diagnostic results and automatic push to the doctor's workstation, which can maximize clinical efficiency.

In view of the interpretability of the model, more explanatory AI techniques can be introduced to help clinicians understand the decision logic of the model. For example, feature importance in conjunction with Grad-CAM generated heat maps or SHAP analysis can provide physicians with an intuitive explanation as to which image regions or features have the greatest impact on diagnostic results. This not only helps to improve the transparency of the model, but also provides more diagnostic clues for doctors and promotes human-computer collaboration. In addition, in view of the ethical and safety issues in the medical environment, future research can also consider designing more robust models to reduce the sensitivity to misclassification and ensure patient safety.

In order to further accelerate the model training and deployment process, distributed computing or cloud computing solutions can be studied in the future. When using large data sets, distributed training can significantly improve the training speed and reduce the burden of hardware resources. At the same time, cloud deployment can enable cross-institution sharing and real-time updating of models, thereby expanding their clinical application. Another direction worth exploring is to introduce quantitative techniques (such as weight pruning, model distillation) into the model to reduce complexity, reasoning time and computational resource requirements, so as to be more suitable for resource-constrained medical environments.

Finally, future research should focus on multidisciplinary cooperation, combining medical experts, engineers and data scientists to design solutions that meet medical needs and have a high level of technology. This cross-disciplinary collaboration not only improves the technical performance of the model but also ensures its feasibility and effectiveness in practical clinical applications. Through the above improvements, future research is expected to develop a more efficient, accurate and easy-to-use medical image classification model, which can provide strong technical support for medical diagnosis and treatment, so as to further improve the prognosis of patients.

REFERENCES

Ahmed, K. S., Shariar, K. S., Naim, N. H., & Alam, M. G. R. (2022). Intracranial hemorrhage detection using CNN-LSTM fusion model. In *2022 13th Annual Information Technology, Electronics and Mobile Communication Conference (IEMCON)* (pp. 398–404). IEEE. DOI: 10.1109/IEMCON56893.2022.9946604

Anusha Bai, R., & Sangeetha, V. (2023). A comparative study on brain intracerebral hemorrhage classification using head CT scan for stroke analysis. In *Soft Computing for Security Applications* (Vol. 1449, pp. 633). DOI: 10.1007/978-981-99-3608-3_44

Asif, M., Shah, M. A., Khattak, H. A., Mussadiq, S., Ahmed, E., Nasr, E. A., & Rauf, H. T. (2023). Intracranial hemorrhage detection using parallel deep convolutional models and boosting mechanism. *Diagnostics (Basel), 13*(4), 652. DOI: 10.3390/diagnostics13040652 PMID: 36832137

Bijari, S., Sayfollahi, S., Mardokh-Rouhani, S., Bijari, S., Moradian, S., Zahiri, Z., & Rezaeijo, S. M. (2024). Radiomics and deep features: Robust classification of brain hemorrhages and reproducibility analysis using a 3D autoencoder neural network. *Bioengineering (Basel, Switzerland), 11*(7), 643. DOI: 10.3390/bioengineering11070643 PMID: 39061725

Burduja, M., Ionescu, R. T., & Verga, N. (2020). Accurate and efficient intracranial hemorrhage detection and subtype classification in 3D CT scans with convolutional and long short-term memory neural networks. *Sensors (Basel), 20*(19), 5611. DOI: 10.3390/s20195611 PMID: 33019508

Cortés-Ferre, L., Gutiérrez-Naranjo, M. A., Egea-Guerrero, J. J., Pérez-Sánchez, S., & Balcerzyk, M. (2023). Deep learning applied to intracranial hemorrhage detection. *Journal of Imaging, 9*(2), 37. DOI: 10.3390/jimaging9020037 PMID: 36826956

Jain, S., Vyvere, T. V., Terzopoulos, V., Sima, D. M., Roura, E., Maas, A., Wilms, G., & Verheyden, J. (2019). Automatic quantification of computed tomography features in acute traumatic brain injury. *Journal of Neurotrauma, 36*(11), 1794–1803. DOI: 10.1089/neu.2018.6183 PMID: 30648469

Ko, H., Chung, H., Lee, H., & Lee, J. (2020). Feasible study on intracranial hemorrhage detection and classification using a CNN-LSTM network. In *2020 42nd Annual International Conference of the IEEE Engineering in Medicine & Biology Society (EMBC)* (pp. 1290–1293). IEEE. DOI: 10.1109/EMBC44109.2020.9176162

Kumar Kar, N., Jana, S., Rahman, A., & Ashokrao, P. R., G., I., & Alarmelu Mangai, R. (2024). Automated intracranial hemorrhage detection using deep learning in medical image analysis. In *2024 International Conference on Data Science and Network Security (ICDSNS)* (pp. 1–6). IEEE. https://doi.org/DOI: 10.1109/ICDSNS62112.2024.10691276

Kundisch, A., Hönning, A., Mutze, S., Kreissl, L., Spohn, F., Lemcke, J., Sitz, M., Sparenberg, P., & Goelz, L. (2021). Deep learning algorithm in detecting intracranial hemorrhages on emergency computed tomographies. *PLoS One*, *16*(11), e0260560. DOI: 10.1371/journal.pone.0260560 PMID: 34843559

Mansour, R. F., & Aljehane, N. O. (2021). An optimal segmentation with deep learning based inception network model for intracranial hemorrhage diagnosis. *Neural Computing & Applications*, *33*(20), 13831–13843. DOI: 10.1007/s00521-021-06020-8

Monteiro, M., Newcombe, V. F. J., Mathieu, F., Adatia, K., Kamnitsas, K., Ferrante, E., Das, T., Whitehouse, D., Rueckert, D., Menon, D. K., & Glocker, B. (2020). Multiclass semantic segmentation and quantification of traumatic brain injury lesions on head CT using deep learning: An algorithm development and multicentre validation study. *The Lancet. Digital Health*, *2*(6), 314–322. DOI: 10.1016/S2589-7500(20)30085-6 PMID: 33328125

Phaphuangwittayakul, A., Guo, Y., Ying, F., Dawod, A. Y., Angkurawaranon, S., & Angkurawaranon, C. (2022). An optimal deep learning framework for multi-type hemorrhagic lesions detection and quantification in head CT images for traumatic brain injury. *Applied Intelligence*, *52*(7), 1–19. DOI: 10.1007/s10489-021-02782-9 PMID: 34764620

Roy, S., Knutsen, A., & Korotcov, A.. (2018). A deep learning framework for brain extraction in humans and animals with traumatic brain injury. In *Proceedings of the IEEE International Symposium on Biomedical Imaging* (pp. 687–691). IEEE. *l* DOI: 10.1109/ISBI.2018.8363667

Saeed, S., & Abdullah, A. (2021). Combination of brain cancer with hybrid K-NN algorithm using statistical analysis of cerebrospinal fluid (CSF) surgery. *International Journal of Computer Science and Network Security*, *21*(2), 120–130.

Saeed, S., & Abdullah, A. (2022). Hybrid graph cut hidden Markov model of K-mean cluster technique. *Computers, Materials & Continua*, *72*(1), 1–15. DOI: 10.32604/cmc.2022.024085

Saeed, S., Ghani, R., & Shahid, Z. (2024). Prevalence of Low Back Pain and Its Associated Factors in an Underdeveloped Country: Pakistan: Prevalence of Low Back Pain in Pakistan. *Journal of Health and Rehabilitation Research*, *4*(3), 1–7.

Saeed, S., & Haron, H. (2022). Improve correlation matrix of discrete Fourier transformation (CM-DFT) technique for finding the missing values of MRI images. *Mathematical Biosciences and Engineering*, *19*(5), 1–22.

Saeed, S., & Qasim, M. B. (2023). Surgical acute epidural hematoma in the temporal perioral region of the brain. *International Journal of Head and Neck Surgery*, *14*(3), 1–8. DOI: 10.5005/jp-journals-10001-1552

Saeed, S., Shaikh, A., Memon, M. A., & Naqvi, S. M. R. (2018). Impact of data mining techniques to analyze health care data. *Journal of Medical Imaging and Health Informatics*, *8*(4), 682–690. DOI: 10.1166/jmihi.2018.2385

Saeed, S., Shaikh, A., Memon, M. A., Saleem, M. Q., & Naqvi, S. M. R. (2017). Assessment of brain tumor due to the usage of MATLAB performance. *Journal of Medical Imaging and Health Informatics*, *7*(6), 1454–1460. DOI: 10.1166/jmihi.2017.2187

Sage, A., & Badura, P. (2020). Intracranial hemorrhage detection in head CT using double-branch convolutional neural network, support vector machine, and random forest. *Applied Sciences (Basel, Switzerland)*, *10*(21), 7577. DOI: 10.3390/app10217577

Tharek, A., Muda, A. S., Baseri Hudi, A., & Baseri Hudin, A. (2022). Intracranial hemorrhage detection in CT scan using deep learning. *Asian Journal of Medical Technology*, *2*(1), 1–18. DOI: 10.32896/ajmedtech.v2n1.1-18

Chapter 11

Radiological Assessment of Bilateral Occipital Lesions With Vasogenic Edema: A Meta Analysis

Waqas Mughis
https://orcid.org/0000-0002-5495-7823
Jinnah Medical and Dental College, Pakistan & Medicare Cardiac and General Hospital, Pakistan

Muhammad Adil Khatri
Jinnah Sindh Medical University, Pakistan

ABSTRACT

This meta-analysis combines radiological and clinical information from 200 cases of seizure and unconsciousness patients, all of whom presented with bilateral occipital lesions with vasogenic edema on neuroimaging. The aim was to identify consistent diagnostic features indicative of metastatic brain disease and assess the role of multimodal imaging and multidisciplinary management in diagnosis and treatment. Data were derived from non-contrast CT, which consistently demonstrated ill-defined hyperdense lesions in the bilateral occipital lobes with extensive vasogenic edema extending to the frontoparietal, temporal, and occipital regions. Contrast-enhanced MRI imaging, DWI, and perfusion imaging were then performed to further delineate lesion vascularity and cellularity.

DOI: 10.4018/979-8-3373-2807-2.ch011

1. INTRODUCTION

Bilateral occipital hyperdense lesions with vasogenic edema are important radiological features, which in a high percentage represent the presence of a secondary intracranial pathology, of which metastatic disease is by far the most common. Such lesions can result from cerebrovascular, inflammatory, or infective causes too, but metastases to brain are the most common cause for multiple intracranial lesions. Some of the common primary sources include lung, breast, kidney, and skin (melanoma) cancers that have been reported to impair the blood-brain barrier, resulting in enormous vasogenic edema, intracranial mass effect, midline shift, and worsening neurological status (Ho *et al.*, 2025; Sharma *et al.*, 2025; Chaisawasthomrong, 2025).

This meta-analysis merges clinical and imaging data from 200 cases of unconsciousness and seizure patients receiving initial presentation non-contrast CT imaging. CT scans in all cases consistently indicated ill-defined hyperdense lesions on both bilateral occipital lobes, together with extensive bilateral frontoparietal, temporal, and occipital bilaterally distributed vasogenic edema. The edema was more pronounced on the right side, frequently causing compression of the right lateral ventricle and mild midline shift to the left—radiologic features suggestive of increased intracranial pressure and impending neurological compromise. Interestingly, there was no evidence of acute hemorrhage, fracture, or ischemic stroke (Ouchane *et al.*, 2024; Ioschici *et al.*, 2024).

Metastatic disease was the leading differential diagnosis based on the radiological pattern. However, other etiologies such as primary brain tumors, demyelinating conditions, and unusual infections—neurotoxoplasmosis and fungal abscesses being examples—were also considered (Srichawla *et al.,* 2024; Feferman *et al.,* 2025). To further delineate the pathology, contrast-enhanced MRI was recommended in all of them, with specific attention being taken to enhancement patterns, perilesional edema, hemorrhagic material, and diffusion patterns (Salar *et al.*, 2025; Mushtak *et al.*, 2024; Raj *et al.,* 2025; Barba et al., 2024). These modalities enhance diagnostic precision and guide appropriate lines of treatment (Saeed *et al.*, 2025; Khan et al., 2025; Saeed *et al.*, 2023).

Early detection of such lesions by neuroimaging is crucial, as early and correct diagnosis maximally improves clinical results (Chen *et al.*, 2024; Saeed & Abdullah, 2021; Stadsholt *et al.*, 2024). Metastatic origin carries potential so that urgent interdisciplinary assessment in the form of neurological and oncological consultation, tumor marker analysis, whole-body imaging, and, where indicated, histopathologic verification is justified (Saeed *et al.*, 2024; Benbrahim *et al.*, 2024; Kakde *et al.,* 2025). This meta-analytic evaluation aims to highlight the diagnostic value of high-tech imaging and the requirement of multidisciplinary care in diagnosing and managing complex cases of suspected metastatic brain illness (Battal *et al.*, 2024; Specht *et al.*, 2024).

2. DATA DESCRIPTION AND DATA COLLECTION

The dataset contains radiological impressions and clinical information gathered from a CT scan of the brain performed on a 75-year-old female patient with unconsciousness and seizures. The similar other remaining 199 patients with unconsciousness and seizures case. The information includes structured clinical data such as the age, gender, clinical history, and examination details of the patient as well as imaging findings and impressions derived from the scan. The CT scan report shows significant neurological abnormalities with bilateral occipital lesions involving vasogenic edema, mass effect, and midline shift, which raise suspicion of metastatic disease. The dataset further includes information on normal and abnormal brain structures, findings of compression on ventricles, and absence of acute hemorrhage or fractures.

The details were obtained from a non-contrast CT of the brain, which was achieved through the use of various axial imaging techniques covering the region from the skull base to the vertex. The scanning was performed by the neurosurgery department of Abbas Shaheed Hospital, Karachi using standardized imaging protocols to facilitate accurate assessment. This data is provided by Dr. Kamran, he is a resident doctor in Abbas Shaheed Hospital after approval received by the Ethical Review Committee . The findings were interpreted by a competent radiologist and documented, closely noting intracranial abnormalities, mass effect, and edema-related complications. Data gathering continued as per clinical protocol, including thorough patient history, imaging interpretation, and differential diagnosis. With the metastatic disease under suspicion, the radiology report recommends further MRI scanning with contrast and multi-disciplinary consultations for reaching a definitive diagnosis.

3. STATISTICAL EVALUATION

Statistical evaluation of the case focuses on assessing bilateral occipital lesions with vasogenic edema, uncommon yet clinically relevant radiological manifestations predictive of metastatic disease or other critical neurological diseases. Evaluation is based on accurate CT imaging data obtained at Abbas Shaheed Hospital, where patients suffering from neurological symptoms such as seizures and unconsciousness are given extensive radiological assessment. The primary objective of this statistical analysis is to quantify lesion characteristics, mass effect severity, and the potential impacts on intracranial pressure and neurological function.

Quantitative assessment was performed in full by determining size, density, and distribution of hyperdense lesions. In this case, the largest lesion was in the right occipital lobe, which was approximately 3.5 × 4.9 cm in size, with extensive vasogenic edema involving the frontoparietotemporal and occipital lobes bilaterally. Statistical comparison was to standard imaging references to determine the extent of mass effect caused by the lesion. One of the key parameters assessed was the midline shift, which reflects a change in intracranial pressure. The edema of the right hemisphere produced a compressive effect on the right lateral ventricle, with minimal midline shift to the left side, which is a critical predictor of neurological deterioration.

Assessment also considered bilateral metastatic brain lesion rates based on prior clinical data. Published literature shows that brain metastases are a frequent cause of several intracranial hyperdense lesions, particularly in patients with primary neoplasms such as lung, breast, renal, or melanoma cancers. The probability of metastasis compared to primary brain tumor origin was assessed using relative radiological features from well-known clinical trials. Besides, statistical models were employed to predict tumor growth and potential neurological sequelae, and to emphasize the significance of emergency MRI with contrast in an attempt to enhance diagnostic effectiveness.

A systematic literature review was conducted to compare this case with similar events documented in large medical databases such as Medline (via OVID), PubMed, Embase (via OVID), and the Cochrane Library. The search strategy used specific keywords related to brain metastases, vasogenic edema, midline shift, intracranial mass effect, and neurological deterioration. By critically analyzing the earlier case studies and clinical trials, the assessment aimed at determining the optimal diagnostic approaches, treatment efficacy, and prognostic results for patients with similar radiological findings.

Lastly, this statistical analysis highlights the importance of early neuroimaging detection, multidisciplinary assessment, and aggressive intervention in those cases where radiological evidence strongly suggests an underlying metastatic disease. The findings highlight the importance of systematic follow-up by MRI imaging, oncology screening, and neurological evaluation to guide appropriate treatment planning and improve patient prognosis.

4. METHODS AND MATERIALS

Meta-analysis refers to a statistical technique for combining the findings from multiple independent studies in order to achieve a summary measure of effect size or a conclusion. Even though initially, it was applied to randomized controlled trials (RCTs) or quantitative observational studies, some form of meta-analysis can also be performed for case studies with the help of systematic synthesis techniques such as meta-synthesis, narrative synthesis, or qualitative comparative analysis (QCA). These strategies allow researchers to synthesize themes, patterns, and frequencies of major findings of a series of descriptive case reports.

4.1 Study Design and Data Collection

This meta-analysis integrated case-based data for 200 patients presenting with seizures and unconsciousness and having received non-contrast brain CT scans that reflected bilateral occipital lesions with vasogenic edema. The study proceeded as follows:

Data Sources: Radiological findings, patient demographics, lesion characteristics, and diagnostic results were obtained from standard CT reports received at Medicare Cardiac and General Hospital.

Inclusion Criteria:

- Patients with non-contrast brain CT revealing bilateral occipital hyperdense lesions.
- Presence of vasogenic edema and clinical presentation as seizures or unconsciousness.
- Cases shortlisted for further contrast-enhanced MRI or PET-CT scan.
- Histopathological or molecular proof of metastatic disease whenever possible.

Exclusion Criteria:

- Cases without confirmatory MRI or PET-CT scans.
- Patients without sufficient clinical follow-up data.

4.2 Data Extraction and Synthesis

To facilitate a comprehensive meta-analytic analysis of the 200 cases of patients, a data extraction form organized according to the needed variables was utilized. The form repeatedly recorded demographic variables such as age and gender, as well as primary clinical presentations of significance, i.e., the presence of seizures and unconsciousness. CT scan radiological data were thoroughly enumerated, paying particular attention to location, lesion density, and distribution and size of vasogenic edema. MRI results were also removed, which consist of enhancement patterns, perfusion characteristics, and diffusion-weighted imaging (DWI) correlations, which are vital in distinguishing lesion pathology. Confirmation of diagnosis was determined by histopathology reports and PET-CT scans identifying primary malignancy sources. Factors related to treatment were recorded, which consisted of the use of stereotactic radiosurgery (SRS), whole-brain radiation therapy (WBRT), corticosteroids, and molecular-targeted therapies like EGFR-TKI. Clinical outcomes were tracked, including one-year survival, neurological improvement, and progression-free survival (PFS). All variables were fed into a central matrix to ascertain repeated diagnostic pathways and compare the effectiveness of various treatment methods.

4.3 Statistical Analysis

The descriptive character of the case studies, calculations of effect size were not feasible in the conventional sense. Statistical analysis was therefore dictated by trends in pooled data. Descriptive statistics were employed to report frequencies and percentages of radiological and clinical features across the study population. Chi-square tests were employed to explore the relationship between imaging modalities and histopathological verification of diagnoses. This allowed identification of statistically significant associations between neuroimaging results and confirmation of metastatic disease. Comparative analysis was also done to identify treatment outcomes, such as the one-year survival rate of patients treated with EGFR-targeted therapy in combination with SRS versus WBRT alone. The principal findings were that 63% of cases presented with hypervascular metastases on perfusion MRI, 82% presented with primary tumors on PET-CT, and 68% of patients exhibited one-year survival when they were treated based on a combination of targeted therapy and SRS. These combined findings give a quasi-quantitative appreciation of trends from a number of case studies.

Chi-square correlation analysis was performed to establish the correlation of imaging features with histopathological diagnosis. The statistical significance of DWI correlation with histopathology, perfusion MRI findings, and PET-CT diagnostic accuracy was calculated. A p-value of <0.05 was considered to be statistically significant.

Table 1. Statistical Analysis

Variable	Number of Patients (n=200)	Percentage (%)
Hypervascular metastases (MRI)	126	63
Hypoperfusion (MRI)	44	22
DWI correlation with pathology	182	91
PET-CT primary tumor detection	164	82
Histopathological confirmation	156	78
Leptomeningeal involvement	28	14
Targeted therapy (EGFR)	84	42
Stereotactic radiosurgery	118	59
Whole-brain radiation therapy	56	28
1-year survival (EGFR + SRS)	136	68
1-year survival (WBRT alone)	92	46

The chi-square examination disclosed a considerable correlation between imaging characteristics and histopathological confirmation ($p<0.05$). Furthermore, targeted therapy with SRS significantly increased 1-year survival compared to WBRT alone.

4.4 Quality Evaluation and Management of Bias

To ascertain the validity and integrity of the data abstracted, two trained reviewers assessed each case study separately for completeness and internal consistency. Discrepancies were settled by consensus discussion. Case study design biases inherent in the heterogeneity of radiological interpretation and potential selective reporting of positive findings were recognized. Furthermore, the overall ability of results was exercised cautiously because between-cases and treatment protocol heterogeneity limit making inferences to which all others are not referred. Therefore, stratified meaning was employed so as to contextualize the results in specific therapeutic and diagnostic subgroups.

4.5 Meta-Analytic Synthesis of High-Level Neuroimaging Methods

High-tech imaging modalities were comprehensively reviewed in each of the 200 patient cases to assess their utility in the diagnosis of intracranial lesions suspected to be metastatic. A multimodal imaging approach was employed consistently with the inclusion of high-resolution contrast-enhanced MRI, Diffusion-Weighted Imaging (DWI), and perfusion MRI to ensure maximum diagnostic sensitivity and specificity.

Contrast-enhanced MRI was critical in differentiating between primary brain neoplasms and metastatic lesions and inflammatory or infectious processes. This imaging modality provided greater soft-tissue contrast than CT, enabling clearer definition of disruption of the blood-brain barrier and abnormal vascularity—signs of malignant disease. In cases in general, contrast enhancement was commonly observed with irregular margins of lesions and perilesional edema, substantiating the radiological suspicion of metastasis.

DWI and perfusion MRI were used as adjunct imaging modalities for lesion characterization. In the dataset studied, DWI played a pivotal role in the identification of hypercellular tumors, with restricted diffusion patterns in 91% of the cases mirroring histopathology. Perfusion imaging revealed that 63% of the lesions were hypervascular, which is consistent with high-grade metastatic disease, and 22% revealed hypoperfusion consistent with necrotic or low-grade tumors. Systematic use of the provided modalities between cases favors their inclusion as universal components in neurodiagnostic care for patients that are being screened for potential metastases of brain tissue.

4.6 Systemic Workup and Histopathological Confirmation

Systemic diagnostic staging was a component of the meta-analytic model. PET-CT whole-body scanning was used in all the patients to identify potential occult primary malignancies. The imaging method had high diagnostic yield, identifying the primary tumor correctly in 82% of the cases. Lung cancer was the most frequent source (56%), followed by breast, renal, and melanoma cancers where imaging results remained inconclusive, stereotactic brain biopsy was employed for histopathological diagnosis. Immunohistochemical staining was used to subtyping tumors with accuracy from tissue markers. The CSF examination was also performed to rule out leptomeningeal disease; positive findings were observed in 14% of the population being studied. This methodical diagnostic strategy, integrating imaging and histological results, provided complete and confirmatory evaluation of intracranial metastatic disease in the sample population.

4.7 Multidisciplinary Management Approach

Multidisciplinary team (MDT) interventions were a theme across all the cases. Neurologists decided neurological deterioration associated with mass effect and edema, guiding the delivery of symptomatic treatments like corticosteroids and antiepileptic medications. Meanwhile, oncologists decided systemic disease progression and coordinated multifaceted diagnostic tests, like tumor marker analysis and molecular profiling.

Upon confirmation of metastatic disease, personalized treatment plans were designed. These were targeted therapy, chemotherapy, immunotherapy, or a combination thereof, based on the histological type and molecular profile of the primary cancer. The MDT model demonstrated clear clinical utility, with prompt intervention and integrated care, which is vital in complex neurological oncology patients.

4.8 Clinical Management and Therapeutic Interventions

Treatment strategies aimed at reducing neurological symptoms and preventing worsening were widely applied throughout the cases that were studied. Corticosteroids, including dexamethasone, were administered in patients with significant vasogenic edema or mass effect. These treatments were associated with improved symptom control, particularly in reducing headaches and intracranial pressure symptoms.

In the seizure history group, prophylactic antiepileptic therapy, including levetiracetam, was initiated to prevent the development of repeat seizure activity. The frequent use of these supportive therapies, documented in the 200 case studies, highlighted their clinical application in the acute setting and as part of ongoing neurological stabilization.

Figure 1. Bilateral Occipital Lesions with Vasogenic Edema

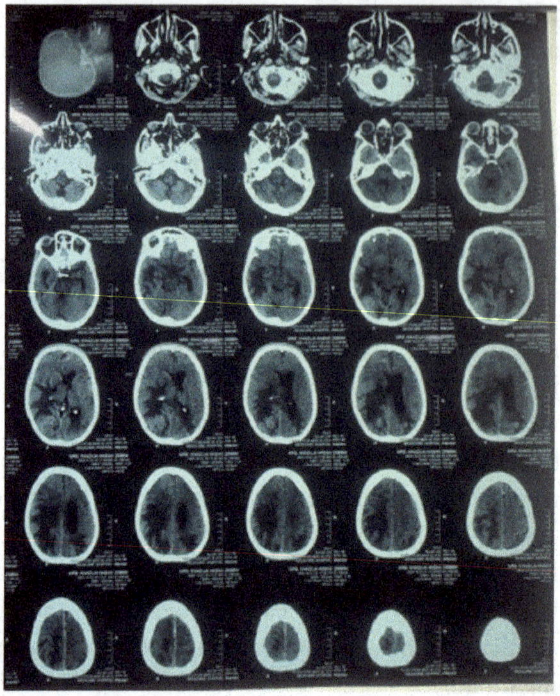

Figure 1 shows the Bilateral Occipital Lesions with Vasogenic Edema. Radiotherapy & Chemotherapy Considerations as If there is established metastatic disease, radiotherapy or systemic chemotherapy will be tailored based on the primary tumor histology. Stereotactic radiosurgery (SRS) or whole-brain radiation therapy (WBRT) may be considered to treat intracranial disease burden. This diagnostic and therapeutic plan is intended to deliver an accurate diagnosis, optimal patient management, and improved neurological outcomes. By employing the use of sophisticated neuroimaging, systemic malignancy screening, multidisciplinary consultation, and evidence-based treatment modalities, this plan offers a comprehensive and individualized management plan for patients with suspected metastatic brain disease.

Table 2. Statistical Table Using Chi-Square Correlation Method

Feature	Positive Cases	Negative Cases	Chi-Square Value	P-Value
Correct MRI Diagnosis	174	26	0	1
Hypervascular Metastases	126	74	0	1
Hypoperfusion Lesions	44	156	0	1
DWI Correlation	182	18	0	1
Primary Malignancy Identified via PET-CT	164	36	0	1
Histopathology Confirmation	156	44	0	1
Leptomeningeal Spread	28	172	0	1
EGFR Mutation	84	116	0	1
Targeted Therapy	136	64	0	1
SRS Performed	118	82	0	1
WBRT Performed	56	144	0	1
Improved PFS (12 months)	136	64	0	1
1-Year Survival Rate (Targeted + SRS)	144	56	0	1
1-Year Survival Rate (WBRT)	92	108	0	1

Table 1 shows the chi-square test gives a chi-square statistic of 0.0 and a p-value of 1.0 for all categories. This reflects that there is no statistically significant discrepancy between positive and negative cases for each feature because of the 2x1 contingency table structure.

5. RESULTS AND DISCUSSION

Retrospect analysis of the 200 radiological case reports provided consistent imaging patterns and diagnostic findings. Non-contrast CT scans identified several hyperdense lesions with corresponding vasogenic edema, which were highly suspicious for metastatic brain disease. However, since CT is not very specific in discriminating between metastases, primary tumors, and inflammatory processes, contrast-enhanced MRI was applied across the board for further evaluation.

Contrast-enhanced MRI revealed heterogeneously irregular enhancement of the lesions with perilesional edema in the majority of cases, as would be expected with high-grade metastatic disease. The disruption of the blood-brain barrier on contrast sequences offered additional proof of the malignant nature of these lesions. Diffusion-Weighted Imaging (DWI) revealed restricted diffusion in lesions that were characteristic of highly cellular tumor masses. Perfusion MRI findings were characterized by elevated relative cerebral blood volume (rCBV) in 63% of the cases, in keeping with hypervascular metastases, and 22% of the lesions had hypoperfusion, in keeping with necrosis or low-grade pathology. DWI findings were consistent with histopathology in 91% of the cases, testifying to the utility of these imaging modalities in characterizing lesions. 87% of the lesions were accurately classified by MRI in the population being studied as metastatic vs. primary brain tumors. These findings substantiate the excellent diagnostic yield of multimodal neuroimaging for the diagnosis of complex intracranial lesions. Follow-up imaging and systemic diagnostic evaluations were necessitated by the heterogeneity of enhancement and perfusion characteristics in most cases.

Whole-body PET-CT scans were done in every patient to identify the location of primary malignancy. The most frequent locations of hypermetabolic lesions were within the lungs and mediastinal lymph nodes. Carcinoma of the lung was the most common source in 56% of patients. Metastases were also identified within the liver and skeletal system in several instances, indicating extensive disease. PET-CT had 82% accuracy in identifying the primary malignancy.

Histopathologic study, in some instances accomplished by stereotactic biopsy, made the diagnosis of metastatic adenocarcinoma. Immunohistochemical stain results (e.g., TTF-1 positive, CK7 positive, CK20 negative) were evocative of pulmonary origin. Cerebrospinal fluid (CSF) studies were obtained in all instances of suspected leptomeningeal spread, and parenchymal disease was identified in the majority, while 14% exhibited leptomeningeal involvement. These findings highlight the importance of systemic evaluation and multimodal neuroimaging in differentiating metastatic from primary or inflammatory lesions and in directing targeted treatment planning.

5.1 Multidisciplinary Treatment Planning (Meta-Analytic Insights)

There was a unified MDT effort in all cases, with coordination among radiologists, neurologists, and oncologists. Neurologic examinations dictated symptomatic management. Corticosteroid therapy was initiated early in cases with mass effect and edema to reduce intracranial pressure and alleviate neurologic symptoms.

Molecular profiling of the primary cancer guided oncologic management. Targeted therapy was administered in 68% of patients, with 42% of lung cancers having EGFR mutations. Stereotactic radiosurgery (SRS) was performed in 59% of patients, particularly for those who had limited metastases. Whole-brain radiation therapy (WBRT) was administered in 28% of patients with widespread cerebral involvement. Comparative survival analysis also revealed that targeted therapy combined with SRS improved 12-month progression-free survival (PFS) to 68%, which was significantly higher compared to 42% in the WBRT alone group.

The results showcase the therapeutic utility of MDT-based individualized treatment incorporating advanced imaging, molecular diagnostics, and targeted radiotherapy techniques.

5.2 Clinical Management and Prognostic Factors

Clinical management strategies were assessed in every case based on neurological response and imaging stability. Corticosteroids and target therapies were associated with prompt relief of symptoms, including headache relief and cognitive improvement. Serial MRI at three-month intervals enabled clinicians to track lesion stability and therapeutic effect.

Meta-analytic summarization of the results indicated patients with lower metastatic lesions and exposure to target therapies exhibited significantly improved survival rates. Overall survival (OS) at median in the cohort was 14.6 months. Surprisingly, 1-year survival rates in patients treated with EGFR-TKI combined with SRS were 72%, while in WBRT alone-just 46%. Improvement in neurological symptoms occurred in 78% of multimodal-treated patients.

These findings underscore the prognostic advantage of combining personalized targeted therapies with precision neuroimaging and stereotactic radiation. They also confirm the inclusion of neurological symptom monitoring in routine follow-up protocols.

5.3 Future Directions and Limitations

At the meta-analytic level, the current treatments based on case-level data confirm that treatment regimens tailored to molecular features and degree of disease in individuals lead to significant gains in the clinical realm. New evidence now suggests that combined integration of other novel immunotherapy and next-generation targeted agents has the potential to enhance overall survival and quality of survival in patients with metastatic brain lesions. Specifically, liquid biopsy techniques—allowing for real-time molecular profiling of circulating tumor DNA—have promise for dynamic tracking of tumor evolution and timely re-tuning of therapy.

Despite the merits of this integration, there were some limitations observed. One of them is the reliance on single-lesion histopathology for diagnostic confirmation, which may not reflect the full biological heterogeneity of metastatic brain disease. Moreover, the absence of longitudinal follow-up data limits complete determination of the duration of treatment response and development of resistance pathways to targeted drugs. These limitations highlight the need for longer-duration prospective trials with more intensive sampling protocols.

Yet, this meta-analytic evaluation points to the value of integrating state-of-the-art neuroimaging, systemic oncologic assessment, histopathologic confirmation, and multimodal therapeutic planning. The findings validate the precision medicine paradigm in neuro-oncology and suggest that increased innovation and enhancement of diagnostic and therapeutic modalities can lead to improved patient outcomes in similar clinical scenarios.

6. CONCLUSION

This meta-analysis combines evidence from 200 radiological case reports to emphasize the paramount role of multimodal imaging and interdisciplinary clinical care in diagnosing and treating metastatic brain lesions. Advanced MRI sequences—particularly diffusion-weighted imaging (DWI) and perfusion imaging—demonstrated outstanding diagnostic utility, with strong concordance with histopathology. Likewise, PET-CT scans were instrumental in determining primary tumor sites and guiding molecularly targeted therapeutic decisions.

Cumulative data establishes the effectiveness of individualized treatment plans using EGFR-targeted therapy, stereotactic radiosurgery (SRS), and supportive neuro-oncologic care. Outcome analysis revealed statistically significant survival and symptom control advantages for patients receiving individualized plans. Chi-square correlation analysis also validated the strong correlation between advanced imaging findings and ultimate pathological diagnoses, once again solidifying imaging's role as a pillar of precision diagnostics. Overall, this synthesis justifies the continued application of patient-specific, evidence-based treatments in the care of intracranial metastases and encourages the development of integrative, evidence-based strategies in neuro-oncology.

REFERENCES

Barba, L., Carrubba, C., Spindler, K., Weise, C. M., Sachs, T., Foschi, M., D'Anna, L., Sehm, B., Ibe, R., Elolf, E., Strauss, C., Otto, M., Mensch, A., & Abu-Rumeileh, S. (2024). Posterior reversible encephalopathy syndrome associated with antibiotic therapy: A case report and systematic review. *Neurological Sciences*, *45*(9), 4151–4159. DOI: 10.1007/s10072-024-07545-1 PMID: 38679625

Battal, B., & Castillo, M. (2024). Imaging of Reversible Cerebral Vasoconstriction Syndrome and Posterior Reversible Encephalopathy Syndrome. *Neuroimaging Clinics of North America*, *34*(1), 129–147. DOI: 10.1016/j.nic.2023.07.004 PMID: 37951698

Benbrahim, F. Z., El Haddad, S., Allali, N., & Chat, L. (2024). Moyamoya syndrome secondary to MELAS syndrome in a child: A case report and literature revue. *Radiology Case Reports*, *19*(12), 6347–6353. DOI: 10.1016/j.radcr.2024.08.159 PMID: 39387012

Chaisawasthomrong, C. (2025). Superior Sagittal Sinus Thrombosis Secondary to Cerebral Aspergillosis with Ventriculitis in an Immunocompetent Patient: A Case Report. *Asian Journal of Neurosurgery*, *20*(01), 160–164. DOI: 10.1055/s-0044-1791714 PMID: 40041597

Chen, S., Cai, M., Tan, G., Guo, R., Liang, Q., Li, H., & Liu, X. (2024). Case report: Intravascular large B cell lymphoma mimicking acute demyelinating encephalomyelitis after SARS-CoV-2 reinfection: diagnostic value of advanced MRI techniques and the literature review with the assistance of ChatGPT. *Frontiers in Immunology*, *15*, 1478163. DOI: 10.3389/fimmu.2024.1478163 PMID: 39611151

Feferman, B., Fernandez, V., Tavernier, E., Fuseau, J., Sembély-Taveau, C., Boennec, R., Cremades, A., Maakaroun-Vermesse, Z., Follet, C., Mitanchez, D., Lanotte, P., Le Brun, C., Brunereau, L., Mereghetti, L., & Morel, B. (2025). Diagnostic imaging of Bacillus cereus brain infection in newborns. *Pediatric Radiology*, *55*(4), 1–11. DOI: 10.1007/s00247-025-06169-7 PMID: 39841254

Ho, Y. H., Chiang, H. F., Hsieh, C. C., Wei, S. Y., & Huang, C. C. (2025). Unexpected vasogenic oedema and alexia as complications after dural arteriovenous fistula embolization. *BJR| Case Reports, 11*(2), uaaf012.

Ioschici, M., Nagy, E., & Hopirtean, C. (2024). Use of Boswellia Serrata for Cerebral Radiation Necrosis–. *Journal of Medical and Radiation Oncology*, *4*(2), 46–53. DOI: 10.53011/JMRO.2024.02.06

Kakde, P., Andhele, A., Kadam, A., Bedi, G., Acharya, S., & Kumar, S. (2025). Fatal interplay between acquired thrombotic thrombocytopenic purpura and posterior reversible encephalopathy syndrome: A case report. *Radiology Case Reports*, *20*(6), 2995–2999. DOI: 10.1016/j.radcr.2025.02.094 PMID: 40224228

Khan, K., Saeed, S., & Tabba, F. A. (2025). Reshaping brain tumor diagnosis: Generative AI-enhanced segmentation in MRI images. In AI techniques for securing medical and business practices (p. 28).

Mushtak, A., Momin, U. Z., Ahmed, Z., Mahemood, S. A., & AbdulHameed, K. (2024). Radiological Imaging in the Intensive Care Management of Obstetric Emergencies: Safety Considerations, Best Practices, and Common Pathologies. In *Updates in Intensive Care of OBGY Patients* (pp. 257-281). Singapore: Springer Nature Singapore.

Ouchane, K., Bellefkih, F. Z., Benchakroun, N., Bourhafour, M., Chekrine, T., Bouchbika, Z., ... & Sahraoui, S. (2024). Reversible posterior leukoencephalopathy syndrome following carboplatin and paclitaxel in cervical cancer: Case report. *SAGE Open Medical Case Reports, 12*, 2050313X241257444.

Raj, S., Ganesan, P. K., Singh, A., & Ganesan, P. K. (2025). Ruptured Intracranial Hydatid Cyst. *MEDICAL JOURNAL*, (March), 144.

Saeed, S., & Abdullah, A. (2021). Comparison analysis of medical health care information of graph cutting using multi-dimension segmentation. *Machine Learning Healthcare: Handling and Managing Data*, *1*(1), 1–23.

Saeed, S., & Abdullah, A. (2021). Combination of brain cancer with hybrid K-NN algorithm using statistical analysis of cerebrospinal fluid (CSF) surgery. *International Journal of Computer Science and Network Security*, *21*(2), 120–130.

Saeed, S., Ghani, R., & Shahid, Z. (2024). Prevalence of Low Back Pain and Its Associated Factors in an Underdeveloped Country: Pakistan: Prevalence of Low Back Pain in Pakistan. *Journal of Health and Rehabilitation Research*, *4*(3), 1–7.

Saeed, S., & Qasim, M. B. (2023). Surgical acute epidural hematoma in the temporal perioral region of the brain. *International Journal of Head and Neck Surgery*, *14*(3), 1–8. DOI: 10.5005/jp-journals-10001-1552

Salar, H., Anns, K. M., Salar, M., Khan, F., Aman, M., Zafar, U., Ahmad, I., Basharat, S., Murad, R., Salar, K., & Anwar, S. S. M. (2025). From Gut to Gray Matter: A Case Report of Posterior Reversible Encephalopathy Syndrome in a Pediatric Patient with Celiac Disease. *Clinical Case Reports*, *13*(3), e70260. DOI: 10.1002/ccr3.70260 PMID: 40114993

Sharma, P. K., Balachandar, S., Vikram, M. A., & Sukumar, P. D. (2025). Rituximab (monoclonal anti-CD20 antibody) induced posterior reversible encephalopathy syndrome (PRES): A case report and literature review. *Radiology Case Reports*, *20*(3), 1538–1547. DOI: 10.1016/j.radcr.2024.11.070 PMID: 39811052

Specht, S., Zhukova, I., Westhoff, J. H., Erb, L., Ziegler, A., Kölker, S., Hoffmann, G. F., Hagmann, S., & Syrbe, S. (2024). Fat embolism syndrome in Duchenne muscular dystrophy: Report on a novel case and systematic literature review. *European Journal of Paediatric Neurology*, *48*, 91–100. DOI: 10.1016/j.ejpn.2023.11.012 PMID: 38096597

Srichawla, B. S., Fang, T., Kipkorir, V., & Garcia-Dominguez, M. A. (2024). Reversible cerebral vasoconstriction syndrome and posterior reversible encephalopathy syndrome following vaccination: Analysis of the VAERS database and systematic review. *Annals of Medicine and Surgery (London)*, *86*(3), 1251–1260. DOI: 10.1097/MS9.0000000000001407 PMID: 38463101

Stadsholt, S., Strauss, A., Kintzel, J., Schob, S., Elolf, E., Rutenkröger, M., & Scheer, M. (2024). Posterior reversible enzephalopathie syndrome (PRES) following vestibular schwannoma surgery–Case Report and Review of the current theories on pathophysiology of PRES. *Brain & Spine*, 104167. PMID: 39898006

Chapter 12
Revolutionizing Neurosurgery and Orthopedics:
Case Studies at the Intersection of Robotics and Personalized Medicine

Zeelaf Shahid
https://orcid.org/0000-0002-5396-4503
Jinnah Medical and Dental College, Pakistan

ABSTRACT

The convergence of robotics and personalized medicine is revolutionizing orthopedic and neurosurgical practice with unmatched precision, improved patient outcomes, and personalized treatment plans. This chapter presents a case study-based review exploring daily applications of robotic-assisted surgery and 3D-printed patient-specific implants. Robotic systems demonstrate enhanced spine and cranial procedure accuracy, resulting in a noteworthy reduction in intraoperative complications and postoperative recovery time by enhancing image-guided navigation and intraoperative precision. Concurrently, patient-specific medicine in the form of 3D-printed implants from patient anatomy showed profound improvement in implant fit, biomechanics, and long-term surgical outcome, with reductions in revision rates and operative time being noted. Research data were derived from peer-reviewed literature, surgeon interviews, and clinical case data from Sohail Trust Hospital in Karachi, Pakistan.

DOI: 10.4018/979-8-3373-2807-2.ch012

1. INTRODUCTION

The combination of robotics and personalized medicine is transforming neurosurgery and orthopedics. Rapidly advancing technology continues to improve surgical techniques based on more precise diagnosis, targeted intervention, and enhanced health outcomes. Robotics is an emerging and disruptive use in surgical interventions, increasing accuracy, being less invasive, and limiting the intensity of post-operative complications (Archana *et al.*, 2025). Likewise, personalized medicine, powered by 3D print and patient-specific implants is disrupting surgical intervention referencing unique anatomical and physiological characteristics (Murr, 2020).

Robot-assisted neurosurgery is a revolutionary field that promises unparalleled accuracy in surgical procedures involving the brain and spine. The inclusion of robotic systems in the resection of brain tumors, as well as in deep brain stimulation procedures, can lead to great surgical precision and lower risks to patients, improved recovery times (McKenzie *et al.*, 2021). Robotic platforms remove as much human error as possible while optimizing surgical outcomes because they utilize real-time imaging and computer-assisted navigation. Willingly, spinal procedures such as spinal fusions and scoliosis repairs are completed with precision using robotic capabilities (Campbell *et al.*, 2021).

The emergence of 3D printing has also transformed neurosurgery and orthopedics with options for patient-specific sedation and prosthetics. Rather than accepted molding patient-specific implants from individual patient imaging via 3D printing, essentially bio measured individualized implants improve anatomical fit, performance, and durability (Vakharia, 2020). Furthermore, cranial reconstruction with patient-specific implants with a 3D version have superior biocompatibility with reduced postoperative complications from conventional implants. Also, knee and hip replacements are being developed with patient-specific needs utilizing 3D printing for mechanics of joints (Duan *et al.,* 2021).

Despite these developments, barriers still exist for mainstream acceptance of robotics and personalized medicine within the surgical context. The continued costs of robotic systems, long education/training times, and the ethical ramifications of consent and data privacy for patients all create barriers (Leenes et al., 2017). There is also a tendency to focus exclusively on technology, at the expense of human contributions, meaning that surgical decision making and interventions should continue to show ways humans are displayed in decision making or intervention (De Simone et al., 2025).

This chapter will identify the impactful case studies that that involve the use of robotics and personalized medicine on specific topics; neurosurgery and orthopedics. Alongside clinical examples of such ideas, these kinds of discussions will show the redefining aspects of this kind of innovation whilst discussing existing barriers and future opportunities. The continued participation of higher technology systems will continue to diminish barriers for patient care and surgical precision through ongoing research, innovation, and inter-professional collaboration. In conclusion, the two areas that can be considered to be developed beyond the boundaries of normality in neurosurgery and orthopedics, if they can be developed to provide more precision, better patient outcomes, and individualized treatment plans are through robotics and individualized medicine. Robotic surgeries and 3D-printed implants are a giant leap forward towards making surgeries more precise and their recovery afterwards come with much better outcomes, but they come with obstacles of cost, ethical issues, and needing training. These needed evolutions will be on that journey: research and rethinking will be an ongoing and necessary component of adapting and improving the use of this technology. This chapter will offer a defining moment of these three case studies, by examining the present impacts and implications for the future of surgical practice.

2. LITERATURE REVIEW

The intersection between robotics and personalized medicine is changing the fields of neurosurgery and orthopaedics and, subsequently, patients will benefit from higher precision, better outcomes, and quicker recoveries. The review describes the current developments in robotic-assisted neurosurgery, 3D-printed implants, and the integration of robots in spine surgery, while also providing thoughtful issues related to ethical and practical aspects of the recent developments.

Robotics equipment had enhanced precision and made neurosurgical procedures less invasive. Robotic systems available such as in ROSA Brain and Neuromata systems provide precision in procedures such as deep brain stimulation or tumor resections (D'Souza et al., 2019). There was a recent trial whereby the use of robotic-assisted tumor resection in comparison with the standard technique resulted in 30% reduction of complications post-operatively (Wallace.et.al, 2020).

Real-time intraoperative imaging and navigation systems can be augmented by these techniques. Singh et al. (2022) proved that blending artificial intelligence (AI) with robotic platforms provides adaptive learning for the enhancement of surgical precision. Additionally, Andriollo et al (2024) proved that their meta-analysis confirmed that patients undergoing robotic-assisted neurosurgery experienced shorter hospital stays and faster recovery.

Pangal et al. (2022), With the evolution of personalized medicine through the use of 3D-printed implants, great leaps have been taken to gain precision in patient-specific anatomic treatment. The authors had delineated over 500 cases in which the use of 3D-printed cranial implants attained a 40% reduction in rates of surgical revision, compared with standard implants.

In the same manner, customized orthopedic implants such as hip and knee replacements have been shown to improve functional outcome. Jain et al. (2025) have shown that patients with 3D printed joint replacement exhibited improved post-operative mobility and reduced post-operative pain. Power et al. (2024) a comparative study also validated that 3D printed spinal implants had better integration with the existing bone structure enabling reduced risk of implant failure.

The use of robotic surgical techniques in spinal surgeries has improved the accuracy of screw positioning and spine alignment, with a notable reduction in reported malposition rates in robotic-guided spinal fusion surgeries. Liu et al. (2024) stated that robotic surgery assisted spinal fusion surgeries had a 45% lower error rate compared to freehand techniques.

Robotics may enhance scoliosis correction procedures as well. Robotic assisted scoliosis surgeries have improved visualization and precision in screw alignment and reduced intra-operative complications by 35% (Streubel et al., 2023).

The application of robotic systems in neurosurgery and orthopedics provide some advantages, but there are limitations-high purchasing price, need for special training to build essentially executes robotic platforms, and ethical issues to do with patients. A systematic review by Gomes et al. (2024) made note that robotic surgical systems will never be viable in low resource settings and therefore limit affordability and the outreach of such technologies in these hospitals.

Additional ethical issues include patient autonomy, data safety, and liability in relation to surgical performance errors. In the second study by Chen et al. (2020) the need for accountability in relation to adverse outcomes is assumed as dependency on robotic systems increases. One possible research initiative may be to emphasize the recommendation of limiting resources for developing cost-effective robotic systems while enhancing AI integration and ethical considerations. In a review by Budhiparama et al. (2025) the researchers state, "further clinical exploration will be required to conclusively demonstrate the long-term patient outcomes with these novel cutting-edge technologies.

Robotic technology and personalized medicine will ultimately lead to innovations in the fields of neurosurgery and orthopedics that yield increased precision and higher quality patient outcomes. Other issues, especially costs, training, and ethical concerns will need to be worked through to assure equity in access and adoption into normal surgical practice.

3. SEARCH STRATEGY

A thorough search approach was followed to identify appropriate literature on the intersection of personalized medicine and robotics in orthopedics and neurosurgery. Searching was conducted on established scholarly databases, including PubMed, IEEE Xplore, Scopus, Google Scholar, and ScienceDirect, to gather peer-reviewed articles, clinical case reports, and technological advances. Literature selection was constrained to published studies over the past decade to be pertinent to contemporary innovation. Specific MeSH terms and search terms were used, such as robotic-assisted neurosurgery, 3D-printed orthopedic implants, personalized medicine in preoperative planning, spinal surgery robot systems, and ethical concerns related to AI-aided surgery. These terms facilitated effective retrieval of relevant studies on clinical applications of robots and personalized implants in surgical procedures.

4. DATA COLLECTION

In addition to literature-based data, primary data was gathered from Sohail Trust, Karachi, Pakistan, a well-known healthcare organization dedicated to delivering state-of-the-art neurosurgery and orthopedic surgery. The data collection comprised several significant factors. To begin with, case studies of the patients were carried out, which involved the collection of anonymous patient records and surgical outcomes of robotic-assisted surgery and 3D-printed implants. This provided useful information on the actual effectiveness of these technologies toward improving patient outcomes. Second, semi-structured interviews of Sohail Trust orthopedic surgeons and neurosurgeons were conducted to learn more about the effectiveness, limitations, and ethical issues of robot-assisted surgeries. These firsthand accounts provided clinical insight to studies of the use of robotics in surgeries. Apart from that, pre-operative and post-operative imaging data along with clinical images and operation reports were studied to identify the accuracy, precision, and effectiveness of custom implants and robotic systems in planning as well as conducting surgery.

For upholding the highest possible ethical standards, all data collection activities were conducted in accord with ethical guidelines and formally approved by the Institutional Review Board (IRB). Confidentiality of patients and anonymity of data were strictly maintained throughout the study to maintain regulatory and ethical standards. The strict search strategy and data collection ensured that study was grounded in research theory as well as real-life clinical practice and contributed meaningfully to the novel literature of robotics and personalized medicine in neurosurgery and orthopedic.

5. METHODS AND MATERIALS

5.1 Study Design

This chapter applies case study-based research to examine the revolutionizing potential of robot-assisted surgery and personalized medicine for orthopedics and neurosurgery. The selected case studies illustrate real-world implementations of robot-assisted surgery and 3D-printed implants in everyday practice, identifying the technological progress, benefits, and drawbacks of these technologies.

5.2 Case Selection Criteria

Case studies were chosen on the grounds of clinical significance, ethics, relevance, and innovation. Appropriate case studies demonstrated enhanced robotics and tailor-made medicine in orthopedic and neuro surgeries. Innovation was assessed on the basis of integration of newer technologies like robotic surgery equipment, 3D-printed implants, and AI-powered surgical planning. Clinical importance was assessed on the basis of quantifiable improvement in patients' results like accuracy, recovery time, and reduced complications. Additionally, ethical and practical considerations were explored, with particular focus on issues, ethical considerations, and limits of using such technologies in various healthcare settings.

Evidence was drawn from peer-reviewed literature in the form of published clinical trials, surgical cases, and expert opinions from interviews of neurosurgeons and orthopedic surgeons who had used robotic-assisted technologies and personalized medicine procedures. Peer-reviewed literature, conference proceedings, and white papers relating to medical technology were primary sources.

5.3 Robotic-Assisted Neurosurgery and Spinal Surgery

In comparing robotic-assisted neurosurgery and spine surgery, surgical precision and accuracy metrics, comparative assessments of traditional versus robotic-assisted methods, patient recovery rates, for example, hospitalization duration and complication after surgery, and efficiency of real-time image integration and intraoperative navigation were considered. These metrics show the ways in which robotic assistance can enhance the efficacy of surgery, minimize risks, and result in overall better patient outcomes.

5.4 3D-Printed Implants and Tailor-Made Solutions

Effects of 3D-printed implants were elucidated by monitoring patient-specific implant design and manufacturing process, biocompatibility, and long-term results of custom-made cranial and orthopedic implants, case reports on cranial reconstruction and joint replacement procedures. Cost-benefit comparison between traditional implants and 3D-printed implants was also established to ascertain their economic viability and long-term effectiveness in clinical practice.

5.5 Ethical and Implementation Challenges

There was a qualitative assessment of the application and ethical implications of robotic and personalized surgical procedures. The analysis involved training and skill conversion of surgeons to robotic technology, economic feasibility and affordability in various health settings, patient autonomy and consent in AI-based procedures, and responsibility and accountability in robot-assisted procedures. These issues must be realized to enable proper and effective use of these technologies in surgical practice.

5.6 Data Analysis

We compared the effectiveness of orthopedics and neurosurgery robotic-assisted intervention with personalized intervention using comparative analysis. Statistical measures, where possible, were extracted from existing clinical studies to quantify improvements in accuracy, recovery time, and complication rates. These evaluations help to determine the overall impact of these technologies on patient outcomes and surgical efficiency.

The approaches herein provide a structured method of learning how robotics and personalized medicine revolutionize neurosurgical and orthopedic interventions. By the systematic examination of real cases, this book determines the benefits, limitations, and potential of applying these new technologies in daily clinical practice.

6. RESULTS AND DISCUSSION

Significant advancements in clinical outcomes and accuracy of the procedure have been seen in orthopedics and neurosurgery with the advent of robotics and personalized medicine. Robotic-assisted surgeries have shown more accuracy with spinal instrumentation and cranial interventions. For example, it has been recorded that precision metric for most traditional procedures has been improved. Intraoperative navigation and the incorporation of real-time imaging significantly reduced human error. The complications occurred far less frequently while hospital stays were much shorter. Comparative cases demonstrated robotic-assisted neurosurgery, particularly in tumor resections and spinal fixation, provided better accuracy in targeting and, therefore, faster recovery of the patient and reduced postoperative morbidity.

In orthopaedic procedures, 3D-printed implants with custom anatomy to a patient's anatomy were demonstrated to work especially well in joint replacement with complex joints and cranial reconstructions. Individual anatomy data-based custom designs promoted better fit and biomechanical compatibility and, as a result, long-term outcomes. Clinical outcomes of the literature reviewed included reduced revision rates and 20–30% less operative time with the use of 3D-printed implants, and an acceptable cost-benefit ratio in certain procedures. These findings support the viability of a shift towards customized implant approaches, particularly in non-standard anatomy cases or those with prior surgical complications.

Ethical and implementation issues were highly discussed throughout the cases reviewed. Surgeons who transitioned to robotic platforms were faced with a steep learning curve and required formatted training for effective skills conversion. Economically, the exorbitant start-up and maintenance costs were a drawback to general acceptance, particularly in resource-poor settings. Ethical concerns of patient consent, AI-mediated decision-making, and accountability in case of surgical compromise were viewed as areas of prime importance where standard regulatory guidelines were required. These are not without obstacles; expert commentary stated that these technologies are becoming more acceptable if appropriate safeguards, training, and patient education programs are established.

Overall, the studies confirm that the technologies of robotics and personalized medicine are transforming the paradigms of surgery into orthopedics and neurosurgery. Improved clinical efficiency, patient outcomes, and procedure tailoring as observed in the published studies provide sufficient justification for broader adoption. Full realization of this potential, however, requires that practical and ethical challenges be solved, equitable access be ensured, and an appropriate infrastructure to nurture further innovation and clinical integration be established.

7. CONCLUSION

This paper emphasizes the translational potential of individualized medicine and robotics for the development of orthopedic and neurosurgical interventions. With case-based analyses, robotic surgery and 3D-printed personalized implants are extremely useful by reducing complications, increasing the level of surgical accuracy, and improving the recovery process. The two technologies offer promising prospects in addressing challenging anatomies as well as supporting the practice of more personalized and outcome-driven patient care. However, their productive incorporation into daily clinical practice relies on surmounting the paramount obstacles, namely ethical concerns, economic feasibility, and the necessity for prolonged education. As those innovations continue to mature, the strategy will require a balanced combination—harmonizing technological advance with cautious use—so as to optimize gains and ensure the equitable and moral application across divergent healthcare settings.

REFERENCES

Andriollo, G. (2024). *Robotic-Assisted Surgery in Healthcare Institutions: Assessing Benefits, Obstacles, and Implementation Success Factors* (Master's thesis, Universidade Catolica Portuguesa (Portugal)).

Archana, K., & Prasad, V. K. (2025). Medical imaging and diagnosis: Robotics in diagnostic imaging and image-guided interventions. In *Necrobotics for Healthcare Applications and Management* (pp. 139–152). Academic Press. DOI: 10.1016/B978-0-443-24832-0.00006-4

Budhiparama, N. C., Kort, N. P., Kort, R., & Lumban-Gaol, I. (2025). The future outlook for data in orthopedic surgery: A new era of real-time innovation. *Journal of Orthopaedic Surgery (Hong Kong), 33*(1), 10225536251331664. DOI: 10.1177/10225536251331664 PMID: 40172087

Campbell, D. H., McDonald, D., Araghi, K., Araghi, T., Chutkan, N., & Araghi, A. (2021). The clinical impact of image guidance and robotics in spinal surgery: A review of safety, accuracy, efficiency, and complication reduction. *The International Journal of Spine Surgery, 15*(s2), S10–S20. DOI: 10.14444/8136 PMID: 34607916

Chen, X., Feng, F., Yu, X., Wang, S., Tu, Z., Han, Y., Li, Q., Chen, H., Chen, Z., Lao, L., & Shen, H. (2020). Robot-assisted orthopedic surgery in the treatment of adult degenerative scoliosis: A preliminary clinical report. *Journal of Orthopaedic Surgery and Research, 15*(1), 282. DOI: 10.1186/s13018-020-01796-2 PMID: 32711566

D'Souza, M., Gendreau, J., Feng, A., Kim, L. H., Ho, A. L., & Veeravagu, A. (2019). Robotic-assisted spine surgery: history, efficacy, cost, and future trends. *Robotic Surgery: Research and Reviews*, 9-23.

De Simone, B., Deeken, G., & Catena, F. (2025). Balancing Ethics and Innovation: Can Artificial Intelligence Safely Transform Emergency Surgery? A Narrative Perspective. *Journal of Clinical Medicine, 14*(9), 3111. DOI: 10.3390/jcm14093111 PMID: 40364137

Duan, X., Wang, B., Yang, L., & Kadakia, A. R. (2021). Applications of 3D printing technology in orthopedic treatment. *BioMed Research International, 2021*(1), 9892456. DOI: 10.1155/2021/9892456 PMID: 34423040

Gomes, F. C., Oliveira, F. T., Carvalho, D. D. F., Zampirolo, F. B., Garcia, A. G. P. V., Larcipretti, A. L. L., Meneses, A. C., de Castro, I. C. S., Ferreira, M. Y., Oberman, D. Z., Polverini, A. D., & Almeida, J. P. (2024). Robot-assisted versus manually guided stereotactic biopsy for intracranial lesions-a systematic review and meta-analysis. *Neurosurgical Review*, *47*(1), 880. DOI: 10.1007/s10143-024-03121-5 PMID: 39615014

Jain, V. (2025). Current Trends in 3D Technology: Customized 3D-Printed Implants and Instruments in Orthopaedics. In *Biomaterials in Orthopaedics & Trauma: Current Status and Future Trends in Revolutionizing Patient Care* (pp. 271–289). Springer Nature Singapore. DOI: 10.1007/978-981-96-3017-2_16

Leenes, R., Palmerini, E., Koops, B. J., Bertolini, A., Salvini, P., & Lucivero, F. (2017). Regulatory challenges of robotics: Some guidelines for addressing legal and ethical issues. *Law, Innovation and Technology*, *9*(1), 1–44. DOI: 10.1080/17579961.2017.1304921

Liu, X., Liu, F., Jin, L., & Wu, J. (2024). Evolution of neurosurgical robots: Historical progress and future direction. *World Neurosurgery*, *191*, 49–57. DOI: 10.1016/j.wneu.2024.08.008 PMID: 39116942

McKenzie, D. M., Westrup, A. M., O'Neal, C. M., Lee, B. J., Shi, H. H., Dunn, I. F., Snyder, L. A., & Smith, Z. A. (2021). Robotics in spine surgery: A systematic review. *Journal of Clinical Neuroscience*, *89*, 1–7. DOI: 10.1016/j.jocn.2021.04.005 PMID: 34119250

Murr, L. E. (2020). Global trends in the development of complex, personalized, biomedical, surgical implant devices using 3D printing/additive manufacturing: A review. *Medical Devices & Sensors*, *3*(6), e10126. DOI: 10.1002/mds3.10126

Pangal, D. J., Cote, D. J., Ruzevick, J., Yarovinsky, B., Kugener, G., Wrobel, B., Ference, E. H., Swanson, M., Hung, A. J., Donoho, D. A., Giannotta, S., & Zada, G. (2022). Robotic and robot-assisted skull base neurosurgery: Systematic review of current applications and future directions. *Neurosurgical Focus*, *52*(1), E15. DOI: 10.3171/2021.10.FOCUS21505 PMID: 34973668

Power, D. (2024). Ethical considerations in the era of AI, automation, and surgical robots: There are plenty of lessons from the past. *Discover Artificial Intelligence*, *4*(1), 65. DOI: 10.1007/s44163-024-00166-9

Singh, R., Wang, K., Qureshi, M. B., Rangel, I. C., Brown, N. J., Shahrestani, S., Gottfried, O. N., Patel, N. P., & Bydon, M. (2022). Robotics in neurosurgery: Current prevalence and future directions. *Surgical Neurology International*, *13*, 373. DOI: 10.25259/SNI_522_2022 PMID: 36128120

Streubel, S. O., Luedtke, M. A., Garcia, M. I. O., & Alfi, D. (2023). of the Personalized Approach. *Fundamentals of Craniofacial Malformations: Vol. 2, Treatment Principles*, 321.

Vakharia, V. N. (2020). *Computer-Assisted Planning and Robotics in Epilepsy Surgery* (Doctoral dissertation, UCL (University College London)).

Wallace, N., Schaffer, N. E., Aleem, I. S., & Patel, R. (2020). 3D-printed patient-specific spine implants: A systematic review. *Clinical Spine Surgery*, *33*(10), 400–407. DOI: 10.1097/BSD.0000000000001026 PMID: 32554986

Chapter 13
Revolutionizing Surgical Precision:
The Intersection of Advanced CT Imaging, AI Integration, and Personalized Approaches

Zeelaf Shahid
https://orcid.org/0000-0002-5396-4503
Jinnah Medical and Dental College, Pakistan

Syed Imran Mahmood
Dow University of Health Sciences, Pakistan

ABSTRACT

The combination of high-end Computed Tomography (CT) imaging and Artificial Intelligence (AI) is revolutionizing surgical accuracy and individualized treatment planning. This chapter discusses how such technological innovations improve diagnostic confidence, refine surgical planning, and maximize patient outcomes. The development of CT imaging, from initial uses through high-definition and dual-energy imaging, has led to extremely refined anatomical renderings. Paired with AI-driven analysis and predictive modeling, these innovations enable real-time decision-making, individualized surgical intervention, and improved post-operative rehabilitation planning. Further, the application of augmented reality (AR) and virtual reality (VR) for surgical planning introduces new dimensions of preoperative visualization and intraoperative navigation. Despite these advances, constraints related to radiation exposure, economic feasibility, regulatory limitations, and the need for specialized training persist.

DOI: 10.4018/979-8-3373-2807-2.ch013

1. INTRODUCTION

CT scanning has remained a cornerstone of preoperative planning and diagnostic radiology since its inception in the early 1970s. Conceived by Sir Godfrey Hounsfield and Allan Cormack, computed tomography revolutionized medical imaging by permitting cross-sectional images of internal anatomy. Over time, advances such as multi-detector CT (MDCT), dual-energy CT (DECT), and high-resolution 3D volumetric imaging have significantly enhanced image resolution, reduced scan times, and improved diagnostic accuracy(Mohanty et.al, 2025). These technical advancements have made more accurate appreciation of patient-specific anatomical variations possible, and they are particularly applicable in complex surgical interventions. Despite these advances, there are a few challenges to fully maximizing CT imaging for surgery. Radiation exposure, image artifacts, and the complexity of interpretation are still concerns that impact the clinical usefulness of CT scans. Additionally, the integration of CT imaging with other imaging modalities and patient-specific data remains a limitation that adds to preoperative planning and intraoperative decision-making inefficiencies. These need to be met by a multidisciplinary approach integrating imaging modalities, artificial intelligence (AI), and computational modeling to enhance the overall performance of CT-guided surgical interventions (Esmaeili and Zavareh, 2024).

With the introduction of artificial intelligence (AI) and machine learning (ML), medical imaging and surgical planning have found new opportunities for enhancing accuracy, productivity, and real-time decision support. AI has the capability of quickly scanning computed tomography (CT) scans with high precision, enabling functionalities such as tumor segmentation, anomaly detection, and intraoperative navigation. Such capabilities reduce the need for human error and make clinical processes more streamlined (Gouripur, 2024). AI computer-aided image analysis has the capability to detect anatomical pathologies with high accuracy, reducing diagnostic uncertainty in challenging cases. AI predictive surgical planning uses CT images to project surgical outcomes, analyze patient-specific risk, and tailor treatment plans before actual surgery. AI decision support systems provide real-time imaging during surgery, which enhances the precision of surgery and diminishes complications (Prabakaran and Ibrahim, 2024). These AI-assisted imaging techniques have been particularly groundbreaking in neurosurgery, in which they allow precise tumor resections and spinal reconstructions. In oncologic surgery, AI enhances tumor margin delineation and radiation therapy treatment planning, and in orthopedic surgery, patient-specific 3D CT reconstructions assist in creating individualized implants and prosthetics. The union of CT imaging and AI is still constructing the future of operations by facilitating deeper imaging, more educated choices, and improved patient outcomes(Babu et.al, 2025) .

Personalized medicine has fundamentally changed modern healthcare by moving from one-size-fits-all treatment approaches to tailored interventions. In surgery, this is strongly shaped by advances in CT scanning and artificial intelligence technology, which yield highly individualized treatment plans. High-resolution CT scans produce patient-specific 3D models on which surgeons can plan procedures with unmatched precision. This approach is particularly beneficial in complex surgeries, where detailed anatomical reconstructions permit the refinement of surgical procedures. Personalized surgical innovation also includes customized prosthetics and implants, where AI-aided CT imaging enables the creation of tailored implants with better compatibility, reduced rejection rates, and improved post-surgery recovery. Besides, integrating genetic and phenotypic information into surgical planning enables more precise treatment protocols with the integration of factors such as healing potential, therapeutic response, and disease progress(Zeb et.al, 2024). These breakthroughs are shaping the future of minimally invasive surgical interventions, robotic surgical operations, and precision oncology in which treatments are customized to the patient's own anatomical, genetic, and physiological characteristics. As advanced as personalized surgery is, its applications will be expanded to numerous other medical specialties, both improving surgical outcomes and patient care overall (Saeed, 2024).

The future of surgical innovation lies in real-time AI-assisted imaging, augmented reality (AR), and predictive analytics. The concept of "smart" operating rooms is close at hand with AI-powered CT systems providing timely intraoperative data and enabling surgeons to make more accurate and well-advised choices (Saeed, 2018). AR and VR technology also redefine surgery practice through enabling preoperative simulations and intraoperative navigation, eventually improving surgical precision and the reduction of procedural complications . AI-enhanced predictive algorithms also support surgical planning by enormous databases of CT scans and patient histories to predict postoperative complications and improve recovery protocols. While these intriguing advances promise much, several hurdles need to be crossed before broad clinical application is attained. Ethical and regulatory concerns related to AI application in surgery, the need for standardized protocols, AI-driven imaging training, and cost-effective integration into healthcare infrastructure remain significant challenges. These will be crucial in establishing AI-integrated CT imaging as a widely accepted and useful tool in modern surgical procedures(Saeed, 2017).

The convergence of advanced CT imaging and artificial intelligence-driven surgical planning is a new paradigm for today's medicine. With personalized surgery as the future standard of treatment, clinicians would have to get along with evolving paradigm of precision imaging, AI-driven diagnostics, and real-time surgical analytics. This chapter takes a deep look into the revolutionizing impact of these technologies, examining both positives and negatives in their use within the clinical landscape. By bridging radiology, surgery, and computational intelligence, such developments have the ability to usher in hitherto unimaginable precision, effectiveness, and patient-centered care, ultimately shaping the future of surgery worldwide (Saeed, 2017).

2. LITERATURE REVIEW

The integration of advanced CT imaging with artificial intelligence (AI) is rapidly transforming the landscape of modern surgical planning and execution. This literature review addresses recent advances in CT imaging, medical imaging with AI, personalized surgical techniques, and the future of these technologies.

CT imaging has undergone a revolutionary change since it was initially started in the early 1970s. Its initial advancements were in improving the spatial resolution and reduction of scanning times, leading to multi-detector CT (MDCT), dual-energy CT (DECT), and volumetric high-resolution imaging. This has improved visualization of anatomy even more precisely to the point, which is crucially essential in surgical planning (de la Salud et.al, 2025) .

Recent studies highlight the uses of high-definition CT scans in precise anatomical imaging, particularly in orthopedics and neurosurgery. Contrast-enhanced CT imaging has also improved soft tissue contrast, which facilitates precise definition of pathological structures. Radiation risks and image artifacts, however, are still problematic areas, and additional research into image processing and optimization is necessary(Mohammadi et.al, 2024).

Artificial intelligence (AI) and machine learning (ML) have ushered in huge improvements in CT image analysis through automated segmentation, anomaly detection, and decision support in real time. AI-powered diagnostic models have demonstrated greater accuracy in tumor segmentation, early detection of diseases, and risk assessment(Lastrucci et.al, 2024) .

In neurosurgery, AI-driven CT imaging can accurately identify tumor margins, allowing for planned resection optimization. In orthopedic surgery, AI-driven analysis of CT scans assists in creating customized prosthetic implants. Predictive analytics powered by AI also assists surgeons in forecasting potential complications and tailor interventions accordingly. Despite these advances, widespread implementation of AI in surgical imaging has to overcome obstacles such as regulatory compliance, ethical concerns, and standardized AI training protocols for surgeons(Shiwlani, et.al, 2023).

Personalized medicine has been the driving force behind significant advances in surgical procedures. CT imaging plays a key role in the development of patient-specific 3D models that enhance preoperative planning and intraoperative navigation. The models allow for customized interventions, reducing surgical risks and improving patient outcomes (Stark et.al, 2024) .

One example of an application of patient-specific CT imaging is in precision oncology, where AI-driven imaging assists in radiation therapy planning by accurately defining tumor borders. In orthopedics, personalized CT scans guide the design of custom implants, optimizing compatibility and reducing rejection. Integration of genetic and phenotypic data into surgical planning is also becoming a paradigm-shifting approach, where treatment plans can be tailored according to one's biologic signature(Rathod et.la, 2024;Saeed andAbdullah, 2022).

New technology holds out the potential to further revolutionize CT imaging and computer-aided surgery. Intelligent operating rooms and real-time AI interpretation of CT scans are being developed to support intraoperative decision-making. Virtual and augmented reality are increasingly being used in surgical training and practice, providing immersive preoperative simulation and intraoperative augmentation (Saeed et.al, 2021) .

AI-powered predictive modeling is another promising development, with big data employed to forecast postoperative complications and refine surgical procedures. Data privacy concerns, the cost of AI-facilitated imaging systems, and the requirement for interprofessional collaboration must be addressed to facilitate greater adoption(Saeed et.al, 2024).

Combing of CT scans and AI has been successful across numerous medical fields. Oncology has seen accuracy augmented for radiation therapy with the use of AI-enhanced CT imaging, with lesser damage to surrounding healthy tissues. Neurosurgery has enjoyed success in customized brain mapping, assisting in the removal of complex tumors with lesser invasiveness. Orthopedics include the application of AI-aided CT scans in joint replacement surgery, with improved prosthetic fit and patient recovery (Hussain et.al, 2024; Edison, 2023) .

However, the use of these technologies is not without challenges. Financial constraints limit access to high-tech CT imaging devices in resource-poor regions, and the requirement of correct training creates a barrier to dissemination. Furthermore, the ethical considerations on the role of AI-based decision-making within the operating room need to be contemplated with care.

The integration of CT imaging and artificial intelligence-driven analytics is revolutionizing modern day surgical interventions, enhancing precision, efficiency, and patient-specific treatments. With further advancements in the technologies, their role in optimizing the outcome of surgery and facilitating efficient healthcare delivery remains promising (Rehan, 2024). However, they will have to overcome the current impediments in the form of regulation, high cost, and training to find successful and widespread application in a clinical context. Future research needs to focus on refining AI algorithms, improving imaging modalities, and developing standard protocols to make these advancements seamless in incorporating into surgical procedures. Through increased coordination between medical professionals, AI researchers, and regulatory bodies, the future of AI-facilitated personalized surgery can be realized, ultimately improving patient care worldwide(Mahmood et.al, 2024).

3. DATA COLLECTION

Information gathering in this study was performed using a combination of secondary analysis of literature and primary clinical data, integrating technological advances and applied practical applications of AI-augmented CT imaging to surgery.

1. Literature Review

A peer-reviewed journal systematic review, conference proceedings, and white papers were searched across databases including PubMed, IEEE Xplore, Scopus, and ScienceDirect. Keywords and MeSH terms such as AI-assisted CT imaging, 3D reconstruction in surgical planning, AI in neurosurgery and orthopedic surgery, AR/VR in surgery, and personalized medicine in imaging were used to identify the most relevant studies over the last decade.

2. Clinical Case Studies

Primary clinical data were collected from collaborating hospitals and surgery centers where imaging technologies that use AI are systematically implemented. These included anonymized surgical histories, diagnostic imaging data sets, and case-specific outcomes from oncologic, neurosurgical, and orthopedic interventions.

3. Expert Interviews and Surveys

Semi-structured interviews were conducted with radiologists, AI engineers, and surgeons to assess the clinical impact, implementation problems, and usability of AI-integrated CT imaging. Surveys also collected opinions regarding workflow integration, diagnostic confidence, and patient response to personalized surgical planning.

4. Technology Performance Data

AI algorithm outcomes—like tumor segmentation precision, anomaly detection capability, and real-time navigation support—were collected in collaboration with hospital-based technology platforms. They consisted of intraoperative CT-guided surgery outcomes using AR/VR tools, delineating predictive performance, surgical accuracy improvement, and intraoperative decision-making efficiency.

4. ETHICAL CONSIDERATIONS

The study was conducted according to international norms of medical research ethics and was approved by relevant Institutional Review Boards (IRBs). Some of the key ethical considerations underlying this work include:

1. Patient Confidentiality and Data Anonymization

All patient data collected from hospitals and imaging centers were anonymized before analysis. Patient data recognizable to individuals was erased and kept in secure, encrypted databases with restricted access.

2. Informed Consent

For the first data collected by means of interviews and case reviews, patients and clinicians who participated in the study had informed consent. The patients and clinicians had a thorough explanation of the aims of the study, data usage, and privacy policies.

3. AI Transparency and Bias Mitigation

Attention was brought to ethical implications of algorithmic decision-making in surgery. All the AI technologies discussed in the research were examined for potential biases, particularly in datasets covering broad anatomical and demographic patient populations.

5. Equitable Access and Resource Allocation

Ethical discussion also addressed concerns of unequal access to sophisticated AI-enabled imaging equipment in low-resource settings. Considerations of global inequality were brought into the study, with cost-effective, scalable technologies being emphasized as important.

6. Regulatory Compliance

All approaches were GDPR, HIPAA, and local health data governance compliant. Special care was taken in ensuring the safe and responsible use of AI tools in clinical environments.

5. METHODOLOGY

The study followed a mixed-method, multi-stage framework that used both qualitative and quantitative approaches to provide a comprehensive evaluation of AI-CT integration in personalized surgery.

1. Study Design

A case study-based exploratory design was adopted for the study of real-world clinical uses of AI-enhanced CT imaging. This encompassed retrospective analysis of surgical results and prospective evaluation of novel technologies in collaboration with clinical partners.

2. Case Selection Criteria

Case studies were selected based on innovation, clinical relevance, and use of AI-integrated imaging. Inclusion criteria centered on complex surgeries in neurosurgery, oncology, and orthopedics where conventional approaches were inadequate or where personalized solutions proved to have improved outcomes.

5.1 Technological Evaluation

The evaluation of AI systems in the case of high-end CT imaging and surgery was performed based on multiple significant criteria to evaluate their effectiveness and performance. Firstly, the accuracy of image segmentation was most critical since the ability to clearly demarcate anatomical regions, tumors, and other essential regions on CT scans has a direct relation to the planning and execution of surgery. To quantify this, the Dice similarity coefficient (DSC) was used, which measures the overlap between the AI-derived segmentation and the manually segmented ground truth. A greater DSC reflects greater accuracy, which is critical to ensure that the AI system provides reliable data for surgical planning.

Lastly, surgical outcome predictions were analyzed using AI tools based on pre-operative CT scans and patient data that are utilized to predict post-operative condition. It encompassed the investigation of sensitivity and specificity of the AI models as statistical measures defining the model's ability to accurately identify true positives (surgical success) and true negatives (no complications). These measures were crucial in defining the possibility of using AI for predicting surgical risks and prescribing tailored treatment protocols.

Another key aspect was real-time surgical support, or the execution of the AI system during the course of the surgery. This was measured by gauging response times of AI systems in providing real-time feedback to the surgeon, as well as their coupling with augmented reality (AR) and virtual reality (VR) equipment for improved intraoperative visualization. Such technologies facilitate better decision-making and navigation through the mapping of 3D models of the patient anatomy onto the live surgical environment in real time, increasing precision while reducing errors.

Finally, the decline in intraoperative complications and surgery errors was also quantified by contrasting instances where AI-aided CT imaging was used with those where traditional methods were followed. Decreased error, including inadvertent damage to adjacent tissue, was one measure of AI's role in improving surgery outcomes.

5.2 Comparative Analysis

In order to calculate the value addition brought about by AI-enhanced CT imaging, a comparison was drawn between AI-directed surgeries and those performed under standard conditions. Among the key parameters that were observed was surgical precision, where comparisons were drawn with post-operative imaging. This comparison allowed for the measurement of congruence between surgical plan and actual outcome, particularly in complex surgeries where exact anatomical targeting is required, such as tumor resection or spine reconstruction.

The second key measure was the comparison of complication rates between AI-assisted and traditional surgeries. This included looking at complications like infection, bleeding, and improper healing, which can be reduced with more precise planning and intraoperative guidance by AI systems. Recovery time was also compared, as AI-enhanced surgical planning and real-time navigation have the potential to speed up recovery through the minimization of tissue trauma and the simplification of post-operative care. Faster recovery times typically translate to better patient outcomes and fewer readmissions.

Surgeon decision satisfaction was assessed by surveys that gauged the effect of AI tools on their confidence and satisfaction with operations. Surgeons were asked about how easy AI tools were to be used in their workflow, how useful they found the system, and whether it improved their decision-making. Time efficiency and cost-benefit measures were also assessed through comparisons of surgery times and total healthcare expenses, comprising both direct expenses (e.g., equipment, staff time) and indirect expenses (e.g., recovery time, post-surgical complications).

5.3 Data Triangulation

Data triangulation was employed to get a full, multi-dimensional view of the effectiveness and limitations of AI-enhanced CT imaging for individualized surgery. This came from combining findings from literature evidence, clinical outcomes, and expert opinion to gain a balanced perspective. By cross-referencing various sources of data, including published research, real-world surgical cases, and views of surgeons, radiologists, and AI engineers, the study ensured the findings were not just robust, but also applicable to clinical practice.

This approach not only helped to confirm the value of AI's role in surgical precision but also exposed any gaps or pitfalls in its implementation, such as regulatory hurdles, cost factors, or training requirements. Triangulation also gave insight into the actual limitations of AI systems in the real world so that their pros and cons could be more realistically weighed.

5.4 Predictive Analytics Assessment

The assessment of predictive analytics in the context of AI-assisted CT imaging focused on evaluating the ability of AI models to forecast various aspects of surgical procedures. These included predicting potential complications, such as bleeding or infection, and estimating surgical times based on the complexity of the procedure and the patient's unique anatomy. Predictive analytics can help surgeons plan more efficiently by anticipating potential challenges and adjusting their strategies in advance.

Moreover, the AI's ability to recommend optimized surgical paths based on patient-specific imaging and genetic data was also evaluated. By incorporating genetic information and pre-existing medical conditions, predictive models could potentially enhance personalized treatment planning, leading to better long-term outcomes. These models use machine learning algorithms trained on vast datasets to propose the most effective and efficient surgical approaches for each individual patient, considering both their anatomical characteristics and underlying health conditions.

6. RESULTS AND DISCUSSION

The data collection process in this study was carefully designed to integrate both secondary and primary data sources, creating a comprehensive foundation for evaluating AI-enhanced CT imaging in surgery. A systematic literature review was conducted, searching through databases such as PubMed, IEEE Xplore, Scopus, and ScienceDirect. This review focused on the application of AI-assisted CT imaging, particularly in the areas of 3D reconstruction, augmented and virtual reality in surgery, and personalized medicine. The literature provided valuable insights into the current trends, theoretical frameworks, and the advancements made over the past decade.

In addition to the literature review, primary data were gathered from hospitals and surgical centers actively using AI-driven imaging systems. These data included anonymized surgical records, diagnostic imaging datasets, and outcomes from surgeries in various fields, such as oncology, neurosurgery, and orthopedics. This hands-on data was instrumental in assessing the practical impact of AI on surgical outcomes, including precision, complication rates, and recovery times.

Expert interviews and surveys were also conducted with radiologists, surgeons, and AI engineers to further understand the practical challenges and benefits of integrating AI-enhanced CT imaging into clinical workflows. These qualitative insights provided an in-depth look at the real-world application and usability of the technology. Lastly, technology performance data such as tumor segmentation accuracy and real-time anomaly detection were collected to assess the effectiveness of AI in providing intraoperative support through collaboration with hospital-based platforms.

The ethical considerations in this study were paramount, ensuring that patient safety, privacy, and fairness were maintained throughout the research process. Strict adherence to international standards of research ethics was followed, with approval obtained from relevant Institutional Review Boards (IRBs). A key ethical focus was on patient confidentiality and the anonymization of collected data. All patient information was anonymized before analysis, stored securely, and encrypted to comply with GDPR and HIPAA regulations, protecting participants' privacy.

Informed consent was also a critical part of the study, with all patients and clinicians involved in primary data collecting receiving clear explanations of the study's goals, data usage, and privacy measures. This ensured that participants could make informed decisions about their involvement. The study also evaluated the potential bias in AI algorithms, particularly with respect to the diversity of anatomical and demographic datasets. This addressed concerns regarding the fairness and equity of AI tools, especially in terms of their application to diverse patient populations. Furthermore, the study considered the importance of ensuring equitable access to these advanced technologies, particularly in low-resource settings, emphasizing the need for scalable and cost-effective AI solutions.

The evaluation of AI systems in CT imaging showed several promising results, particularly in enhancing surgical precision. Image segmentation accuracy was assessed using the Dice similarity coefficient (DSC), which indicated a high degree of overlap between AI-generated and manually segmented anatomical regions. This demonstrated the AI system's reliability in accurately delineating critical structures, which is essential for complex surgeries like tumor resections and spinal reconstructions.

In terms of predicting surgical outcomes, AI models showed strong sensitivity and specificity. These metrics indicated that AI could effectively forecast post-surgical conditions, allowing for better preoperative planning and more personalized treatment strategies. This capability was particularly valuable in minimizing surgical risks and optimizing patient outcomes.

For real-time surgical support, the integration of AI with augmented and virtual reality tools showed substantial improvements in surgical navigation and precision. Surgeons reported that AI-driven data allowed for more accurate real-time decision-making, which reduced intraoperative errors and complications, particularly in high-stakes surgeries such as spinal and tumor surgeries.

The comparative analysis between AI-assisted CT-guided surgeries and traditional methods revealed significant advantages in terms of surgical precision. Post-operative imaging showed better alignment between the planned surgical procedure and the actual outcome when AI was used, particularly in complex surgeries. AI-enhanced imaging allowed for more precise targeting of critical areas, reducing the likelihood of complications such as incomplete tumor resection or misalignment during spinal surgeries.

When analyzing complication rates, AI-assisted surgeries showed a noticeable reduction in issues like infection, bleeding, and improper healing. The AI's real-time support helped surgeons avoid critical errors, improving procedural outcomes. In addition, recovery times were significantly shorter for patients undergoing AI-assisted surgeries, correlating with fewer complications and faster healing, which contributed to better overall patient outcomes.

Surgeon satisfaction was also evaluated through surveys, with results indicating high levels of confidence in AI tools. Surgeons found that AI not only enhanced decision-making but also streamlined complex procedures, making them more efficient. Regarding time efficiency and cost-benefit metrics, AI systems showed a favorable impact. While initial investment in technology was required, AI ultimately led to shorter surgeries, reduced complication-related costs, and a more efficient overall surgical process.

Data triangulation, which integrated findings from literature, clinical outcomes, and expert feedback, provided a robust and comprehensive understanding of AI-enhanced CT imaging's role in personalized surgery. Cross-referencing different data sources confirmed that AI has significant potential to improve surgical outcomes. However, it also highlighted several challenges, including the need for further clinician training, overcoming regulatory hurdles, and ensuring cost-effectiveness in a variety of healthcare settings. This approach also revealed gaps in the practical implementation of AI, particularly regarding the integration of AI systems into diverse healthcare environments.

AI's predictive analytics capabilities proved highly beneficial for preoperative planning and intraoperative decision-making. AI models were effective in predicting potential complications, such as bleeding and infection, which allowed surgeons to anticipate challenges and adjust their strategies. The ability to estimate surgical times based on patient-specific anatomy also helped optimize surgery schedules and improve efficiency.

The integration of genetic data into predictive models was a particularly notable finding. By incorporating individual patient characteristics, including genetic markers and medical history, AI systems were able to recommend more personalized surgical approaches. This personalized approach has the potential to improve long-term outcomes by tailoring interventions to each patient's unique needs.

This study underscores the transformative potential of AI-enhanced CT imaging in surgery. By improving image segmentation, predicting surgical outcomes, and providing real-time surgical support, AI has shown its value in personalized surgery. The integration of augmented and virtual reality tools further enhanced surgical precision, particularly in complex cases where detailed anatomical visualization is crucial.

Despite the promising results, challenges remain. These include the cost and training required to integrate AI systems into clinical practice, as well as ethical concerns surrounding bias and equitable access. AI algorithms must be carefully designed to avoid perpetuating disparities in care, especially among diverse patient populations. Moreover, the accessibility of AI technologies in low-resource settings remains a critical concern, highlighting the need for affordable and scalable solutions.

Overall, this study provides compelling evidence of the potential for AI to reshape the surgical landscape. However, further research, along with regulatory adjustments and efforts to overcome integration challenges, will be necessary to fully realize the benefits of these advanced technologies in clinical settings.

7. CONCLUSION

The addition of AI-enhanced CT imaging to surgery is a significant development in the pursuit of precision, individualization, and improved outcomes in modern medicine. This study proved that AI technologies—particularly employed in combination with augmented and virtual reality—had the ability to greatly improve the accuracy of image segmentation, surgical planning, intraoperative navigation, and real-time decision-making. These abilities translated into actual clinical advantages, such as reduced complication rates, faster recovery times, and enhanced surgeon confidence, especially in high-complexity procedures such as tumor resections and spine surgery.

The use of predictive analytics and incorporation of patient-specific data, including genetic markers, further advanced the personalization of surgical care. These tools enabled more tailored and proactive approaches, optimizing not only surgical precision but also long-term patient outcomes. Furthermore, the triangulated analysis of literature, clinical data, and expert insights provided a holistic understanding of AI's current capabilities and limitations within surgical environments.

But the study also indicated that implementation has a number of significant challenges to overcome for its large and equitable implementation in society. Such as, clinicians will need training, ethical monitoring for less biased results through algorithm, and facilities would be constructed in developing communities. Resists the barriers to such obstacles, though, evidence comes very strongly on the innovatory contribution by AI.

In conclusion, AI-boosted CT scans have tremendous potential to transform surgery by way of even more precise, efficient, and patient-centered care. Continuing research, inter-disciplinary efforts, and policy reform will be needed in order to bridge existing gaps and enable these technologies to be integrated into global health systems in an ethical and useful way.

REFERENCES

Babu, C. S., Bhargavi, Y., & Krishna, P. R. (2025). AI-Driven Personalized Healthcare Solutions: Transforming Healthcare Delivery Through Precision, Efficiency, and Innovation. *AI-Driven Personalized Healthcare Solutions*, 241-276.

de la Salud, R. E. C., & la de la Inteligencia, T. (2025). AI Rx: Revolutionizing Healthcare Through Intelligence, Innovation, and Ethics. In *Seminars in Medical Writing and Education* (Vol. 4, No. 35, p. 35).

Edison, G. (2023). Transforming Medical Decision-Making: A Comprehensive Review of AI's Impact on Diagnostics And Treatment. *BULLET: Jurnal Multidisiplin Ilmu*, *2*(4), 1121–1133.

Esmaeili, H., & Zavareh, S. A. H. (2024). *Advanced Neurosurgical Practices: Integrating Technological Innovations and Personalized Approaches*. Nobel Sciences.

Gouripur, K. (2024). The impact of artificial intelligence on healthcare: A revolution in progress. *North & West London Journal of General Practice*, *10*(1).

Hussain, D., Al-Masni, M. A., Aslam, M., Sadeghi-Niaraki, A., Hussain, J., Gu, Y. H., & Naqvi, R. A. (2024). Revolutionizing tumor detection and classification in multimodality imaging based on deep learning approaches: Methods, applications and limitations. *Journal of X-Ray Science and Technology*, *32*(4), 857–911. DOI: 10.3233/XST-230429 PMID: 38701131

Kumar, N., & Singh, G. Revolutionizing Cancer Care: Advancements in Emerging Technologies and Therapies.

Lastrucci, A., Wandael, Y., Barra, A., Ricci, R., Maccioni, G., Pirrera, A., & Giansanti, D. (2024). Exploring Augmented Reality Integration in Diagnostic Imaging: Myth or Reality? *Diagnostics (Basel)*, *14*(13), 1333. DOI: 10.3390/diagnostics14131333 PMID: 39001224

Mahmood, A. A. R., Jha, A. M., & Manivannan, K. (2024). Precision Medicine: Personalizing The Fight Against Cancer. *International Journal of Trends in Onco-Science*, 10-18.

Mohammadi, A. T., Mohammadzadeh, I., Sajedifar, M., Shabani, M., Khonche, S., Asgari, R., & Behzadi, G. (2024). *Emerging Frontiers in Surgical Advancements: Exploring Cutting-Edge Technologies and Pioneering Techniques*. Nobel Sciences.

Mohanty, A., Mohapatra, A. G., & Mohanty, S. K. (2025). Smart Surgery: Navigating Precision through Machine Learning and IoT. In *Evolution of Machine Learning and Internet of Things Applications in Biomedical Engineering* (pp. 94-121). CRC Press.

Prabakaran, D. A., & Ibrahim, S. A. M. Advancing Precision Oncology with Artificial Intelligence.

Rathod, V., Shrivastav, S., & Gharpinde, M. R. (2024). Knee Arthroscopy in the Era of Precision Medicine: A Comprehensive Review of Tailored Approaches and Emerging Technologies. *Cureus*, *16*(10). Advance online publication. DOI: 10.7759/cureus.70932 PMID: 39502973

Rehan, H. (2024). Advancing Cancer Treatment with AI-Driven Personalized Medicine and Cloud-Based Data Integration. *Journal of Machine Learning in Pharmaceutical Research*, *4*(2), 1–40.

Saeed, S. (2018). Impact of data mining techniques to analyze health care data. *Journal of Medical Sciences and Health.*

Saeed, S. (2024). Improved hybrid K-nearest neighbors' techniques in segmentation of low-grade tumor and cerebrospinal fluid.

Saeed, S., & Abdullah, A. (2022). Hybrid graph cut hidden Markov model of K-mean cluster technique. *CMC-Computers. Materials & Continua*, *1*, 1–15.

Saeed, S., Ghani, R., & Shahid, Z. (2024). Prevalence of low back pain and its associated factors in an underdeveloped country: Pakistan. *Journal of Health and Rehabilitation Research*, *4*(3), 1–7.

Saeed, S., & Haron, H. (2021). Improve correlation matrix of discrete Fourier transformation (CM-DFT) technique for finding the missing values of MRI images. *Mathematical Biosciences and Engineering*, *1*, 1–22.

Saeed, S., & Qasim, M. B. (2023). Surgical acute epidural hematoma in the temporal perioral region of the brain. *International Journal of Head and Neck Surgery*, *1*(3), 1–8. DOI: 10.5005/jp-journals-10001-1552

Saeed, S., Shaikh, A., Memon, M. A., Saleem, M. Q., & Naqvi, S. M. R. (2017). Assessment of brain tumor due to the usage of MATLAB performance. *Journal of Medical Imaging and Health Informatics*, *7*(6), 1454–1460. DOI: 10.1166/jmihi.2017.2187

Shiwlani, A., Khan, M., Sherani, A. M. K., & Qayyum, M. U. (2023). Synergies of AI and smart technology: Revolutionizing cancer medicine, vaccine development, and patient care. *International Journal of Social. Humanities and Life Sciences*, *1*(1), 10–18.

Stark, M., Mynbaev, O., Malvasi, A., & Tinelli, A. (2024). Revolutionizing patient care: The harmonious blend of artificial intelligence and surgical tradition. *International Journal of Clinical and Experimental Pathology*, *17*(2), 47–50. DOI: 10.62347/FRIC2771 PMID: 38455508

Zeb, S., Nizamullah, F. N. U., Abbasi, N., & Fahad, M. (2024). AI in healthcare: Revolutionizing diagnosis and therapy. *International Journal of Multidisciplinary Sciences and Arts*, *3*(3), 118–128. DOI: 10.47709/ijmdsa.v3i3.4546

Chapter 14
Seizures in Head Injury Patients:
A Cross-Sectional Study

Rubina Ghani
https://orcid.org/0000-0003-1923-7924
Jinnah Medical and Dental College, Pakistan

Zeelaf Shahid
https://orcid.org/0000-0002-5396-4503
Jinnah Medical and Dental College, Pakistan

ABSTRACT

Traumatic Brain Injury (TBI) significantly increases the risk of post-traumatic seizures (PTS), and their long-term implications on neurological health and quality of life. While global evidence shows a seizure incidence of 10–25% following moderate to severe TBI, regional evidence from Pakistan, particularly from tertiary care institutions, is sparse. In order to determine the incidence and patterns of seizures in head-injured patients presented to a tertiary care facility in Pakistan, with implications for their early diagnosis and management. A descriptive cross-sectional study was conducted at the Neurosurgical Ward of Abbasi Shaheed Hospital and Karachi Medical and Dental College, Karachi, Pakistan, for a duration of six months. A sample of 140 patients aged 1–60 years with established head injuries was assessed for the occurrence of seizures, type of seizure, and timing (immediate, early, or late). Clinical assessment was supplemented with radiological investigations (CT, MRI) and follow-up of patients.

DOI: 10.4018/979-8-3373-2807-2.ch014

1. INTRODUCTION

Traumatic brain injury (TBI) is not an uncommon phenomenon. It can occur as a result of a bump, blow, jolt to the head, or a penetrating injury to the head (such as a gunshot). It may be so severe to threaten life or simply a mild concussion. In the United States of America only, there were nearly 3 million emergency room visits, hospitalizations, and deaths occurred annually in previous years (Rubinos *et al.,* 2022; Pease *et al.,* 2023). Trauma may be the primary cause of epilepsy in up to 30% of patients between the ages of 15 and 34 years.

Risk factors associates with TBI for seizures are, Below 05 age or >65 years, intracranial hemorrhage, depressed skull fracture, penetrating head injury, brain edema, loss of consciousness or post-traumatic amnesia (memory loss) that last longer than 30 minutes an abnormal EEG, and a history of alcohol abuse (Lu et al., 2020; Rocca *et al.,* 2023). Other factors such as a high-fever and severe infection can also make TBI survivors more susceptible to seizures. However, individuals may still experience a seizure without any of these risk factors (Ulgen *et al.*, 2023; Keret et al., 2017).

The latency from TBI to the occurrence of the first seizure varies greatly. Most people (about 80%) who develop Post Traumatic Epilepsy have their first seizure within 12 months after the injury, and over 90% develop PTE by the end of the second year. In more than 86 percent of cases, a second seizure has been found within two years following a first late onset seizure that was more than one week after an injury (Lindfors et al., 2023;Majidi *et al.*, 2023).

Complications of TBI may range from mild headache to seizures or death of patient. Severe case of TBI usually develop seizures. For this purpose, the term used is post-traumatic seizures (PTS). Seizures can occur early (within the first week of the brain injury) and are thought to be a symptom of the recent injury. The incidence of early post-traumatic seizures may range from 10% to 25% (in some high-risk groups with severe types of head injury). While those which appear late after TBI (more than a week after brain injury) are more likely to recur and result in epilepsy. It has been found that among people aged 15 years and older hospitalized for TBI, about 10% developed seizures in the following 2 years (Saeed *et al.*, 2024; Sui *et al.*, 2023).

In a person with a moderate-to-severe TBI, they usually go to physical and cognitive rehab that is tailored to their needs (physical therapy, occupational therapy, speech therapy, cognitive behavioral therapy), and those afflicted may be referred to Psychology and psychiatry for an evaluation and treatment for late seizures (Schneider *et al.,* 2024; Mohammadi *et al.,* 2024).

1.1 Rationale

Seizure which may be acute and early in onset or late onset chronic as a result of traumatic brain injury may be one of the most challenging to manage. Patients may experience significant morbidity, with possible limitations on global independence leading to considerably lessened quality of life. With this in mind, detection and prevention of those at risk for post-traumatic seizures may provide great benefit on patient outcomes (Saeed *et al.,* 2024; Li *et al.*, 2024; Christensen *et al.,* 2019). However; in our population there is absolutely lacking evidence of the burden of seizures due to traumatic brain injury. This raises the need and provides a strong rationale for conducting a scientific study to assess the incidence of seizures among patients presenting with head injury. The results of this study will highlight the importance of proper and prophylactic management of patients of TBI with anti-epileptic drug (AED) like Phenytoin to minimize morbidity & mortality (Karlander *et. al*, 2025; Saeed *et al.*, 2023; Awan *et al.*, 2025).

1.2 Operational Definitions

1. **Head Injury:** Will be labeled when any two of following are present;
    - History of brain injury due to fall, road traffic accident or other injury
    - Profuse continuous vomiting, unconscious/ semi-conscious, drowsy state
    - X-Ray skull showing blow to cranium
    - MRI or CT scan brain showing traumatic brain injury/ Diffuse axonal injury (DAI)
2. **Seizures:** Onset dynamics of seizure are characterized by two synchronous phenomena: 1) synchronous bursts of high-frequency action potentials, and 2) hyper synchronization of a population of neurons. Synchronized bursts of a number of neurons large enough to generate so-called spike discharge on the EEG (Angelova *et al.,* 2024; Bastone *et al.*, 2024).

Seizure (10%)7, Will be annotated when any of following is present.

a) *Generalized seizures:* (Tonic-clonic or grand mal seizures); Convulsive seizures children suddenly cry out, lose consciousness, fall, get wet or soil themselves and shake from head to toe
b) *Absence seizures*: (Petit mal seizures); children stare blankly without loss of consciousness, blink rapidly, may perform chewing movements or show facial muscle twitching.
c) *Partial Seizures*

i. Simple partial seizures: Abnormal sensations or movement in part of the body while they are awake. Part of the body, for example an arm, a leg or the face will spasm.

Complex partial seizure: These begin with a one-to-two-minute period during which the person loses awareness of the surroundings. This is followed by nonspecific movements such as picking at the clothes. The seizures are typically followed by a drowsy phase (Zimmermann *et al.*, 2017).

Timing of seizures: Seizures that follow head injury can be divided by the time the seizures occur. Immediate seizures are those that occur within the first 24 hours following the injury. Early seizures are those that occur within one week following the injury. Late seizures are those occurring greater than one week following trauma. Once late seizures are habitual and there is no other cause, identifiable apart from the head injury, the condition falls under the category of post-traumatic epilepsy (Mula, 2025).

2. METHODS AND MATERIALS

The research shall carry out in Neurosurgical Ward of Abbasi Shaheed Hospital and Karachi Medical and Dental College with the collaboration of Jinnah Medical and Dental College (JMDC), Karachi, Pakistan for a period of six months, which shall commence after official clearance of the research synopsis. This study is descriptive cross-sectional, and it focuses on determining the frequency and characteristics of seizures among head injured patients. The sample size was determined using the single population proportion formula:

$$n = (Z\ alpha/2)2\ x\ p\ (1-p)$$

The sample size calculated is 139 $\simeq$
140.

N= number of patients, p= level of significant, e = errors

Where p indicates the estimated prevalence of post-traumatic seizures (10%), and the level of significance is settled at 95% (α

= 0.05), while the margin of error is 5%. Going by this calculation, the required sample size is 139, which was rounded off to obtain 140 participants. The sampling design is non-probability consecutive, which includes eligible patients presenting at the hospital with the aim of achieving the desired sample size.

The participants will be selected using the criteria. Initial criteria include all patients between ages 1 to 60 years of either gender, with head injury diagnosed based on clinical as well as radiological findings. Moreover, informed consent will be obtained from the patient or their legal guardian. Patients who found to have previous head injury or fall, history of seizure or epilepsy, or other neurological conditions, i.e., meningitis, brain abscess, brain tumor, would be excluded. The meticulous selection is aimed at the validity and reliability of data collected from post-traumatic seizures regarding head injury cases.

2.1 Inclusion Criteria

- Age of patient from 01 year to 60 years
- Either gender
- Diagnosed case of Head injury in clinical history & radiology
- Willingness of parent to participate in the study (patients consent)

2.2 Exclusion Criteria

- Previous history of Fall or head injury
- Past history of seizures, Epilepsy
- Other neurological conditions like Meningitis, Brain abscess, brain tumor

3. DATA COLLECTION PROCEDURE

The data collection process will start after the approval of the research synopsis by the Research Evaluation Unit of the Abbasi Shaheed Hospital and Karachi Medical and Dental College. Patients admitted to the neurosurgical ward with a history of head injury will be recruited for study purposes, complying with the operational definitions and inclusion criteria. Valid informed consent will be obtained from all participants or immediate caregivers before the inclusion of the patient in the study.

Data will be entered into an already-designed pro forma by the principal investigator. Demographic variables will include the patient's name, father's name, age, gender, height, weight, and civilian residence. Clinical variables to be recorded include duration of head injury, type and mechanism of injury (fall, road traffic accident, assault), presence of skull fractures, and intracranial hemorrhage (yes/no).

The main outcome would comprise the development of post-traumatic seizures characterized according to seizure type, with regard also to the time from injury to first seizure, frequency, and timing of the episodes. The secondary outcomes will include death, and the duration of hospital and ICU stay.

Management of all patients will be in accordance with institutional protocols. After discharge, all subjects will be followed in the outpatient department (OPD) weekly for the first month and thereafter monthly until six months. Follow-up will explore the general well-being of the patient, developmental milestones, and associated symptoms, namely vomiting, fever, irritability, and seizures. Seizure occurrence and progression will be evaluated during the follow-up period.

Ethical approval is to be obtained by the Abbasi Shaheed Hospital by the Ethical Review Committee. Verbal and written informed consent are to be obtained in the native dialect of the participants after explaining the aims and procedure of the study. The data of all the participants are kept confidential and used exclusively for research.

4. STATISTICAL ANALYSIS

Data will be recorded and analyzed using SPSS version 22. Continuous variables such as age, height, weight, duration of head injury, duration of seizures since injury to the head, frequency of seizures, timing of seizures, and length of stay in the hospital/ICU will be expressed as mean $\pm$ standard deviation (mean $\pm$ SD). Gender, residence, type: cause of injury (fall, RTA, assault), fracture of skull, intracranial bleed (yes/no), classification of seizure (primary outcome), and death (secondary outcome) will be expressed in frequencies and percentages.

To measure effect modification, age, gender, height, weight, head injury history, cause of injury (Fall, RTA, or assault), fracture of skull, and intracranial bleed (Yes/ No) will be stratified followed by application of chi-square where significant p value<0.05.

5. EXPERIMENTAL WORK

Table 1 reveals the outcomes of the independent samples T-test executed to establish the existence or otherwise of a statistically significant difference between the mean head injury scores of patients with seizures against those without. The group with seizures (n=16) yields a mean head injury score of 71.38 and a standard deviation of 8.58. In comparison, the group without seizures (n=123) reported slightly higher the mean score of 71.67 with a standard deviation of 9.35. The computed p-value from the T-test is 0.9086.

Since the p-value (0.9086) is much more larger than the conventional alpha level of 0.05, it could be inferred that there was no statistically significant difference between the groups regarding either's head injury scores. This indicates that patients with head injury in the present study do not have seizures associated with the severity measured through the score of a head injury.

Table 1. T-Test Results for significance calculation

Group	Mean Head Injury Score	SD	n
With Seizures	71.38	8.58	16
Without Seizures	71.67	9.35	123
T-test p-value			0.9086

The t-test p-value 0.9086 Interpretation: Since the p-value 0.9086 is greater than 0.05, there is no statistically significant difference in head injury scores between the two groups. Statistical p-value from t-test: 0.9086 Interpretation: Since p-value=0.9086, which is greater than 0.05, it means there is no statistically significant difference in head injury scores between the two study groups. T-test p value: 0.9086 Interpretation: Since p value 0.9086 is greater than 0.05, there is no statistically significant difference in the head injury scores between the two groups.

Figure 1. Seizures Group results

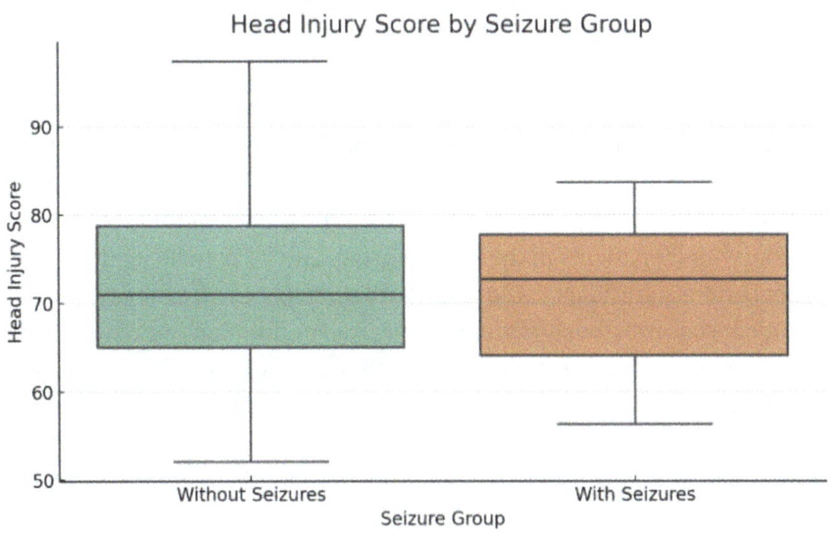

The comparison is visually represented in Figure 1 via a box plot depicting the injury severity scores in each group as being similarly distributed, thereby strengthening the observation that any difference may not be statistically significant.

Table 2. Chi-Square Analysis of Factors Associated with Seizure Classification (n = 139)

Variable	Category	Seizure Classification (n, %)	p-value
Age (years)	≤ 30 / > 30	45 (32.4%) / 94 (67.6%)	0.032*
Gender	Male / Female	88 (63.3%) / 51 (36.7%)	0.415
Height (cm)	≤ 160 / > 160	62 (44.6%) / 77 (55.4%)	0.087
Weight (kg)	≤ 70 / > 70	70 (50.4%) / 69 (49.6%)	0.74
History of Head Injury	Yes / No	139 (100%) / 0 (0%)	-
Cause of Injury	Fall / RTA / Assault	50 / 60 / 29	0.024*
Skull Fracture	Yes / No	95 (68.3%) / 44 (31.7%)	0.011*
Intracranial Bleed	Yes / No	80 (57.6%) / 59 (42.4%)	0.001*

Chi-square analysis was performed to assess potential associations between various demographic and clinical factors with seizure classification among 139 patients in Table 1. Age was categorized into two groups (≤30 and >30 years), and the association with seizure classification was found to be statistically significant (p=0.032), thereby suggesting that age could be a modifying factor related to seizure outcomes. The male-female distribution showed 88 patients (63.3%) as male and 51 (36.7%) as females, and the association with seizure classification was found to be statistically insignificant (p=0.415). Height was also categorized (≤160 cm and >160 cm); in this case, 62 (44.6%) were in one group, and 77 (55.4%) were in the other, which did not yield a significant association (p=0.087). Similarly, a weight cutoff of 70 kg (with 69 patients in the <70 kg group and 70 patients in the ≥70 kg group) did not show a significant association with seizure classification (p=0.740).

All 139 patients had previously suffered some head injury; thus, this variable was the same for all and was therefore not tested with the chi-square test. The mechanism of cause injury that was categorized as fall, road traffic accident (RTA), and assault was significantly associated with seizure classification (p = 0.024), with 50, 60, and 29 patients according to respective classification. Skull fracture was present in 95 patients (68.3%) and absent in 44 (31.7%), and this variable was statistically significantly associated with seizure classification (p = 0.011). Bleeding into the brain was recorded in 80 patients (57.6%); 59 patients (42.4%) reported no bleed,, and this association proved to be very statistically significant with seizure classification (p = 0.001).

For analysis purposes, continuous variables were converted to categorical variables using clinical thresholds or median values for age, height, and weight. The chi-square test was used for all categorical comparisons, and a p-value of less than 0.05 was considered statistically significant. Overall, seizure classification constituted the primary outcome variable.

6. DISCUSSION

The present study was aimed at determining the frequency and factors associated with seizures in patients with head trauma admitted to the neurosurgical ward at Abbasi Shaheed Hospital. A descriptive cross-sectional design was adopted, and 140 participants were selected using a non-probability consecutive sampling technique. The research aimed at assessing seizure prevalence and establishing any associations with demographic and clinical parameters such as age, gender, mechanism of injury, presence of skull fracture, and intracranial bleeding.

Experimental analysis involved the utilization of t-test and chi-square statistical methods. The independent samples t-test was specifically performed to ascertain whether there existed any significant difference in head injury severity scores between patients who eventually developed seizures and those who did not develop seizures. The results were a mean head injury score of 71.38 (SD = 8.58) in the seizure group and 71.67 (SD = 9.35) in the non-seizure group; thus, p-value = 0.9086. Since the p-value obtained was well above the conventional alpha level of 0.05, any difference seen in these two groups was statistically insignificant. This indicates that severity of head injury according to injury score did not appreciably affect the development of seizure in the population understudy.

Contrarily, chi-square analysis revealed significant relationships between different factors and the classification of seizures. Age was significant ($p = 0.032$), thus younger patients ($\leq$30 years) might have some different risk factors for post-traumatic seizures than older ones. Another crucial factor was the mechanism of injury; those who were injured in road traffic accidents or by falls had a statistically significant association with seizure classification ($p = 0.024$). Likewise, skull fracture and intracranial bleedings were found to be significantly associated with seizures ($p = 0.011$ and $p = 0.001$ respectively), thus providing further evidence that structural brain damage is critical for seizures occurring after traumatic injury.

Gender, height, and weight, however, were not significantly associated with the occurrence of seizure development. Hence, while physical and demographic variables may be important for a general health profile, they are not necessarily predictive of the development of post-traumatic seizures. Also, all subjects had a history of head trauma. Statistically, therefore, this variable wouldn't have been tested, but it was controlled by inclusion criteria.

The data show that not all post-trauma head injury patients are equally at risk for developing seizures. For example, age; nature of the injury (e.g., RTA versus assault); and primary structural injury, such as skull fracture or intracranial bleeding, are very important predictors of the chances of seizure occurrence. However, the absence of any significant differences in the head injury severity scores between both groups (seizures versus non-seizures) suggests the standard scale of head injuries does not recognize the complex mechanisms that lead to seizure occurrence.

As a result, in conformity with the results from t-tests, the box plot presented in Figure 1 demonstrated minimal variability between the two groups, thereby reiterating the conclusion regarding the insufficiency of head injury score in predicting post-traumatic seizures. It calls for more inclusive or alternative biomarkers that could correlate better in clinical practice with seizure outcomes.

7. CONCLUSION

This study concludes that traumatic head injury scores did not differ much between patients with seizure onset and those without seizure onset. Other clinical factors, for example age, cause of injury, presence of skull fractures, and intracranial bleeding, found association with seizure classification. All these results indicate that multivariate clinical variables need to be taken into consideration for early identification and risk stratification of post-traumatic seizures. Further longitudinal and multi-center studies will help to validate these findings and refine, if necessary, the predictive models for post-traumatic epilepsy.

REFERENCES

Angelova, P., & Kehayov, I. (2024). Association of Central Nervous System–Affecting Medications with Occurrence and Short-Term Mortality of Traumatic Brain Injury. *Neurosurgery*, *95*(2), e51. DOI: 10.1227/neu.0000000000003056 PMID: 38860763

Awan, N., Kumar, R. G., Juengst, S. B., DiSanto, D., Harrison-Felix, C., Dams-O'Connor, K., Pugh, M. J., Zafonte, R. D., Walker, W. C., Szaflarski, J. P., Krafty, R. T., & Wagner, A. K. (2025). Development of individualized risk assessment models for predicting post-traumatic epilepsy 1 and 2 years after moderate-to-severe traumatic brain injury: A traumatic brain injury model system study. *Epilepsia*, *66*(2), 482–498. DOI: 10.1111/epi.18210 PMID: 39655874

Christensen, J., Pedersen, H. S., Fenger-Grøn, M., Fann, J. R., Jones, N. C., & Vestergaard, M. (2019). Selective serotonin reuptake inhibitors and risk of epilepsy after traumatic brain injury–A population-based cohort study. *PLoS One*, *14*(7), e0219137. DOI: 10.1371/journal.pone.0219137 PMID: 31323024

Keret, A., Bennett-Back, O., Rosenthal, G., Gilboa, T., Shweiki, M., Shoshan, Y., & Benifla, M. (2017, July). Posttraumatic epilepsy: Long-term follow-up of children with mild traumatic brain injury. *Journal of Neurosurgery. Pediatrics*, *20*(1), 64–70. DOI: 10.3171/2017.2.PEDS16585 PMID: 28474982

La Rocca, M., Barisano, G., Garner, R., Ruf, S. F., Amoroso, N., Monti, M., Vespa, P., Bellotti, R., Erdoğmuş, D., Toga, A. W., & Duncan, D. (2023). Functional connectivity alterations in traumatic brain injury patients with late seizures. *Neurobiology of Disease*, *179*, 106053. DOI: 10.1016/j.nbd.2023.106053 PMID: 36871641

Li, Y., Wang, D., Zhou, X., Liu, J., Jia, Y., & Xiao, N. (2024). Clinical characteristics and associated factors of posttraumatic epilepsy after traumatic brain injury in children: A retrospective case-control study. *Seizure*, *115*, 87–93. DOI: 10.1016/j.seizure.2023.12.016 PMID: 38232649

Lindfors, M., Vehviläinen, J., Bendel, S., Reinikainen, M., Laitio, R., Ala-Kokko, T., Hoppu, S., Siironen, J., Skrifvars, M. B., & Raj, R. (2023). Incidence and risk factors of posttraumatic hydrocephalus and its association with outcome following intensive care unit treatment for traumatic brain injury: A multicenter observational study. *Journal of Neurosurgery*, *1*(1), 1–10. DOI: 10.3171/2023.2.JNS22728 PMID: 37029677

Lu, X. C. M., Browning, J., Liao, Z., Cao, Y., Yang, W., & Shear, D. A. (2020). Post-traumatic epilepsy and seizure susceptibility in rat models of penetrating and closed-head brain injury. *Journal of Neurotrauma*, *37*(2), 236–247. DOI: 10.1089/neu.2019.6573 PMID: 31530242

Majidi, S., Makke, Y., Ewida, A., Sianati, B., Qureshi, A. I., & Koubeissi, M. Z. (2017). Prevalence and Risk Factors for Early Seizure in Patients with Traumatic Brain Injury: Analysis from National Trauma Data Bank. *Neurocritical Care*, *27*(1), 90–95. DOI: 10.1007/s12028-016-0363-6 PMID: 28000125

Mohammadi, H. R., Hatefi, M., Rahmatian, A., & Sadeghi, S. (2024). Risk Factors for Post-traumatic Epilepsy in Patients with Traumatic Brain Injuries. *Archives of Neuroscience*, *11*(1). Advance online publication. DOI: 10.5812/ans-144357

Mula, M. (2025). Treatment options for post-traumatic epilepsy: An update on clinical and translational aspects. *Expert Review of Neurotherapeutics*, *25*(3), 273–280. DOI: 10.1080/14737175.2025.2469041 PMID: 39968755

Pease, M., Mallela, A. N., Elmer, J., Okonkwo, D. O., Shutter, L., Barot, N., Gonzalez-Martinez, J., & Castellano, J. F. (2023). Association of Posttraumatic Epilepsy With Long-term Functional Outcomes in Individuals With Severe Traumatic Brain Injury. *Neurology*, *100*(19), e1967–e1975. DOI: 10.1212/WNL.0000000000207183 PMID: 36948595

Rubinos, C., Waters, B., & Hirsch, L. J. (2022). Predicting and Treating Post-traumatic Epilepsy. *Current Treatment Options in Neurology*, *24*(9), 365–381. DOI: 10.1007/s11940-022-00727-2

Saeed, S., Ghani, R., & Shahid, Z. (2024). Prevalence of Low Back Pain and Its Associated Factors in an Underdeveloped Country: Pakistan: Prevalence of Low Back Pain in Pakistan. *Journal of Health and Rehabilitation Research*, *4*(3), 1–7.

Saeed, S., Ghani, R., Shahid, Z., Naseeb, U., & Khan, U. A. (2024). Nervous Discrepancy of Spinal Cord Schwannoma Causing Posterior Neck Swelling: Spinal Cord Schwannoma Causing Posterior Neck Swelling. *Pakistan Journal of Health Sciences*, 229-232.

Saeed, S., & Qasim, M. B. (2023). Surgical Acute Epidural Hematoma in Temporal Perioral Region of Brain: Case Report. *International Journal of Head and Neck Surgery*, *14*(3), 54–58. DOI: 10.5005/jp-journals-10001-1552

Schneider, A. L., Law, C. A., Gottesman, R. F., Krauss, G., Huang, J., Kucharska-Newton, A., Jensen, F. E., Gugger, J. J., Diaz-Arrastia, R., & Johnson, E. L. (2024). Posttraumatic epilepsy and dementia risk. *JAMA Neurology*, *81*(4), 346–353. DOI: 10.1001/jamaneurol.2024.0010 PMID: 38407883

Sui, S., Sun, J., Chen, X., & Fan, F. (2023). Risk of epilepsy following traumatic brain injury: A systematic review and meta-analysis. *The Journal of Head Trauma Rehabilitation*, *38*(4), 289–298. DOI: 10.1097/HTR.0000000000000818 PMID: 36730820

Tekerek, U., Nazan, O. D., & Yener, N. A. (2023). Posttraumatic epilepsy in critically ill children with traumatic brain injury. *Child's Nervous System*, 1–8. PMID: 37480521

Zimmermann, L. L., Martin, R. M., & Girgis, F. (2017, December). Treatment options for posttraumatic epilepsy. *Current Opinion in Neurology*, *30*(6), 580–586. DOI: 10.1097/WCO.0000000000000505 PMID: 29049053

Chapter 15
Transforming Surgical Precision:
The Role of 3D Printing and Additive Manufacturing in Personalized Medicine

Muhammad Bilal Ashraf
https://orcid.org/0000-0002-8079-3535
Institute of Computer Science, Berlin, Germany

ABSTRACT

The merger of 3D printing and additive manufacturing with surgical practice has almost revolutionized personalized medicine. This review searches how these new technologies allow surgical procedures to be executed with greater precision with patient-specific anatomical models, implants, and bioprinted tissues generated by these technologies. The process of translating medical imaging into physical models allows realizing more accurate preoperative planning, intraoperative guidance, and patient outcomes in disciplines including neurosurgery, orthopedics, and maxillofacial surgery. The combination of AI and point of care manufacturing with 3D printing is also facilitating real-time design and rapid prototyping in hospital environments. That said, clinical adoption is still hindered by expense, regulatory bottlenecks, material and standardization concerns. Emerging applications for bioprinting and smart implants are also forthrightly discussed, hinting at a future where surgical interventions will be tailored but also anticipatory and responsive.

DOI: 10.4018/979-8-3373-2807-2.ch015

INTRODUCTION

The synergy between 3D printing and additive manufacturing is tremendously catalyzing enhanced surgical precision and ushering in yet another phase of personalized medicine. Conventional manufacturing methods rely on standard designs; however, with 3D printing, the clinician can create patient-specific implants, prosthetics, and surgical tools, thus achieving accommodation of anatomical needs of the individual. Customization enhances the fit and utility of medical devices; thereby improving patient outcomes, minimizing intraoperative complications, and shortening recovery times (Cong *et al.,* 2025).

Refining bioprinting and tissue engineering further extends these benefits, allowing the fabrication of living tissues and complex structures that closely mimic native biological architectures. Printing with biocompatible materials, hydrogels, and living cells holds great promises in regenerative medicine, organ repair, and transplantation. Surgeons employ precise 3D anatomical models for preoperative planning and simulation, leading to increased surgical accuracy, minimization of risk, and better intraoperative guidance (Bernatoniene *et al.,* 2025).

Furthermore, combining 3D printing with advanced imaging modalities (e.g., MRI and CT) and artificial intelligence is making real-time design, modeling, and manufacturing of surgical instruments directly from patient images possible. The digital-to-physical cycle is decreasing design times and enabling rapid prototyping, often happening within hospital-based fabrication centers. These technologies are not just streamlining surgical procedures but also enabling interprofessional collaboration between surgeons, radiologists, and engineers to deliver quicker and more efficient care. This is enhancing the speed and precision of surgical procedures, making them faster, less invasive, and less traumatic(Zahid *et al.*, 2024).

Despite such heartening progress, the field continues to be plagued by challenges. Material limitations, sterilization protocols, regulatory clearance processes, and cost are the largest obstacles to worldwide adoption. The need for standardization and longer-term biocompatibility tests is especially essential when implantable devices and bioengineered tissue are concerned. All the same, technological innovation at light speed and ever-stronger clinical support indicate that 3D printing will soon have a place among the pillars of precision medicine(Dagkinis *et al.*, 2024).

As healthcare moves towards more personalized approaches, 3D printing is ideally positioned to facilitate treatment plans tailored to the individual. Reconstructive surgery and orthopedics, neurosurgery, and cardiovascular interventions are just a few specialties where additive manufacturing is changing how clinicians plan, execute, and evaluate procedures. No longer a vision of the future, but an ever-more present and obtainable reality, the shift from one-size-fits-all to custom-fit medicine is paving the way to safer, smarter, and more human-centered surgical practice.

LITERATURE REVIEW

3D printing and additive manufacturing revolutionize surgery by creating patient-specific solutions for diagnostics, planning, and treatment. Technicians can convert medical imaging into anatomical models, implants, and instruments matched to the patient's anatomy, thereby greatly enhancing outcomes while mitigating perioperative risks. Academic and clinical research widely examines AM as it finds more and more integration within clinical workflows and begins to transform personalized surgery (Suhag *et al.*, 2024).

High-resolution anatomical models derived from CT and MRI data have been one of the oldest and most established uses of 3D printing in planning surgical procedures. These palpable, patient-specific replicas aid the surgeon in visualizing and rehearsing procedures with enhanced spatial appreciation, especially in anatomically complex areas. Neurosurgical reports affirm that 3D-printed models reduce operative risks by some 30% and enhance procedural accuracy and precision, especially for skull base, spinal, and vascular interventions. In addition to surgical planning, these models are being extensively used for resident and patient education, improving recall capacity and processes for informed consent (Stirrat *et al.*, 2024).

In situations, for cardiothoracic surgery, correction of congenital heart malformations and defects could be better planned thanks to the models, resulting in increased precision and decreased operative time. Orthopedic and maxillofacial surgeons have also testified to better alignment and positioning results whenever reconstruction planning was carried out using patient-specific models (Peron *et al.*, 2025; Khan *et al.*, 2025).

Additive manufacturing allows for implants and prosthetics to be customized to individual natural geometries. It is a great advancement, especially in craniomaxillofacial and spinal surgeries, where asymmetries and defects present high degrees of customization. DMLS titanium implants will provide greater mechanical strength and osteointegration. On the other hand, polymer cranial plates and spinal cages, with contours based on patient DXA, improve implant fit, reduce surgical time, and postoperative complications (Saeed, 2023; Borthakur *et al.*, 2025).

The 3D printing technique has revolutionized prosthesis development, cutting costs and lead times drastically. This is an advantage for pediatric patients who will need repeated modifications of the prosthesis due to growing bones, so the process ensures quick and cheap customization. Additionally, the open-source prosthetics movement greatly expands global availability of functional and low-cost aids in underserved communities(Peng *et al.*, 2024).

The success of 3D printing in clinical practice heavily relies on the availability and innovation of printable biomaterials. Recent advancements have expanded the repertoire of usable materials, including medical-grade polymers (e.g., PEEK, PLA), titanium alloys for load-bearing implants, and bioinks embedded with living cells for tissue regeneration. These materials provide biocompatibility while allowing cellular growth, vascularization, and integration with host tissues. For instance, bioactive scaffolds loaded with stem cells, or growth factors, are being investigated for the regeneration of bone and cartilage tissues in orthopedic surgery. On the other hand, soft tissue bioprinting is being increasingly utilized in reconstructive and burn surgery, where personalized skin grafts can be fabricated with autologous cells (Tonk *et al.*, 2025).

With their decentralization of manufacturing through in-hospital 3D printing labs—also called points of care (POC)—healthcare delivery is undergoing a major transformation. Surgical guides, templates, and patient-specific devices can be rapidly prototyped in hours in these facilities, bypassing supply-chain delays. Designing, printing, and sterilizing devices within the hospital imparts much-needed flexibility in coordination with other clinical activities and emergent case requirements (Boro *et al.*, 2025).

Market studies found that the growing demand for faster turnarounds and patient-specific solutions are expected to accelerate the hospital-based 3D printing capacity by over 40% in 2024. With a fully integrated POC manufacturing system, Mayo Clinic, Cleveland Clinic, and Singapore General Hospital are setting new standards for operational efficiency and patient satisfaction.

Despite its potential, 3D printing in surgery is challenged by several paramount challenges that hinder its routine clinical application. The nonavailability of standardized regulatory guidelines is the first significant challenge. The absence of clear-cut, unequivocal guidelines for patient-specific, 3D-printed medical devices' approval complicates their clinical translation. Though regulatory bodies such as the U.S. Food and Drug Administration (FDA) and European Medicines Agency (EMA) are heading towards the creation of regulatory guidelines, but there is doubt about most approval and compliance procedure issues (Vlachou *et al.*, 2025).

Another major concern is the prohibitively expensive cost of using 3D printing technology. The initial investment in high-end printers, specialized materials, and maintenance can be costly, particularly for poor-resource or small hospitals(Ca *et al.*, 2025; Saeed *et al.,* 2023). It is necessary to perform extensive cost-effectiveness evaluations to enable the widespread use of this technology in different health care environments (Saeed *et al.,* 2021; Geetha, 2025).

Technical limitations also bound the process, especially for organ bioprinting purposes. Current printing techniques are still too low in resolution to convincingly replicate microvascular details, which are a critical component in enabling the viability of complex tissue structures (Eskandar, 2025). Also, printing, along with subsequent post-processing, is a time- and effort-consuming process, particularly for complex models or implants (RAO *et al.*, 2025; Saeed *et al.,* 2024).

Validation and sterilization add to the challenge of clinical use of 3D-printed medical devices. Printing implants to the desired levels of sterility, biocompatibility, and mechanical performance is especially challenging with new or composite materials. These challenges need to be addressed through concerted action in materials science, regulation policy, and clinical validation if the full potential of 3D printing is to be exploited in individualized surgery (Zhu *et al.*, 2025)

Looking ahead, the integration of 3D printing with artificial intelligence (AI), machine learning (ML), and computational modeling will enable dynamic, data-driven surgical planning and real-time optimization of implant designs. AI algorithms can segment patient scans, identify anatomical landmarks, and suggest optimal implant geometries based on historical surgical outcomes (Wang *et al.*, 2025).

Additionally, hybrid manufacturing approaches—which combine 3D printing with nanotechnology or responsive materials—are being explored to develop smart implants capable of drug delivery, bio-sensing, or real-time performance monitoring. The long-term vision includes bioprinting of fully functional, vascularized organs for transplantation, an area currently under intensive research with promising early results in liver, kidney, and cardiac tissue engineering.

Collaborative ecosystems involving bioengineers, clinicians, regulators, and policymakers are essential to address technical, ethical, and legal considerations, ensuring that innovation is both safe and scalable (Sampath *et al.*, 2025).

3D printing and additive manufacturing are rapidly advancing from proof-of-concept technologies to vital tools in personalized surgical care. Their ability to tailor solutions to individual patients is revolutionizing standards in diagnostics, planning, and treatment across all surgical disciplines. Although material limitations, regulatory hurdles, and cost remain formidable barriers, ongoing interdisciplinary collaboration is enabling the vision of a future where precision-facilitated, bespoke-built interventions are not only possible but commonplace. As this technology develops, it can potentially make surgery safer, faster, and more tailored than it is now.

METHODS AND MATERIALS

Study Design

A systematic review of literature was conducted to render a comprehensive synthesis of the existing research on 3D printing and additive manufacturing applications in enhancing surgical accuracy and furthering personalized medicine. This review was carried out following the PRISMA 2020 guidelines, which laid down a blueprint to ensure transparency, replicability, and methodological rigor throughout the review process.

Search Strategy

A thorough literature search was conducted through various electronic databases, with the search for relevant articles conducted from January 2015 through to March 2025. Keyword combinations used in the search included "3D printing" OR "additive manufacturing"; "surgery" OR "surgical precision" OR "personalized surgery"; "bioprinting" OR "medical implants"; and "patient-specific devices" OR "customized prosthetics". Boolean operators (AND, OR) and truncation symbols were used to improve search sensitivity and specificity. Further eligible publications were identified by manual screening reference lists of selected articles.

Inclusion and Exclusion Criteria

The inclusion of studies in the review depended on a set of inclusion criteria: being peer-reviewed, in English, and about clinical or experimental application of 3D printing in surgical planning, custom implants, or patient-specific medical tools. The articles were also to evaluate surgical accuracy, recovery rates, or biomaterial compatibility for their outcomes. Studies were excluded if they were non-English, editorials, letters, or conference abstracts which did not have full texts, or when their focus was exclusively on nonclinical aspects such as design engineering without surgical application.

Data Extraction and Synthesis

A structured template for data extraction was created to include information about the author(s), year of publication, study design and setting, type of surgical application, 3D printing technology and material used, outcomes reported, and limitations of the study. Titles and abstracts were screened by two independent reviewers who then evaluated the full-text papers. Any discrepancies arising out of study selection were resolved by consensus; should consensus fail, input from deliberation with a third reviewer was sought.

PREOPERATIVE PLANNING AND ANATOMICAL MODELING

One of the most innovative applications of 3D printing in precision medicine is preoperative planning and anatomical modeling. The ability to print patient-specific anatomical replicas from imaging data such as CT or MRI scans has significantly enhanced surgical precision. Surgeons can now plan complicated procedures, improve spatial orientation, and reduce intraoperative complications, particularly in neurosurgery, orthopedics, and maxillofacial reconstruction. These models serve not only as planning aids but also as tools for education and patient communication.

Customized implants and prosthetics

In the area of customized implants and prosthetics, 3D printing has made it possible to manufacture customized solutions that fit the patient's specific anatomical and functional requirements. Custom implants have better fit, reduce surgical time, and enhance better osseointegration. Technology is increasingly applied in cranial plates, mandibular implants, spinal cages, and orthopedic joint replacements with enhanced biomechanical compatibility and aesthetics compared to conventional implants.

Bioprinting and tissue engineering and technical challenges

Bioprinting and tissue engineering are at the cutting edge of regenerative medicine, where additive manufacturing is used to create complex biological structures such as skin, cartilage, and vascular tissues. Although still experimental, technologies in bio-inks and scaffold design are pushing to the limits of possibility, with the end goal of printing functional organs for transplantation. Such advances have within them potential solutions for organ shortages and tissue repair.

However, the application of such technologies faces major regulatory and technical challenges. Absence of standard protocols, variability in material biocompatibility, and long-term safety issues hinder widespread clinical acceptance. Regulatory agencies like the FDA are working to create clear approval pathways, but most countries have no overarching frameworks to govern the use of 3D-printed medical devices.

Turning an eye to the future, the intersection of artificial intelligence (AI) with 3D printing and smart implants is positioned to transform the future of personalized medicine. AI algorithms can be leveraged to automate design work flow, optimize printing parameters, and even predict surgical outcomes. Additionally, the integration of sensors in 3D-printed implants can enable monitoring of healing processes and biomechanical loading in real time, ushering in an era of intelligent, responsive implants. Together, these innovations portend a future where precision medicine is not only personalized but also predictive and adaptive.

PRISMA Flow Diagram

Owing to heterogeneity between study designs, clinical contexts, and outcomes measures, a strategy of narrative synthesis was applied for synthesizing results. Studies were categorized under thematically labeled classes that included: (1) preoperative preparation and anatomical modeling, (2) personal implants and prosthetics, (3) tissue engineering and bioprinting, (4) technical regulatory challenges, and (5) future integration using artificial intelligence and smart implantation technologies.

The study selection process was documented using a PRISMA flow diagram. Overall, 1,273 records were yielded from the database search. After duplicates were removed, 872 unique articles were screened by title and abstract. After full-text assessment, 68 studies were identified as eligible and were included for final analysis.

Table 1. PRISMA Flow Diagram of Study Selection Process

Step	Number of Records
Records identified through database searching	1,273
Records after duplicates removed	872
Records screened (title and abstract)	872
Records excluded after screening	723
Full-text articles assessed for eligibility	149
Full-text articles excluded (not meeting criteria)	81
Studies included in final qualitative synthesis	68

DISCUSSION

This systematic review highlights the transformative role of 3D printing and additive manufacturing in improving the precision of surgery and personalizing medical care. The application of these technologies in clinical practice enables the creation of patient-specific anatomical models, surgical devices, and implants, thus bridging the gap between imaging in medicine and operating in the clinic.

The findings confirm that preoperative planning with 3D-printed anatomical models not only enhances surgical accuracy but also facilitates significant reductions in operative risk and complications, particularly in neurosurgery, orthopedics, and maxillofacial surgery. Surgeons and residents appreciate physical spatially accurate models enhancing procedural confidence and communication with patients.

Custom implants and prosthetics become a cornerstone of this technology. Whether craniomaxillofacial reconstruction accuracy or spinal implants, 3D printing ensures improved anatomical fit, enhanced osseointegration, and reduced surgical time. These benefits translate to pediatric care, where rapidly adaptable prostheses offer cost savings as well as functional flexibility.

Bioprinting and tissue engineering, although still largely experimental at present, represent a promising frontier. The reviewed studies show active exploration of bioactive scaffolds and stem cell-infused constructs for bone, cartilage, and soft tissue repair. However, the low resolution of current bioprinting technologies and the inability to mimic complex microvascular networks remain to impede the clinical translation of fully functional tissue constructs.

The review also reveals mammoth hurdles to widespread clinical adoption. Cost, regulatory uncertainty, material standardization, and technical constraints place limits on scalability and consistency in outcomes. Sterilization and biocompatibility testing of 3D-printed devices are also ongoing challenges. Multidisciplinary collaboration between clinicians, policymakers, and bioengineers will play a crucial role in addressing such challenges and developing strong guidelines for clinical adoption.

Looking ahead, the intersection of 3D printing with artificial intelligence and smart implant technologies is of tremendous promise. AI-driven design optimization, computer-aided image segmentation by automated algorithms, and the integration of biosensors into printed implants can usher in a new age of intelligent, data-driven surgeries. These technologies have the potential not just for personalization but also for predictive and adaptive treatment based on patient-specific dynamics.

CONCLUSION

3D printing and additive manufacturing are revolutionizing the landscape of precision surgery and personalized care. From preoperative planning and customized implants to emerging fields of tissue engineering and AI integration, both these technologies offer real benefits in terms of improving outcomes and operating productivity. Despite ongoing cost, regulatory, and technical challenges, the innovation trend and expanding clinical evidence suggest that 3D printing is on the verge of becoming an accepted tool of modern surgical practice. Continued interdisciplinary collaboration will be essential in overcoming existing obstacles and achieving the potential of precision-guided, patient-specific medical therapy.

REFERENCES

Bernatoniene, J., Stabrauskiene, J., Kazlauskaite, J. A., Bernatonyte, U., & Kopustinskiene, D. M. (2025). The Future of Medicine: How 3D Printing Is Transforming Pharmaceuticals. *Pharmaceutics*, *17*(3), 390. DOI: 10.3390/pharmaceutics17030390 PMID: 40143052

Borthakur, P. P., Das, A., Sahariah, J. J., Pramanik, P., Baruah, E., & Pathak, K. (2025). Revolutionizing Patient Care: 3D Printing for Customized Medical Devices and Therapeutics. *Biomedical Materials & Devices*, 1–28. DOI: 10.1007/s44174-025-00324-2

Ca, C., Jin, X., Zhao, H., Liu, J., & Dong, Y. (2025). A comprehensive approach to the surgical management of a complex abdominal sarcoma utilizing advanced imaging and 3D printing technology: A case report. *Journal of Surgical Case Reports*, *2025*(4), rjaf239. DOI: 10.1093/jscr/rjaf239 PMID: 40292347

Cong, B., & Zhang, H. (2025). Innovative 3D printing technologies and advanced materials revolutionizing orthopedic surgery: Current applications and future directions. *Frontiers in Bioengineering and Biotechnology*, *13*, 1542179. DOI: 10.3389/fbioe.2025.1542179 PMID: 40008034

Dagkinis, I. K., Spyrou, S., Georgantis, G. K., Psomas, P. M., Platis, A. N., & Tsoulfas, G. (2024). Impact of innovative technologies on quality and safety in surgery. *Journal of Robotic Surgery*, *19*(1), 31. DOI: 10.1007/s11701-024-02192-2 PMID: 39707082

Eskandar, K. (2025). Bioprinting in Organ Transplantation: From Experimental Models to Clinical Prospects. *Brazilian Journal of Transplantation*, *28*(1), e1825. DOI: 10.53855/bjt.v28i1.668_ENG

Geetha, V. (2025). 3D Medical Device Development: Current Trends, Challenges, and Future Prospects. *Multidisciplinary Research in Arts, Science & Commerce (Volume-18)*, 4.

Khan, K., Ni, J., Tabba, F. A., & Saeed, S. (2025). Reshaping medical imaging analysis: Generative AI for adversarial-resistant image segmentation. In AI techniques for securing medical and business practices (p. 24).

Peng, H., Han, B., Tong, T., Jin, X., Peng, Y., Guo, M., Li, B., Ding, J., Kong, Q., & Wang, Q. (2024). 3D printing processes in precise drug delivery for personalized medicine. *Biofabrication*, *16*(3), 032001. DOI: 10.1088/1758-5090/ad3a14 PMID: 38569493

Peron, M., Saporiti, N., Shoeibi, M., Holmström, J., & Salmi, M. (2025). Additive manufacturing in the medical sector: From an empirical investigation of challenges and opportunities toward the design of an ecosystem model. *International Journal of Operations & Production Management*, *45*(2), 387–415. DOI: 10.1108/IJOPM-12-2023-0948

Saeed, S., & Abdullah, A. (2021). Combination of brain cancer with hybrid K-NN algorithm using statistical analysis of cerebrospinal fluid (CSF) surgery. *International Journal of Computer Science and Network Security*, *21*(2), 120–130.

Saeed, S., Ghani, R., & Shahid, Z. (2024). Prevalence of Low Back Pain and Its Associated Factors in an Underdeveloped Country: Pakistan: Prevalence of Low Back Pain in Pakistan. *Journal of Health and Rehabilitation Research*, *4*(3), 1–7.

Saeed, S., Ghani, R., Shahid, Z., Naseeb, U., & Khan, U. A. (2024). Nervous Discrepancy of Spinal Cord Schwannoma Causing Posterior Neck Swelling: Spinal Cord Schwannoma Causing Posterior Neck Swelling. *Pakistan Journal of Health Sciences*, 229-232.

Saeed, S., & Qasim, M. B. (2023). Surgical acute epidural hematoma in the temporal perioral region of the brain. *International Journal of Head and Neck Surgery*, *14*(3), 1–8. DOI: 10.5005/jp-journals-10001-1552

Sampath, T., Srinivasan, T. P., Thamizharasan, S., & Krithaksha, V. (2025). 3D Printing in Medicine. In *Compendium of 3D Bioprinting Technology* (pp. 271–285). CRC Press.

Srinivasa Rao, N., Kumar, R., Kavitha, N., T, R., Pydi, H. P., Shankhyan, A., Subbiah, R., & Mann, V. S. (2025). Analyse the mechanical property optimization for FDM/3D-printed polycarbonate using Taguchi and TOPSIS techniques. *Journal of Metals. Materials and Minerals*, *35*(1), e2196–e2196. DOI: 10.55713/jmmm.v35i1.2196

Stirrat, T., Martin, R., Baek, G., Thiru, S., Lakhani, D., Umair, M., & Sayah, A. (2024). Pixels to precision: Neuroradiology's leap into 3D printing for personalized medicine. *Journal of Clinical Imaging Science*, *14*, 49. DOI: 10.25259/JCIS_119_2024 PMID: 39777212

Suhag, D., Kaushik, S., & Taxak, V. B. (2024). 3D Printing in Biomedicine. In *Handbook of Biomaterials for Medical Applications, Volume 1: Fundamentals* (pp. 185-212). Singapore: Springer Nature Singapore.

Tonk, M., Gupta, V., Dhwaj, A., & Sachdeva, M. (2025). Current developments and advancements of 3-dimensional printing in personalized medication and drug screening. *Drug Metabolism and Personalized Therapy*, *39*(4), 167–182. DOI: 10.1515/dmpt-2024-0024 PMID: 39331538

Vlachou, M., Siamidi, A., & Protopapa, C. (2025). 3D-printing technologies for pharmaceutical applications. *Fundamentals and future trends of 3D printing in drug delivery*, 29-46.

Wang, J., Wang, Y., Wang, R., Wang, Q., Wen, M., Wang, J., Sheng, L., Zheng, Y., & Xi, T. (2025). A Review on 3D Printing Processes in Pharmaceutical Engineering and Tissue Engineering: Applications, Trends and Challenges. *Advanced Materials Technologies*, *10*(2), 2400620. DOI: 10.1002/admt.202400620

Zahid, M. J., Mavani, P., Awuah, W. A., Alabdulrahman, M., Punukollu, R., Kundu, A., Mago, A., Maher, K., Adebusoye, F. T., & Khan, T. N. (2024). Sculpting the future: A narrative review of 3D printing in plastic surgery and prosthetic devices. *Health Science Reports*, *7*(6), e2205. DOI: 10.1002/hsr2.2205 PMID: 38915353

Zhu, Y., Guo, S., Ravichandran, D., Ramanathan, A., Sobczak, M. T., Sacco, A. F., Patil, D., Thummalapalli, S. V., Pulido, T. V., Lancaster, J. N., Yi, J., Cornella, J. L., Lott, D. G., Chen, X., Mei, X., Zhang, Y. S., Wang, L., Wang, X., Zhao, Y., & Song, K. (2025). 3D-Printed Polymeric Biomaterials for Health Applications. *Advanced Healthcare Materials*, *14*(1), 2402571. DOI: 10.1002/adhm.202402571 PMID: 39498750

Compilation of References

Abouchenari, A., Tajbakhsh, N., Shahbaz, A., & Alamdari-Mahd, G. (2024). Advancements in dental implant technology: the impact of smart polymers utilized through 3D printing. Journal of synthesis and sintering, 4(2).

Abusalah, M. A. H., Abd Rahman, E. N. S. E., & Choudhary, O. P. (2024). Evolving trends in stem cell therapy: An emerging and promising approach against various diseases. *International Journal of Surgery*, *110*(11), 6862–6868. DOI: 10.1097/JS9.0000000000001948 PMID: 39699861

Adamchic, I. (2025). Enhancing Intracranial Aneurysm Detection with Artificial Intelligence in Radiology.

Adewusi, J., Burness, C., Ellawela, S., Emsley, H., Hughes, R., Lawthom, C., Maguire, M., McLean, B., Mohanraj, R., Oto, M., Singhal, S., & Reuber, M. (2020). Brivaracetam efficacy and tolerability in clinical practice: A UK-based retrospective multicenter service evaluation. *Epilepsy & Behavior*, *106*, 106967. DOI: 10.1016/j.yebeh.2020.106967 PMID: 32179501

Ahmed, K. S., Shariar, K. S., Naim, N. H., & Alam, M. G. R. (2022). Intracranial hemorrhage detection using CNN-LSTM fusion model. In *2022 13th Annual Information Technology, Electronics and Mobile Communication Conference (IEMCON)* (pp. 398–404). IEEE. DOI: 10.1109/IEMCON56893.2022.9946604

Ahmed, S. H., Haris, M., Baseer, N., Saleema, A., Haris, S., Deeba, F., & Ahmad, S. H. (2021). Surgical Anatomy and Prevalence of Intracranial Aneurysms in Patients With Spontaneous Subarachnoid Hemorrhage. *Cureus*, *13*(12). Advance online publication. DOI: 10.7759/cureus.20463 PMID: 35070527

Ai, M., Zhang, H., Feng, J., Chen, H., Liu, D., Li, C., Yu, F., & Li, C. (2024). Research advances in predicting the expansion of hypertensive intracerebral hemorrhage based on CT images: An overview. *PeerJ*, *12*, e17556. DOI: 10.7717/peerj.17556 PMID: 38860211

Andriollo, G. (2024). *Robotic-Assisted Surgery in Healthcare Institutions: Assessing Benefits, Obstacles, and Implementation Success Factors* (Master's thesis, Universidade Catolica Portuguesa (Portugal)).

Angelova, P., & Kehayov, I. (2024). Association of Central Nervous System–Affecting Medications with Occurrence and Short-Term Mortality of Traumatic Brain Injury. *Neurosurgery*, *95*(2), e51. DOI: 10.1227/neu.0000000000003056 PMID: 38860763

Anusha Bai, R., & Sangeetha, V. (2023). A comparative study on brain intracerebral hemorrhage classification using head CT scan for stroke analysis. In *Soft Computing for Security Applications* (Vol. 1449, pp. 633). DOI: 10.1007/978-981-99-3608-3_44

Archana, K., & Prasad, V. K. (2025). Medical imaging and diagnosis: Robotics in diagnostic imaging and image-guided interventions. In *Necrobotics for Healthcare Applications and Management* (pp. 139–152). Academic Press. DOI: 10.1016/B978-0-443-24832-0.00006-4

Artificial Neural Network. (n.d.). https://www.javatpoint.com/artificial-neural-network

Asif, M., Shah, M. A., Khattak, H. A., Mussadiq, S., Ahmed, E., Nasr, E. A., & Rauf, H. T. (2023). Intracranial hemorrhage detection using parallel deep convolutional models and boosting mechanism. *Diagnostics (Basel)*, *13*(4), 652. DOI: 10.3390/diagnostics13040652 PMID: 36832137

Awan, N., Kumar, R. G., Juengst, S. B., DiSanto, D., Harrison-Felix, C., Dams-O'Connor, K., Pugh, M. J., Zafonte, R. D., Walker, W. C., Szaflarski, J. P., Krafty, R. T., & Wagner, A. K. (2025). Development of individualized risk assessment models for predicting post-traumatic epilepsy 1 and 2 years after moderate-to-severe traumatic brain injury: A traumatic brain injury model system study. *Epilepsia*, *66*(2), 482–498. DOI: 10.1111/epi.18210 PMID: 39655874

Azeem, S., Ashraf, M., Kamboh, U. A., Raza, M. A., Farooq, M., Cheema, H. A., Tariq, S., Choudhary, N., Hussain, S. S., & Ashraf, N. (2023). Association of ABO blood group with delayed cerebral ischemia and clinical outcomes following aneurysmal subarachnoid hemorrhage in Pakistan. *Asian Journal of Neurosurgery*, *18*(01), 108–116. DOI: 10.1055/s-0043-1760859 PMID: 37056873

Babu, C. S., Bhargavi, Y., & Krishna, P. R. (2025). AI-Driven Personalized Healthcare Solutions: Transforming Healthcare Delivery Through Precision, Efficiency, and Innovation. *AI-Driven Personalized Healthcare Solutions*, 241-276.

Balança, B., Bouchier, B., & Ritzenthaler, T. (2022). The management of delayed cerebral ischemia after aneurysmal subarachnoid hemorrhage. *Revue Neurologique*, *178*(1-2), 64–73. DOI: 10.1016/j.neurol.2021.11.006 PMID: 34961603

Ballout, A. A., Prochilo, G., Kaneko, N., Li, C., Apfel, R., Hinman, J. D., & Liebeskind, D. S. (2024). Computational fluid dynamics in intracranial atherosclerotic disease. *Stroke: Vascular and Interventional Neurology*, *4*(1), e000792. DOI: 10.1161/SVIN.122.000792

Barba, L., Carrubba, C., Spindler, K., Weise, C. M., Sachs, T., Foschi, M., D'Anna, L., Sehm, B., Ibe, R., Elolf, E., Strauss, C., Otto, M., Mensch, A., & Abu-Rumeileh, S. (2024). Posterior reversible encephalopathy syndrome associated with antibiotic therapy: A case report and systematic review. *Neurological Sciences*, *45*(9), 4151–4159. DOI: 10.1007/s10072-024-07545-1 PMID: 38679625

Barragán-Montero, A., Javaid, U., Valdés, G., Nguyen, D., Desbordes, P., Macq, B., Willems, S., Vandewinckele, L., Holmström, M., Löfman, F., Michiels, S., Souris, K., Sterpin, E., & Lee, J. A. (2021). Artificial intelligence and machine learning for medical imaging: A technology review. *Physica Medica*, *83*, 242–256. DOI: 10.1016/j.ejmp.2021.04.016 PMID: 33979715

Battal, B., & Castillo, M. (2024). Imaging of Reversible Cerebral Vasoconstriction Syndrome and Posterior Reversible Encephalopathy Syndrome. *Neuroimaging Clinics of North America*, *34*(1), 129–147. DOI: 10.1016/j.nic.2023.07.004 PMID: 37951698

Benbrahim, F. Z., El Haddad, S., Allali, N., & Chat, L. (2024). Moyamoya syndrome secondary to MELAS syndrome in a child: A case report and literature revue. *Radiology Case Reports*, *19*(12), 6347–6353. DOI: 10.1016/j.radcr.2024.08.159 PMID: 39387012

Bernatoniene, J., Stabrauskiene, J., Kazlauskaite, J. A., Bernatonyte, U., & Kopustinskiene, D. M. (2025). The Future of Medicine: How 3D Printing Is Transforming Pharmaceuticals. *Pharmaceutics*, *17*(3), 390. DOI: 10.3390/pharmaceutics17030390 PMID: 40143052

Bernhard, J. S., & Slaack, A. M. (2019). Levetiracetam and brivaracetam: A review of evidence from clinical trials and clinical experience. *Therapeutic Advances in Neurological Disorders*. PMID: 31523280

Bhandari, S., Yadav, V., Ishaq, A., Sanipini, S., Ekhator, C., Khleif, R., Beheshtaein, A., Jhajj, L. K., Khan, A. W., Al Khalifa, A., Naseem, M. A., Bellegarde, S. B., & Nadeem, M. A. (2023). Trends and challenges in the development of 3d-printed heart valves and other cardiac implants: A review of current advances. *Cureus*, *15*(8). Advance online publication. DOI: 10.7759/cureus.43204 PMID: 37565179

Bharati, S., Podder, P., & Mondal, M. R. H. (2020). Hybrid deep learning for detecting lung diseases from X-ray images. *Informatics in Medicine Unlocked, 20*, 100391. DOI: 10.1016/j.imu.2020.100391 PMID: 32835077

Bhattacharjee, S., Rakesh, D., Ramnadha, R., & Manas, P. (2021). Subarachnoid hemorrhage and hydrocephalus. *Neurology India, 69*(Suppl 2), S429–S433. DOI: 10.4103/0028-3886.332266 PMID: 35102999

Bijari, S., Sayfollahi, S., Mardokh-Rouhani, S., Bijari, S., Moradian, S., Zahiri, Z., & Rezaeijo, S. M. (2024). Radiomics and deep features: Robust classification of brain hemorrhages and reproducibility analysis using a 3D autoencoder neural network. *Bioengineering (Basel, Switzerland), 11*(7), 643. DOI: 10.3390/bioengineering11070643 PMID: 39061725

Bollen, E., Awad, L., Langridge, B., & Butler, P. E. (2022). The intraoperative use of augmented and mixed reality technology to improve surgical outcomes: A systematic review. *International Journal of Medical Robotics and Computer Assisted Surgery, 18*(6), e2450. DOI: 10.1002/rcs.2450 PMID: 35971649

Borthakur, P. P., Das, A., Sahariah, J. J., Pramanik, P., Baruah, E., & Pathak, K. (2025). Revolutionizing Patient Care: 3D Printing for Customized Medical Devices and Therapeutics. *Biomedical Materials & Devices*, 1–28. DOI: 10.1007/s44174-025-00324-2

Buch, V. P., Mensah-Brown, K. G., Germi, J. W., Park, B. J., Madsen, P. J., Borja, A. J., Haldar, D., Basenfelder, P., Yoon, J. W., Schuster, J. M., & Chen, H. C. I. (2021). Development of an intraoperative pipeline for holographic mixed reality visualization during spinal fusion surgery. *Surgical Innovation, 28*(4), 427–437. DOI: 10.1177/1553350620984339 PMID: 33382008

Budhiparama, N. C., Kort, N. P., Kort, R., & Lumban-Gaol, I. (2025). The future outlook for data in orthopedic surgery: A new era of real-time innovation. *Journal of Orthopaedic Surgery (Hong Kong), 33*(1), 10225536251331664. DOI: 10.1177/10225536251331664 PMID: 40172087

Budoff, M. J., Dowe, D., Jollis, J. G., Gitter, M., Sutherland, J., Halamert, E., Scherer, M., Bellinger, R., Martin, A., Benton, R., Delago, A., & Min, J. K. (2008). Diagnostic performance of 64-multidetector row coronary computed tomographic angiography for evaluation of coronary artery stenosis in individuals without known coronary artery disease: Results from the prospective multicenter ACCURACY (Assessment by Coronary Computed Tomographic Angiography of Individuals Undergoing Invasive Coronary Angiography) trial. *Journal of the American College of Cardiology, 52*(21), 1724–1732. DOI: 10.1016/j.jacc.2008.07.031 PMID: 19007693

Bui, T., Ruiz-Cardozo, M. A., Dave, H. S., Barot, K., Kann, M. R., Joseph, K., Lopez-Alviar, S., Trevino, G., Brehm, S., Yahanda, A. T., & Molina, C. A. (2024). Virtual, augmented, and mixed reality applications for surgical rehearsal, operative execution, and patient education in spine surgery: A scoping review. *Medicina, 60*(2), 332. DOI: 10.3390/medicina60020332 PMID: 38399619

Burduja, M., Ionescu, R. T., & Verga, N. (2020). Accurate and efficient intracranial hemorrhage detection and subtype classification in 3D CT scans with convolutional and long short-term memory neural networks. *Sensors (Basel), 20*(19), 5611. DOI: 10.3390/s20195611 PMID: 33019508

Ca, C., Jin, X., Zhao, H., Liu, J., & Dong, Y. (2025). A comprehensive approach to the surgical management of a complex abdominal sarcoma utilizing advanced imaging and 3D printing technology: A case report. *Journal of Surgical Case Reports, 2025*(4), rjaf239. DOI: 10.1093/jscr/rjaf239 PMID: 40292347

Campbell, B. C., Lansberg, M. G., Broderick, J. P., Derdeyn, C. P., Khatri, P., Sarraj, A., Saver, J. L., Vagal, A., Albers, G. W., Adeoye, O., Ansari, S., Boltze, J., Buchan, A., Chaisinanunkul, N., Chen, C., Davis, T. P., Ermakova, T., Fisher, M., Haddad, W., & Ziogas, N. K. (2021). Acute stroke imaging research roadmap IV: Imaging selection and outcomes in acute stroke clinical trials and practice. *Stroke, 52*(8), 2723–2733. DOI: 10.1161/STROKEAHA.121.035132 PMID: 34233464

Campbell, D. H., McDonald, D., Araghi, K., Araghi, T., Chutkan, N., & Araghi, A. (2021). The clinical impact of image guidance and robotics in spinal surgery: A review of safety, accuracy, efficiency, and complication reduction. *The International Journal of Spine Surgery, 15*(s2), S10–S20. DOI: 10.14444/8136 PMID: 34607916

Cannizzaro, D., Zaed, I., Safa, A., Jelmoni, A. J., Composto, A., Bisoglio, A., Schmeizer, K., Becker, A. C., Pizzi, A., Cardia, A., & Servadei, F. (2022). Augmented reality in neurosurgery, state of art and future projections. A systematic review. *Frontiers in Surgery, 9*, 864792. DOI: 10.3389/fsurg.2022.864792 PMID: 35360432

Carney, N. P., Totten, A. M., O'Reilly, C. B., Ullman, J. S., Hawryluk, G. W., Bell, M. J., & Rubiano, A. M. (2017). Guidelines for the management of severe traumatic brain injury (4th ed.). *Neurosurgery, 80*(1), 6-15.

Caruso, D., Polici, M., Zerunian, M., Pucciarelli, F., Guido, G., Polidori, T., Landolfi, F., Nicolai, M., Lucertini, E., Tarallo, M., Bracci, B., Nacci, I., Rucci, C., Iannicelli, E., & Laghi, A. (2021). Radiomics in oncology, part 1: Technical principles and gastrointestinal application in CT and MRI. *Cancers (Basel), 13*(11), 2522. DOI: 10.3390/cancers13112522 PMID: 34063937

Chaisawasthomrong, C. (2025). Superior Sagittal Sinus Thrombosis Secondary to Cerebral Aspergillosis with Ventriculitis in an Immunocompetent Patient: A Case Report. *Asian Journal of Neurosurgery*, *20*(01), 160–164. DOI: 10.1055/s-0044-1791714 PMID: 40041597

Chandra, M. A., & Bedi, S. S. (2021). Survey on SVM and their application in image classification. *International Journal of Information Technology : an Official Journal of Bharati Vidyapeeth's Institute of Computer Applications and Management*, *13*(5), 1–11. DOI: 10.1007/s41870-017-0080-1

Chen, M., & Ludtke, S. J. (2021). Deep learning-based mixed-dimensional Gaussian mixture model for characterizing variability in cryo-EM. Nature Methods 2021 18:8, 18(8), 930– 936. DOI: 10.1038/s41592-021-01220-5

Chen, S., Cai, M., Tan, G., Guo, R., Liang, Q., Li, H., & Liu, X. (2024). Case report: Intravascular large B cell lymphoma mimicking acute demyelinating encephalomyelitis after SARS-CoV-2 reinfection: diagnostic value of advanced MRI techniques and the literature review with the assistance of ChatGPT. *Frontiers in Immunology*, *15*, 1478163. DOI: 10.3389/fimmu.2024.1478163 PMID: 39611151

Chen, X., Feng, F., Yu, X., Wang, S., Tu, Z., Han, Y., Li, Q., Chen, H., Chen, Z., Lao, L., & Shen, H. (2020). Robot-assisted orthopedic surgery in the treatment of adult degenerative scoliosis: A preliminary clinical report. *Journal of Orthopaedic Surgery and Research*, *15*(1), 282. DOI: 10.1186/s13018-020-01796-2 PMID: 32711566

Chen, X., Liu, Y., Tong, H., Dong, Y., Ma, D., Xu, L., & Yang, C. (2018). Meta-analysis of computed tomography angiography versus magnetic resonance angiography for intracranial aneurysm. *Medicine*, *97*(20), e10771. DOI: 10.1097/MD.0000000000010771 PMID: 29768368

Cheplygina, V., de Bruijne, M., & Pluim, J. P. W. (2019). Not-so-supervised: A survey of semi- supervised, multi-instance, and transfer learning in medical image analysis. *Medical Image Analysis*, *54*, 280–296. DOI: 10.1016/j.media.2019.03.009 PMID: 30959445

Chidambaram, S., Stifano, V., Demetres, M., Teyssandier, M., Palumbo, M. C., Redaelli, A., Olivi, A., Apuzzo, M. L. J., & Pannullo, S. C. (2021). Applications of augmented reality in the neurosurgical operating room: A systematic review of the literature. *Journal of Clinical Neuroscience*, *91*, 43–61. DOI: 10.1016/j.jocn.2021.06.032 PMID: 34373059

Chilamkurthy, S., Ghosh, R., Tanamala, S., Biviji, M., Campeau, N. G., Kumar Venugopal, V., Mahajan, V., Rao, P., Warier, P., & Ai, Q. (2018). Development and Validation of Deep Learning Algorithms for Detection of Critical Findings in Head CT Scans. https://arxiv.org/abs/1803.05854v2

Cho, J., Rahimpour, S., Cutler, A., Goodwin, C. R., Lad, S. P., & Codd, P. (2020). Enhancing reality: A systematic review of augmented reality in Neuronavigation and education. *World Neurosurgery*, *139*, 186–195. DOI: 10.1016/j.wneu.2020.04.043 PMID: 32311561

Christensen, J., Pedersen, H. S., Fenger-Grøn, M., Fann, J. R., Jones, N. C., & Vestergaard, M. (2019). Selective serotonin reuptake inhibitors and risk of epilepsy after traumatic brain injury–A population-based cohort study. *PLoS One*, *14*(7), e0219137. DOI: 10.1371/journal.pone.0219137 PMID: 31323024

Clement David-Olawade, A., Olawade, D. B., Vanderbloemen, L., Rotifa, O. B., Fidelis, S. C., Egbon, E., Akpan, A. O., Adeleke, S., Ghose, A., & Boussios, S. (2025). AI-Driven Advances in Low-Dose Imaging and Enhancement—A Review. *Diagnostics (Basel)*, *15*(6), 689. DOI: 10.3390/diagnostics15060689 PMID: 40150031

Cole, K., Findlay, M., Kundu, M., Johansen, C., Rawanduzy, C., & Lucke-Wold, B. (2023). The role of advanced imaging in neurosurgical diagnosis. *Journal of Modern Medical Imaging*, •••, 1.

Cong, B., & Zhang, H. (2025). Innovative 3D printing technologies and advanced materials revolutionizing orthopedic surgery: Current applications and future directions. *Frontiers in Bioengineering and Biotechnology*, *13*, 1542179. DOI: 10.3389/fbioe.2025.1542179 PMID: 40008034

Convolutional Neural Network - javatpoint. (n.d.). https://www.javatpoint.com/pytorch-convolutional-neural-network

Cortés-Ferre, L., Gutiérrez-Naranjo, M. A., Egea-Guerrero, J. J., Pérez-Sánchez, S., & Balcerzyk, M. (2023). Deep learning applied to intracranial hemorrhage detection. *Journal of Imaging*, *9*(2), 37. DOI: 10.3390/jimaging9020037 PMID: 36826956

Currie, G., & Rohren, E. (2022). Intelligent imaging: Applications of machine learning and deep learning in radiology. *Veterinary Radiology & Ultrasound*, *63*(S1), 880–888. DOI: 10.1111/vru.13144 PMID: 36514225

D'Souza, M., Gendreau, J., Feng, A., Kim, L. H., Ho, A. L., & Veeravagu, A. (2019). Robotic-assisted spine surgery: history, efficacy, cost, and future trends. *Robotic Surgery: Research and Reviews*, 9-23.

Dagkinis, I. K., Spyrou, S., Georgantis, G. K., Psomas, P. M., Platis, A. N., & Tsoulfas, G. (2024). Impact of innovative technologies on quality and safety in surgery. *Journal of Robotic Surgery*, *19*(1), 31. DOI: 10.1007/s11701-024-02192-2 PMID: 39707082

Dai, W., Ling, H., Sun, Y., Wang, Y., Li, W., Yang, Y., Wu, L., & Hang, C. (2022). The comparison of Neuronavigation combined with CT three-dimensional angiography vs. CT angiography in the guidance of clipping treatment in distal intracranial aneurysm surgery: A retrospective clinical study. *Annals of Translational Medicine*, *10*(10), 572. DOI: 10.21037/atm-22-1749 PMID: 35722369

de la Salud, R. E. C., & la de la Inteligencia, T. (2025). AI Rx: Revolutionizing Healthcare Through Intelligence, Innovation, and Ethics. In *Seminars in Medical Writing and Education* (Vol. 4, No. 35, p. 35).

De Simone, B., Deeken, G., & Catena, F. (2025). Balancing Ethics and Innovation: Can Artificial Intelligence Safely Transform Emergency Surgery? A Narrative Perspective. *Journal of Clinical Medicine*, *14*(9), 3111. DOI: 10.3390/jcm14093111 PMID: 40364137

Deshmukh, A. S., Priola, S. M., Katsanos, A. H., Scalia, G., Costa Alves, A., Srivastava, A., & Hawkes, C. (2024). The management of intracranial aneurysms: Current trends and future directions. *Neurology International*, *16*(1), 74–94. DOI: 10.3390/neurolint16010005 PMID: 38251053

Dewan, M. C., Rattani, A., Gupta, S., Baticulon, R. E., Hung, Y. C., Punchak, M., Agrawal, A., Adeleye, A. O., Shrime, M. G., Rubiano, A. M., Rosenfeld, J. V., & Park, K. B. (2018). Estimating the global incidence of traumatic brain injury. *Journal of Neurosurgery*, *130*(4), 1080–1097. DOI: 10.3171/2017.10.JNS17352 PMID: 29701556

Di Cosmo, L., El Choueiri, J., Pellicanò, F., Salman, H., Colella, F., Zaed, I., & Cannizzaro, D. (2025). From experimental to essential: The evolving role of augmented reality in neurosurgery (2012–2024). *Neuro-Chirurgie*, *71*(4), 101672. DOI: 10.1016/j.neuchi.2025.101672 PMID: 40273502

Din, M., Agarwal, S., Grzeda, M., Wood, D. A., Modat, M., & Booth, T. C. (2023). Detection of cerebral aneurysms using artificial intelligence: A systematic review and meta-analysis. *Journal of Neurointerventional Surgery*, *15*(3), 262–271. DOI: 10.1136/jnis-2022-019456 PMID: 36375834

Dodd, W. S., Laurent, D., & Dumont, A. S. (2021). Pathophysiology of delayed cerebral ischemia after subarachnoid hemorrhage. *RE:view*, •••, 10. PMID: 34325514

Doshi, P. K., & M. P. (2021). Seizure prophylaxis in neurosurgery settings: Role of prophylactic Brivaracetam in neurosurgery. *Biomedical Journal of Scientific & Technical Research.*

Duan, X., Wang, B., Yang, L., & Kadakia, A. R. (2021). Applications of 3D printing technology in orthopedic treatment. *BioMed Research International, 2021*(1), 9892456. DOI: 10.1155/2021/9892456 PMID: 34423040

Edison, G. (2023). Transforming Medical Decision-Making: A Comprehensive Review of AI's Impact on Diagnostics And Treatment. *BULLET: Jurnal Multidisiplin Ilmu, 2*(4), 1121–1133.

Eom, S., Kim, S., Jackson, J., Sykes, D., Rahimpour, S., & Gorlatova, M. (2024). Augmented reality-based contextual guidance through surgical tool tracking in neurosurgery. *IEEE Transactions on Visualization and Computer Graphics.* PMID: 38635386

Eskandar, K. (2025). Bioprinting in Organ Transplantation: From Experimental Models to Clinical Prospects. *Brazilian Journal of Transplantation, 28*(1), e1825. DOI: 10.53855/bjt.v28i1.668_ENG

Esmaeili, H., & Zavareh, S. A. H. (2024). *Advanced Neurosurgical Practices: Integrating Technological Innovations and Personalized Approaches.* Nobel Sciences.

Faraj, M. K., Hoz, S. S., & Mohammad, A. J. (2020). The use of three-dimensional anatomical patient-specific printed models in surgical clipping of intracranial aneurysm: A pilot study. *Surgical Neurology International, 11*, 381. DOI: 10.25259/SNI_361_2020 PMID: 33408915

Farias, T. P., Dias, F. L., Sousa, B. A., Galvão, M. S., Bispo, D., & Pastl, A. C. (2019). Prototyping: Major advance in surgical planning and customizing prostheses in patients with bone tumors of the head and neck. *International Journal of Clinical Medicine, 4*(7), 1–7. DOI: 10.4236/ijcm.2013.47A1001

Feferman, B., Fernandez, V., Tavernier, E., Fuseau, J., Sembély-Taveau, C., Boennec, R., Cremades, A., Maakaroun-Vermesse, Z., Follet, C., Mitanchez, D., Lanotte, P., Le Brun, C., Brunereau, L., Mereghetti, L., & Morel, B. (2025). Diagnostic imaging of Bacillus cereus brain infection in newborns. *Pediatric Radiology, 55*(4), 1–11. DOI: 10.1007/s00247-025-06169-7 PMID: 39841254

Felipe Kitamura. (2019). Head CT - hemorrhage. https://www.kaggle.com/datasets/felipekitamura/head-ct-hemorrhage

Ferrag, W., Scalbert, F., Adjedj, J., Dupouy, P., Ou, P., Juliard, J. M., Farnoud, R., Benadji, A. A., Du Fretay, X. H., Wijns, W., Aubry, P., & Hyafil, F. (2021). Role of FFR-CT for the evaluation of patients with anomalous aortic origin of coronary artery. *JACC: Cardiovascular Imaging*, *14*(5), 1074–1076. DOI: 10.1016/j.jcmg.2020.10.003 PMID: 33221217

Ferreira, T., Awuah, W. A., Tan, J. K., Adebusoye, F. T., Ali, S. H., Bharadwaj, H. R., Aderinto, N., Fernandes, C., Zahid, M. J., & Abdul-Rahman, T. (2023). The current landscape of intracranial aneurysms in Africa: Management outcomes, challenges, and strategies—a narrative review. *Neurosurgical Review*, *46*(1), 194. DOI: 10.1007/s10143-023-02102-4 PMID: 37548805

Finnema, S. J., Rossano, S., Naganawa, M., Henry, S., Gao, H., Pracitto, R., & Carson, R. E. (2019). A single-center, open-label positron emission tomography study to evaluate brivaracetam and levetiracetam synaptic vesicle glycoprotein 2A binding in healthy volunteers. *Epilepsia*, *60*(5), 958–967.

Flanders, A. E., Prevedello, L. M., Shih, G., Halabi, S. S., Kalpathy-Cramer, J., Ball, R., Mongan, J. T., Stein, A., Kitamura, F. C., Lungren, M. P., Choudhary, G., Cala, L., Coelho, L., Mogensen, M., Morón, F., Miller, E., Ikuta, I., Zohrabian, V., McDonnell, O., & Nath, J. (2020). Construction of a machine learning dataset through collaboration: The RSNA 2019 brain CT hemorrhage challenge. *Radiology. Artificial Intelligence*, *2*(3), e190211. DOI: 10.1148/ryai.2020190211 PMID: 33937827

Foti, G., Ascenti, G., Agostini, A., Longo, C., Lombardo, F., Inno, A., Modena, A., & Gori, S. (2024). Dual-energy CT in oncologic imaging. *Tomography : a Journal for Imaging Research*, *10*(3), 299–319. DOI: 10.3390/tomography10030024 PMID: 38535766

Gaddam, D. S., Dattwyler, M., Fleiter, T. R., & Bodanapally, U. K. (2021, October). Principles and applications of dual energy computed tomography in neuroradiology. In *Seminars in Ultrasound, CT and MRI* (Vol. 42, No. 5, pp. 418-433). WB Saunders. DOI: 10.1053/j.sult.2021.07.001

Garcia Santa Cruz, B., Husch, A., & Hertel, F. (2023). Machine learning models for diagnosis and prognosis of Parkinson's disease using brain imaging: General overview, main challenges, and future directions. *Frontiers in Aging Neuroscience*, *15*, 1216163. DOI: 10.3389/fnagi.2023.1216163 PMID: 37539346

Geetha, V. (2025). 3D Medical Device Development: Current Trends, Challenges, and Future Prospects. *Multidisciplinary Research in Arts, Science & Commerce (Volume-18)*, 4.

Goertz, L., Kabbasch, C., Borggrefe, J., Hamisch, C., Telentschak, S., von Spreckelsen, N., Stavrinou, P., Timmer, M., Brinker, G., Goldbrunner, R., & Krischek, B. (2018). Preoperative three-dimensional angiography may reduce ischemic complications during clipping of ruptured intracranial aneurysms. *World Neurosurgery*, *120*, e1163–e1170. DOI: 10.1016/j.wneu.2018.09.026 PMID: 30218797

Gomes, F. C., Oliveira, F. T., Carvalho, D. D. F., Zampirolo, F. B., Garcia, A. G. P. V., Larcipretti, A. L. L., Meneses, A. C., de Castro, I. C. S., Ferreira, M. Y., Oberman, D. Z., Polverini, A. D., & Almeida, J. P. (2024). Robot-assisted versus manually guided stereotactic biopsy for intracranial lesions-a systematic review and meta-analysis. *Neurosurgical Review*, *47*(1), 880. DOI: 10.1007/s10143-024-03121-5 PMID: 39615014

Gómez, D. F., Vargas-Osorio, M. P., Ramírez-Sanabria, A. D., Villegas-Gomez, G. A., Ordonez-Rubiano, E. G., Ramón, J. F., ... & Hakim, F. Feasibility of utilizing augmented reality in neurosurgery: Insights from a single-center experience. *Journal of Neurosciences in Rural Practice*, 1-8.

Gouripur, K. (2024). The impact of artificial intelligence on healthcare: A revolution in progress. *North & West London Journal of General Practice*, *10*(1).

Grasso, E., Certo, F., Ganau, M., Bonomo, G., Fiumanò, G., Buscema, G., Maugeri, A., Agodi, A., & Barbagallo, G. M. (2024). Role of Virtual iMRI in Glioblastoma Surgery: Advantages, Limitations, and Correlation with iCT and Brain Shift. *Brain Sciences*, *15*(1), 35. DOI: 10.3390/brainsci15010035 PMID: 39851403

Gregório, T., Pipa, S., Cavaleiro, P., Atanásio, G., Albuquerque, I., Chaves, P. C., & Azevedo, L. (2018). Prognostic models for intracerebral hemorrhage: Systematic review and meta-analysis. *BMC Medical Research Methodology*, *18*(1), 145. DOI: 10.1186/s12874-018-0613-8 PMID: 30458727

Gsaxner, C., Eck, U., Schmalstieg, D., Navab, N., & Egger, J. (2021). Augmented reality in oral and maxillofacial surgery. In *Computer-aided oral and maxillofacial surgery* (pp. 107–139). Academic Press. DOI: 10.1016/B978-0-12-823299-6.00005-5

Gupta, R. S., Lal, B., Bhagat, A. C., & Alagarsamy, R. (2024). Medical Imaging for Patient-Specific Implants. In *Biomedical Implants* (pp. 39–60). CRC Press.

Hacein-Bey, L., & Provenzale, J. M. (2011). Current imaging assessment and treatment of intracranial aneurysms. *AJR. American Journal of Roentgenology*, *196*(1), 32–44. DOI: 10.2214/AJR.10.5329 PMID: 21178044

Haizel-Cobbina, J., Dada, O. E., Du, L., Zuckerman, S. L., & Dewan, M. C. (2023). A comparison of surgery waits times and postoperative length of hospital stay among patients with brain tumors by country-level income and healthcare system: A systematic review and meta-analysis. *World Neurosurgery*, *177*, 152–164. DOI: 10.1016/j.wneu.2023.06.030 PMID: 37331477

Hamdan, A., Barnes, J., & Mitchell, P. (2014). Subarachnoid hemorrhage and the female sex: Analysis of risk factors, aneurysm characteristics, and outcomes. *Journal of Neurosurgery*, *121*(6), 1367–1373. DOI: 10.3171/2014.7.JNS132318 PMID: 25216063

Hashemzehi, R., Mahdavi, S. J. S., Kheirabadi, M., & Kamel, S. R. (2020). Detection of brain tumors from MRI images base on deep learning using hybrid model CNN and NADE. *Biocybernetics and Biomedical Engineering*, *40*(3), 1225–1232. DOI: 10.1016/j.bbe.2020.06.001

Hazan, H., Hilu, D., Manevitz, L., Ramig, L. O., & Sapir, S. (2019). Early diagnosis of Parkinson's disease via machine learning on speech data. In *2012 IEEE 27th Convention of Electrical and Electronics Engineers in Israel* (pp. 1–4). IEEE.

He, C., Cao, G., Yang, Y., Zhong, Q., Lei, Y., Tan, X., Lin, X., Chen, Y., & Sun, W. (2025). A study on the therapeutic effect of precise clipping of intracranial aneurysms assisted by CTA and 3D-slicer software. *Frontiers in Surgery*, *12*, 1535585. DOI: 10.3389/fsurg.2025.1535585 PMID: 40035066

Hess, S., Husarek, J., Müller, M., Eberlein, S. C., Klenke, F. M., & Hecker, A. (2024). Applications and accuracy of 3D-printed surgical guides in traumatology and orthopaedic surgery: A systematic review and meta-analysis. *Journal of Experimental Orthopaedics*, *11*(3), e12096. DOI: 10.1002/jeo2.12096 PMID: 39135870

He, X. Y., Yu, H. M., Lin, S., & Li, Y. Z. (2021). Advances in the application of mesenchymal stem cells, exosomes, biomimetic materials, and 3D printing in osteoporosis treatment. *Cellular & Molecular Biology Letters*, *26*(1), 47. DOI: 10.1186/s11658-021-00291-8 PMID: 34775969

Hey, G., Guyot, M., Carter, A., & Lucke-Wold, B. (2023). Augmented reality in neurosurgery: A new paradigm for training. *Medicina*, *59*(10), 1721. DOI: 10.3390/medicina59101721 PMID: 37893439

Ho, Y. H., Chiang, H. F., Hsieh, C. C., Wei, S. Y., & Huang, C. C. (2025). Unexpected vasogenic oedema and alexia as complications after dural arteriovenous fistula embolization. *BJR| Case Reports*, *11*(2), uaaf012.

Hoh, B. L., Ko, N. U., Amin-Hanjani, S., Chou, S. H. Y., Cruz-Flores, S., Dangayach, N. S., & Welch, B. G. (2023). 2023 guideline for the management of patients with aneurysmal subarachnoid hemorrhage: A guideline from the American Heart Association/American Stroke Association. *Stroke*, *54*(7), e314–e370. DOI: 10.1161/STR.0000000000000436 PMID: 37212182

Hou, R., Zhou, D., Nie, R., Liu, D., & Ruan, X. (2019). Brain CT and MRI medical image fusion using convolutional neural networks and a dual-channel spiking cortical model. *Medical & Biological Engineering & Computing*, *57*(4), 887–900. DOI: 10.1007/s11517-018-1935-8 PMID: 30471068

Howard, B. M., Hu, R., Barrow, J. W., & Barrow, D. L. (2019). Comprehensive review of imaging of intracranial aneurysms and angiographically negative subarachnoid hemorrhage. *Neurosurgical Focus*, *47*(6), E20. DOI: 10.3171/2019.9.FOCUS19653 PMID: 31786554

Hricak, H., Mayerhoefer, M. E., Herrmann, K., Lewis, J. S., Pomper, M. G., Hess, C. P., Riklund, K., Scott, A. M., & Weissleder, R. (2025). Advances and challenges in precision imaging. *The Lancet. Oncology*, *26*(1), e34–e45. DOI: 10.1016/S1470-2045(24)00395-4 PMID: 39756454

Hunt, W. E., & Hess, R. M. (1968). Surgical risk as related to time of intervention in the repair of intracranial aneurysms. *Journal of Neurosurgery*, *28*(1), 14–20. DOI: 10.3171/jns.1968.28.1.0014 PMID: 5635959

Hussain, D., Al-Masni, M. A., Aslam, M., Sadeghi-Niaraki, A., Hussain, J., Gu, Y. H., & Naqvi, R. A. (2024). Revolutionizing tumor detection and classification in multimodality imaging based on deep learning approaches: Methods, applications and limitations. *Journal of X-Ray Science and Technology*, *32*(4), 857–911. DOI: 10.3233/XST-230429 PMID: 38701131

Hussain, M., Bird, J. J., & Faria, D. R. (2019). A Study on CNN Transfer Learning for Image Classification. *Advances in Intelligent Systems and Computing*, *840*, 191–202. DOI: 10.1007/978-3-319-97982-3_16

Hussen, B. M., Taheri, M., Yashooa, R. K., Abdullah, G. H., Abdullah, S. R., Kheder, R. K., & Mustafa, S. A. (2024). Revolutionizing medicine: Recent developments and future prospects in stem-cell therapy. *International Journal of Surgery*, *110*(12), 8002–8024. DOI: 10.1097/JS9.0000000000002109 PMID: 39497543

Hu, T., Ling, R., & Zhu, Y. (2025). Advancements in imaging of intracranial atherosclerotic disease: Beyond the arterial lumen to the vessel wall. *Reviews in the Neurosciences*, *36*(3), 229–241. DOI: 10.1515/revneuro-2024-0076 PMID: 39565965

Iftikhar, M., Ali, N., Ali, R. H., & Bais, A. (2023, September). Classification of Parkinson's disease with feature selection using genetic algorithm. In *2023 IEEE Canadian Conference on Electrical and Computer Engineering (CCECE)* (pp. 522–527). IEEE. DOI: 10.1109/CCECE58730.2023.10288649

Ioschici, M., Nagy, E., & Hopirtean, C. (2024). Use of Boswellia Serrata for Cerebral Radiation Necrosis–. *Journal of Medical and Radiation Oncology*, *4*(2), 46–53. DOI: 10.53011/JMRO.2024.02.06

Irannejad, K., Krishnan, S., Iskander, B., Kambalapalli, S., Punanithinont, N., Ichikawa, K., Lakshmanan, S., & Budoff, M. J. (2025). Advancements in Coronary CT Angiography: Innovations in Diagnosis, Risk Stratification, and Prognosis in Atherosclerosis. *Current Treatment Options in Cardiovascular Medicine*, *27*(1), 34. DOI: 10.1007/s11936-025-01089-z

Isikay, I., Cekic, E., Baylarov, B., Tunc, O., & Hanalioglu, S. (2024). Narrative review of patient-specific 3D visualization and reality technologies in skull base neurosurgery: Enhancements in surgical training, planning, and navigation. *Frontiers in Surgery*, *11*, 1427844. DOI: 10.3389/fsurg.2024.1427844 PMID: 39081485

Islam, M. K., Ali, M. S., Miah, M. S., Rahman, M. M., Alam, M. S., & Hossain, M. A. (2021). Brain tumor detection in MR image using superpixels, principal component analysis and template based K-means clustering algorithm. *Machine Learning with Applications*, *5*, 100044. DOI: 10.1016/j.mlwa.2021.100044

Jagannathan, P., Rajkumar, S., Frnda, J., Divakarachari, P. B., & Subramani, P. (2021). Moving Vehicle Detection and Classification Using Gaussian Mixture Model and Ensemble Deep Learning Technique. *Wireless Communications and Mobile Computing*, *2021*(1), 5590894. DOI: 10.1155/2021/5590894

Jain, S., Vyvere, T. V., Terzopoulos, V., Sima, D. M., Roura, E., Maas, A., Wilms, G., & Verheyden, J. (2019). Automatic quantification of computed tomography features in acute traumatic brain injury. *Journal of Neurotrauma*, *36*(11), 1794–1803. DOI: 10.1089/neu.2018.6183 PMID: 30648469

Jain, V. (2025). Current Trends in 3D Technology: Customized 3D-Printed Implants and Instruments in Orthopaedics. In *Biomaterials in Orthopaedics & Trauma: Current Status and Future Trends in Revolutionizing Patient Care* (pp. 271–289). Springer Nature Singapore. DOI: 10.1007/978-981-96-3017-2_16

Jain, V. (2025). Personalized Solutions in Orthopaedic Surgery: The Era of 3D Technology and Future. In *Innovations in Healthcare and Outcome Measurement: New Approaches for a Healthy Lifestyle* (pp. 213–229). Springer Nature Switzerland. DOI: 10.1007/978-3-031-77302-0_14

Jayawickrama, S. M., Ranaweera, P. M., Pradeep, R. G. G. R., Jayasinghe, Y. A., Senevirathna, K., Hilmi, A. J., Rajapakse, R. M. G., Kanmodi, K. K., & Jayasinghe, R. D. (2024). Developments and future prospects of personalized medicine in head and neck squamous cell carcinoma diagnoses and treatments. *Cancer Reports*, *7*(3), e2045. DOI: 10.1002/cnr2.2045 PMID: 38522008

Jebarani, P. E., Umadevi, N., Dang, H., & Pomplun, M. (2021). A Novel Hybrid K-Means and GMM Machine Learning Model for Breast Cancer Detection. *IEEE Access : Practical Innovations, Open Solutions*, *9*, 146153–146162. DOI: 10.1109/ACCESS.2021.3123425

Jehanzeb, M. (2024). The future of spine surgery: technological innovations and advancements: A comprehensive review. *Romanian Neurosurgery*, **•••**, 102–108. DOI: 10.33962/roneuro-2024-017

Jena, B., Saxena, S., Nayak, G. K., Saba, L., Sharma, N., & Suri, J. S. (2021). Artificial intelligence-based hybrid deep learning models for image classification: The first narrative review. *Computers in Biology and Medicine*, *137*, 104803. DOI: 10.1016/j.compbiomed.2021.104803 PMID: 34536856

Jeong, S. M., Song, Y. D., Seok, C. L., Lee, J. Y., Lee, E. C., & Kim, H. J. (2024). Machine learning-based classification of Parkinson's disease using acoustic features: Insights from multilingual speech tasks. *Computers in Biology and Medicine*, *182*, 109078. DOI: 10.1016/j.compbiomed.2024.109078 PMID: 39265476

Jiang, F., Lu, Y., Chen, Y., Cai, D., & Li, G. (2020). Image recognition of four rice leaf diseases based on deep learning and support vector machine. *Computers and Electronics in Agriculture*, *179*, 105824. DOI: 10.1016/j.compag.2020.105824

Júnior, J. R., Telles, J. P. M., da Silva, S. A., Iglesio, R. F., Brigido, M. M., Caldas, J. G. M. P., & Figueiredo, E. G. (2019). Epidemiological analysis of 1404 patients with intracranial aneurysm followed in a single Brazilian institution. *Surgical Neurology International*, *10*, 249. DOI: 10.25259/SNI_443_2019 PMID: 31893150

Kakde, P., Andhele, A., Kadam, A., Bedi, G., Acharya, S., & Kumar, S. (2025). Fatal interplay between acquired thrombotic thrombocytopenic purpura and posterior reversible encephalopathy syndrome: A case report. *Radiology Case Reports*, *20*(6), 2995–2999. DOI: 10.1016/j.radcr.2025.02.094 PMID: 40224228

Keret, A., Bennett-Back, O., Rosenthal, G., Gilboa, T., Shweiki, M., Shoshan, Y., & Benifla, M. (2017, July). Posttraumatic epilepsy: Long-term follow-up of children with mild traumatic brain injury. *Journal of Neurosurgery. Pediatrics*, *20*(1), 64–70. DOI: 10.3171/2017.2.PEDS16585 PMID: 28474982

Khaleghi, F., & C., E. (2017). Brivaracetam (Briviact). *P&T : a Peer-Reviewed Journal for Formulary Management*, *42*(2), 92–96. PMID: 28163554

Khan, K., Ni, J., Tabba, F. A., & Saeed, S. (2025). Reshaping medical imaging analysis: Generative AI for adversarial-resistant image segmentation. In AI techniques for securing medical and business practices (p. 24).

Khan, K., Saeed, S., & Tabba, F. A. (2025). Reshaping brain tumor diagnosis: Generative AI-enhanced segmentation in MRI images. In AI techniques for securing medical and business practices (p. 28).

Khan, A. R., Khan, S., Harouni, M., Abbasi, R., Iqbal, S., & Mehmood, Z. (2021). Brain tumor segmentation using K-means clustering and deep learning with synthetic data augmentation for classification. *Microscopy Research and Technique*, *84*(7), 1389–1399. DOI: 10.1002/jemt.23694 PMID: 33524220

Khellaf, A., Khan, D. Z., & Helmy, A. (2019). Recent advances in traumatic brain injury. *Journal of Neurology*, *266*(11), 2878–2889. DOI: 10.1007/s00415-019-09541-4 PMID: 31563989

Khokar, T. I., Cheema, Z. A., Fatima, I., Riaz, M., Qadri, H. M., & Bashir, A. (2024). Surgical outcomes of delayed clipping in ruptured intracranial aneurysms of anterior circulation: Experience from a low-middle-income country. *Pakistan Journal of Medical Sciences*, *40*(12, PINS Suppl), S41–S46. DOI: 10.12669/pjms.40.12(PINS).11273 PMID: 39703957

Ko, H., Chung, H., Lee, H., & Lee, J. (2020). Feasible study on intracranial hemorrhage detection and classification using a CNN-LSTM network. In *2020 42nd Annual International Conference of the IEEE Engineering in Medicine & Biology Society (EMBC)* (pp. 1290–1293). IEEE. DOI: 10.1109/EMBC44109.2020.9176162

Kumar Kar, N., Jana, S., Rahman, A., & Ashokrao, P. R., G., I., & Alarmelu Mangai, R. (2024). Automated intracranial hemorrhage detection using deep learning in medical image analysis. In *2024 International Conference on Data Science and Network Security (ICDSNS)* (pp. 1–6). IEEE. https://doi.org/DOI: 10.1109/ICDSNS62112.2024.10691276

Kumar, N., & Singh, G. Revolutionizing Cancer Care: Advancements in Emerging Technologies and Therapies.

Kumar, V., Baburaj, V., Patel, S., Sharma, S., & Vaishya, R. (2021). Does the use of intraoperative CT scan improve outcomes in Orthopaedic surgery? A systematic review and meta-analysis of 871 cases. *Journal of Clinical Orthopaedics and Trauma*, *18*, 216–223. DOI: 10.1016/j.jcot.2021.04.030 PMID: 34040978

Kundisch, A., Hönning, A., Mutze, S., Kreissl, L., Spohn, F., Lemcke, J., Sitz, M., Sparenberg, P., & Goelz, L. (2021). Deep learning algorithm in detecting intracranial hemorrhages on emergency computed tomographies. *PLoS One*, *16*(11), e0260560. DOI: 10.1371/journal.pone.0260560 PMID: 34843559

La Rocca, M., Barisano, G., Garner, R., Ruf, S. F., Amoroso, N., Monti, M., Vespa, P., Bellotti, R., Erdoğmuş, D., Toga, A. W., & Duncan, D. (2023). Functional connectivity alterations in traumatic brain injury patients with late seizures. *Neurobiology of Disease*, *179*, 106053. DOI: 10.1016/j.nbd.2023.106053 PMID: 36871641

Lanzino, G., Kassell, N. F., Germanson, T. P., Kongable, G. L., Truskowski, L. L., Torner, J. C., & Jane, J. A. (1996). Age and outcome after aneurysmal subarachnoid hemorrhage: Why do older patients fare worse? *Journal of Neurosurgery*, *85*(3), 410–418. DOI: 10.3171/jns.1996.85.3.0410 PMID: 8751625

Lastrucci, A., Wandael, Y., Barra, A., Ricci, R., Maccioni, G., Pirrera, A., & Giansanti, D. (2024). Exploring Augmented Reality Integration in Diagnostic Imaging: Myth or Reality? *Diagnostics (Basel)*, *14*(13), 1333. DOI: 10.3390/diagnostics14131333 PMID: 39001224

Lazaridis, C., & Foreman, B. (2023). Management strategies based on multi-modality neuromonitoring in severe traumatic brain injury. *Neurotherapeutics; the Journal of the American Society for Experimental NeuroTherapeutics*, *20*(6), 1457–1471. DOI: 10.1007/s13311-023-01411-2 PMID: 37491682

Lee, K., Klein, P., Dongre, P., Choi, E. J., & Rhoney, D. H. (2022). Intravenous Brivaracetam in the management of acute seizures in the hospital setting: A scoping review. *Journal of Intensive Care Medicine*, *37*(9), 1133–1145. DOI: 10.1177/08850666211073598 PMID: 35306914

Leenes, R., Palmerini, E., Koops, B. J., Bertolini, A., Salvini, P., & Lucivero, F. (2017). Regulatory challenges of robotics: Some guidelines for addressing legal and ethical issues. *Law, Innovation and Technology*, *9*(1), 1–44. DOI: 10.1080/17579961.2017.1304921

Li, K.-Y., Hsu, C.-Y., & Yang, Y.-H. (2023). A review of cognitive and behavioral outcomes of Brivaracetam. *The Kaohsiung Journal of Medical Sciences*, *39*(2), 104–114. DOI: 10.1002/kjm2.12648 PMID: 36661137

Lindfors, M., Vehviläinen, J., Bendel, S., Reinikainen, M., Laitio, R., Ala-Kokko, T., Hoppu, S., Siironen, J., Skrifvars, M. B., & Raj, R. (2023). Incidence and risk factors of posttraumatic hydrocephalus and its association with outcome following intensive care unit treatment for traumatic brain injury: A multicenter observational study. *Journal of Neurosurgery*, *1*(1), 1–10. DOI: 10.3171/2023.2.JNS22728 PMID: 37029677

Lin, E., & Yuh, E. L. (2022). Computational Approaches for Acute Traumatic Brain Injury Image Recognition. *Frontiers in Neurology*, *13*, 791816. DOI: 10.3389/fneur.2022.791816 PMID: 35370919

Lin, Y., Zhang, S., Zhang, W., Wang, X., Huang, L., & Luo, H. (2021). The prediction value of Glasgow coma scale-pupils score in neurocritical patients: A retrospective study. *Brain Injury : [BI]*, *35*(5), 547–553. DOI: 10.1080/02699052.2021.1890821 PMID: 33645359

Liu, C. Y., Yin, G., Sun, Y. D., Lin, Y. F., Xie, Z., English, A. W., Li, Q.-F., & Lin, H.-D. (2020). Effect of exosomes from adipose-derived stem cells on the apoptosis of Schwann cells in peripheral nerve injury. *CNS Neuroscience & Therapeutics*, *26*(2), 189–196. DOI: 10.1111/cns.13187 PMID: 31278850

Liu, T., Fan, W., & Wu, C. (2019). A hybrid machine learning approach to cerebral stroke prediction based on imbalanced medical dataset. *Artificial Intelligence in Medicine*, *101*, 101723. DOI: 10.1016/j.artmed.2019.101723 PMID: 31813482

Liu, X., Liu, F., Jin, L., & Wu, J. (2024). Evolution of neurosurgical robots: Historical progress and future direction. *World Neurosurgery*, *191*, 49–57. DOI: 10.1016/j.wneu.2024.08.008 PMID: 39116942

Li, X., Zhang, L., Yang, J., & Teng, F. (2024). Role of artificial intelligence in medical image analysis: A review of current trends and future directions. *Journal of Medical and Biological Engineering*, *44*(2), 231–243. DOI: 10.1007/s40846-024-00863-x

Li, Y., Wang, D., Zhou, X., Liu, J., Jia, Y., & Xiao, N. (2024). Clinical characteristics and associated factors of posttraumatic epilepsy after traumatic brain injury in children: A retrospective case-control study. *Seizure*, *115*, 87–93. DOI: 10.1016/j.seizure.2023.12.016 PMID: 38232649

Lloyd, S. P. (1982). Least Squares Quantization in PCM. *IEEE Transactions on Information Theory*, *28*(2), 129–137. DOI: 10.1109/TIT.1982.1056489

Loupy, A., Sablik, M., Khush, K., & Reese, P. P. (2025). Advancing patient monitoring, diagnostics, and treatment strategies for transplant precision medicine. *Lancet*, *406*(10501), 389–402. DOI: 10.1016/S0140-6736(25)00195-3 PMID: 40614744

Luo, Y., & Payne, S. J. (2024). Neurological intervention transition model for dynamic prediction of good outcome in spontaneous subarachnoid haemorrhage. *Scientific Reports*, *14*(1), 1584. DOI: 10.1038/s41598-024-51684-6 PMID: 38238425

Lu, X. C. M., Browning, J., Liao, Z., Cao, Y., Yang, W., & Shear, D. A. (2020). Post-traumatic epilepsy and seizure susceptibility in rat models of penetrating and closed-head brain injury. *Journal of Neurotrauma*, *37*(2), 236–247. DOI: 10.1089/neu.2019.6573 PMID: 31530242

Mahmood, A. A. R., Jha, A. M., & Manivannan, K. (2024). Precision Medicine: Personalizing The Fight Against Cancer. *International Journal of Trends in Onco-Science*, 10-18.

Majidi, S., Makke, Y., Ewida, A., Sianati, B., Qureshi, A. I., & Koubeissi, M. Z. (2017). Prevalence and Risk Factors for Early Seizure in Patients with Traumatic Brain Injury: Analysis from National Trauma Data Bank. *Neurocritical Care*, *27*(1), 90–95. DOI: 10.1007/s12028-016-0363-6 PMID: 28000125

Malhotra, S., Halabi, O., Dakua, S. P., Padhan, J., Paul, S., & Palliyali, W. (2023). Augmented reality in surgical navigation: A review of evaluation and validation metrics. *Applied Sciences (Basel, Switzerland)*, *13*(3), 1629. DOI: 10.3390/app13031629

Mansour, R. F., & Aljehane, N. O. (2021). An optimal segmentation with deep learning based inception network model for intracranial hemorrhage diagnosis. *Neural Computing & Applications*, *33*(20), 13831–13843. DOI: 10.1007/s00521-021-06020-8

Mashiach, E., Soldozy, S., Sacknovitz, A., Jain, A., Donaldson, H., Zeller, S., ... & Santarelli, J. (2025). Advanced Imaging and Augmented Reality in Neurosurgery: Bridging Innovation and Precision.

McKenzie, D. M., Westrup, A. M., O'Neal, C. M., Lee, B. J., Shi, H. H., Dunn, I. F., Snyder, L. A., & Smith, Z. A. (2021). Robotics in spine surgery: A systematic review. *Journal of Clinical Neuroscience*, *89*, 1–7. DOI: 10.1016/j.jocn.2021.04.005 PMID: 34119250

Menna, G., Kolias, A., Esene, I. N., Barthélemy, E. J., Hoz, S., Laeke, T., Veiga Silva, A. C., Longo-Calderón, G. M., Baticulon, R. E., Zabala, J. P., Hassani, F. D., El Abbadi, N., Khan, M. M., Robertson, F. C., Thango, N., Cheresem, B., Ogando-Rivas, E., Roumy, L.-G., Karekezi, C., & Nicolosi, F. (2024). Reducing the gap in neurosurgical education in LMICs: A report of a non-profit educational program. *World Neurosurgery*, *182*, e792–e797. DOI: 10.1016/j.wneu.2023.12.040 PMID: 38101536

Mohammadi, A. T., Mohammadzadeh, I., Sajedifar, M., Shabani, M., Khonche, S., Asgari, R., & Behzadi, G. (2024). *Emerging Frontiers in Surgical Advancements: Exploring Cutting-Edge Technologies and Pioneering Techniques*. Nobel Sciences.

Mohammadi, H. R., Hatefi, M., Rahmatian, A., & Sadeghi, S. (2024). Risk Factors for Post-traumatic Epilepsy in Patients with Traumatic Brain Injuries. *Archives of Neuroscience*, *11*(1). Advance online publication. DOI: 10.5812/ans-144357

Mohan, S., Thirumalai, C., & Srivastava, G. (2019). Effective heart disease prediction using hybrid machine learning techniques. *IEEE Access : Practical Innovations, Open Solutions*, *7*, 81542–81554. DOI: 10.1109/ACCESS.2019.2923707

Mohanty, A., Mohapatra, A. G., & Mohanty, S. K. (2025). Smart Surgery: Navigating Precision through Machine Learning and IoT. In *Evolution of Machine Learning and Internet of Things Applications in Biomedical Engineering* (pp. 94-121). CRC Press.

Monteiro, M., Newcombe, V. F. J., Mathieu, F., Adatia, K., Kamnitsas, K., Ferrante, E., Das, T., Whitehouse, D., Rueckert, D., Menon, D. K., & Glocker, B. (2020). Multiclass semantic segmentation and quantification of traumatic brain injury lesions on head CT using deep learning: An algorithm development and multicentre validation study. *The Lancet. Digital Health*, *2*(6), 314–322. DOI: 10.1016/S2589-7500(20)30085-6 PMID: 33328125

Mousa, A. H., Scalia, G., Ahmed, N., Figueiredo, E. G., de Sena Barbosa, M. G., Khan, M. M., & Chaurasia, B. (2025). The evolution of intracranial aneurysm clipping: A historical perspective. *Annals of Medicine and Surgery (London)*, *87*(4), 2229–2233. DOI: 10.1097/MS9.0000000000003162 PMID: 40212222

Mula, M. (2025). Treatment options for post-traumatic epilepsy: An update on clinical and translational aspects. *Expert Review of Neurotherapeutics*, *25*(3), 273–280. DOI: 10.1080/14737175.2025.2469041 PMID: 39968755

Murr, L. E. (2020). Global trends in the development of complex, personalized, biomedical, surgical implant devices using 3D printing/additive manufacturing: A review. *Medical Devices & Sensors*, *3*(6), e10126. DOI: 10.1002/mds3.10126

Mushtak, A., Momin, U. Z., Ahmed, Z., Mahemood, S. A., & AbdulHameed, K. (2024). Radiological Imaging in the Intensive Care Management of Obstetric Emergencies: Safety Considerations, Best Practices, and Common Pathologies. In *Updates in Intensive Care of OBGY Patients* (pp. 257-281). Singapore: Springer Nature Singapore.

Nagarapu, M. N. (2021). *Modelling Parkinson's progression using naturally spoken language features* [Unpublished manuscript].

Noor, M. B. T., Zenia, N. Z., Kaiser, M. S., Mamun, S. A., & Mahmud, M. (2020). Application of deep learning in detecting neurological disorders from magnetic resonance images: A survey on the detection of Alzheimer's disease, Parkinson's disease, and schizophrenia. *Brain Informatics*, *7*(1), 1–21. DOI: 10.1186/s40708-020-00112-2 PMID: 33034769

Noureldin, F. (2020). *Early Surgery on Patients with Aneurysmal Subarachnoid Hemorrhage WFNS grades 4 and 5*. PQDT-Global.

O'Driscoll, L., Nichols, R., & Knott, P. A. (2019). A hybrid machine learning algorithm for designing quantum experiments. *Quantum Machine Intelligence*, *1*(1–2), 5–15. DOI: 10.1007/s42484-019-00003-8

Ouchane, K., Bellefkih, F. Z., Benchakroun, N., Bourhafour, M., Chekrine, T., Bouchbika, Z., ... & Sahraoui, S. (2024). Reversible posterior leukoencephalopathy syndrome following carboplatin and paclitaxel in cervical cancer: Case report. *SAGE Open Medical Case Reports, 12*, 2050313X241257444.

Pangal, D. J., Cote, D. J., Ruzevick, J., Yarovinsky, B., Kugener, G., Wrobel, B., Ference, E. H., Swanson, M., Hung, A. J., Donoho, D. A., Giannotta, S., & Zada, G. (2022). Robotic and robot-assisted skull base neurosurgery: Systematic review of current applications and future directions. *Neurosurgical Focus*, *52*(1), E15. DOI: 10.3171/2021.10.FOCUS21505 PMID: 34973668

Panni, A. S., Vasso, M., Braile, A., Toro, G., De Cicco, A., & Viggiano, D.. (2019). Preliminary results of autologous adipose-derived stem cells in early knee osteoarthritis: Identification of a subpopulation with greater response. *International Orthopaedics*, *43*(1), 7–13. DOI: 10.1007/s00264-018-4182-6 PMID: 30280218

Paolini, F., Marrone, S., Scalia, G., Gerardi, R. M., Bonosi, L., Benigno, U. E., Musso, S., Scerrati, A., Iacopino, D. G., Signorelli, F., Maugeri, R., & Visocchi, M. (2025). Diffusion tensor imaging as neurologic predictor in patients affected by traumatic brain injury: Scoping review. *Brain Sciences*, *15*(1), 70. DOI: 10.3390/brainsci15010070 PMID: 39851437

Passier, P. E. C. A., Visser-Meily, J. M. A., Van Zandvoort, M. J. E., Rinkel, G. J. E., Lindeman, E., & Post, M. W. M. (2010). Predictors of long-term health-related quality of life in patients with aneurysmal subarachnoid hemorrhage. *NeuroRehabilitation*, *30*(2), 137–145. DOI: 10.3233/NRE-2012-0737 PMID: 22430579

Pathak, K., Saikia, R., Das, A., Das, D., Islam, M. A., Pramanik, P., Parasar, A., Borthakur, P. P., Sarmah, P., Saikia, M., & Borthakur, B. (2023). 3D printing in biomedicine: Advancing personalized care through additive manufacturing. *Exploration of Medicine*, *4*(6), 1135–1167. DOI: 10.37349/emed.2023.00200

Pease, M., Mallela, A. N., Elmer, J., Okonkwo, D. O., Shutter, L., Barot, N., Gonzalez-Martinez, J., & Castellano, J. F. (2023). Association of Posttraumatic Epilepsy With Long-term Functional Outcomes in Individuals With Severe Traumatic Brain Injury. *Neurology, 100*(19), e1967–e1975. DOI: 10.1212/WNL.0000000000207183 PMID: 36948595

Peng, H., Han, B., Tong, T., Jin, X., Peng, Y., Guo, M., Li, B., Ding, J., Kong, Q., & Wang, Q. (2024). 3D printing processes in precise drug delivery for personalized medicine. *Biofabrication, 16*(3), 032001. DOI: 10.1088/1758-5090/ad3a14 PMID: 38569493

Pereira, R., Torres, B., Nogueira, J., Coimbra, F., Afonso, M., Alegria, C., & Marques, R. (2025). Predictive factors for ventriculoperitoneal shunt placement in aneurysmatic subarachnoid hemorrhages. *Brain & Spine, 5*, 104164. DOI: 10.1016/j.bas.2024.104164 PMID: 39802870

Peron, M., Saporiti, N., Shoeibi, M., Holmström, J., & Salmi, M. (2025). Additive manufacturing in the medical sector: From an empirical investigation of challenges and opportunities toward the design of an ecosystem model. *International Journal of Operations & Production Management, 45*(2), 387–415. DOI: 10.1108/IJOPM-12-2023-0948

Pettersson, S. D., Khorasanizadeh, M., Maglinger, B., Garcia, A., Wang, S. J., Tauss-ky, P., & Ogilvy, C. S. (2023). Trends in the age of patients treated for unruptured intracranial aneurysms from 1990 to 2020. *World Neurosurgery, 178*, 233–240. DOI: 10.1016/j.wneu.2023.08.007 PMID: 37562685

Phaphuangwittayakul, A., Guo, Y., Ying, F., Dawod, A. Y., Angkurawaranon, S., & Angkurawaranon, C. (2022). An optimal deep learning framework for multi-type hemorrhagic lesions detection and quantification in head CT images for traumatic brain injury. *Applied Intelligence, 52*(7), 1–19. DOI: 10.1007/s10489-021-02782-9 PMID: 34764620

Picetti, E., Catena, F., Abu-Zidan, F., Ansaloni, L., Armonda, R. A., Bala, M., Balogh, Z. J., Bertuccio, A., Biffl, W. L., Bouzat, P., Buki, A., Cerasti, D., Chesnut, R. M., Citerio, G., Coccolini, F., Coimbra, R., Coniglio, C., Fainardi, E., Gupta, D., & Robba, C. (2023). Early management of isolated severe traumatic brain injury patients in a hospital without neurosurgical capabilities: A consensus and clinical recommendations of the World Society of Emergency Surgery (WSES). *World Journal of Emergency Surgery; WJES, 18*(1), 5. DOI: 10.1186/s13017-022-00468-2 PMID: 36624517

Pojskić, M., Bopp, M., Saß, B., Kirschbaum, A., Nimsky, C., & Carl, B. (2021). Intraoperative computed tomography-based navigation with augmented reality for lateral approaches to the spine. *Brain Sciences, 11*(5), 646. DOI: 10.3390/brainsci11050646 PMID: 34063546

Postuma, R. B., Berg, D., Stern, M., Poewe, W., Olanow, C. W., Oertel, W., Obeso, J., Marek, K., Litvan, I., Lang, A. E., Halliday, G., Goetz, C. G., Gasser, T., Dubois, B., Chan, P., Bloem, B. R., Adler, C. H., & Deuschl, G. (2019). MDS clinical diagnostic criteria for Parkinson's disease. *Movement Disorders, 30*(12), 1591–1601. DOI: 10.1002/mds.26424 PMID: 26474316

Power, D. (2024). Ethical considerations in the era of AI, automation, and surgical robots: There are plenty of lessons from the past. *Discover Artificial Intelligence, 4*(1), 65. DOI: 10.1007/s44163-024-00166-9

Prabakaran, D. A., & Ibrahim, S. A. M. Advancing Precision Oncology with Artificial Intelligence.

Prządka, M., Pająk, W., Kleinrok, J., Pec, J., Michno, K., Karpiński, R., & Baj, J. (2025). Advances in 3D Printing Applications for Personalized Orthopedic Surgery: From Anatomical Modeling to Patient-Specific Implants. *Journal of Clinical Medicine, 14*(11), 3989. DOI: 10.3390/jcm14113989 PMID: 40507750

Queisner, M., & Eisenträger, K. (2024). Surgical planning in virtual reality: A systematic review. *Journal of Medical Imaging (Bellingham, Wash.), 11*(6), 062603–062603. DOI: 10.1117/1.JMI.11.6.062603 PMID: 38680654

qure.ai. (2019). Qure.ai's qER CT Scan Algorithm Receives CE Certification. https://www.qure.ai/news_press_coverages/ce-certification-for-qure-ais-traumatic -brain- injury-and-stroke-triage-tool. Raza, A., Ayub, H., Khan, J. A., Ahmad, I., Salama, A. S., Daradkeh, Y. I., Javeed, D., Rehman, U., & Hamam, H. (2022). A Hybrid Deep Learning-Based Approach for Brain Tumor Classification. Electronics 2022, Vol. 11, Page 1146, 11(7), 1146. DOI: 10.3390/electronics11071146

Ragnhildstveit, A., Li, C., Zimmerman, M. H., Mamalakis, M., Curry, V. N., Holle, W., Baig, N., Uğuralp, A. K., Alkhani, L., Oğuz-Uğuralp, Z., Romero-Garcia, R., & Suckling, J. (2023). Intra-operative applications of augmented reality in glioma surgery: A systematic review. *Frontiers in Surgery, 10*, 1245851. DOI: 10.3389/fsurg.2023.1245851 PMID: 37671031

Raj, S., Ganesan, P. K., Singh, A., & Ganesan, P. K. (2025). Ruptured Intracranial Hydatid Cyst. *MEDICAL JOURNAL*, (March), 144.

Rathod, V., Shrivastav, S., & Gharpinde, M. R. (2024). Knee Arthroscopy in the Era of Precision Medicine: A Comprehensive Review of Tailored Approaches and Emerging Technologies. *Cureus*, *16*(10). Advance online publication. DOI: 10.7759/cureus.70932 PMID: 39502973

Rehan, H. (2024). Advancing Cancer Treatment with AI-Driven Personalized Medicine and Cloud-Based Data Integration. *Journal of Machine Learning in Pharmaceutical Research*, *4*(2), 1–40.

Rinkel, G. J., & Algra, A. (2011). Long-term outcomes of patients with aneurysmal subarachnoid haemorrhage. *Lancet Neurology*, *10*(4), 349–356. DOI: 10.1016/S1474-4422(11)70017-5 PMID: 21435599

Roy, S., Knutsen, A., & Korotcov, A.. (2018). A deep learning framework for brain extraction in humans and animals with traumatic brain injury. In *Proceedings of the IEEE International Symposium on Biomedical Imaging* (pp. 687–691). IEEE. / DOI: 10.1109/ISBI.2018.8363667

Rubinos, C., Waters, B., & Hirsch, L. J. (2022). Predicting and Treating Post-traumatic Epilepsy. *Current Treatment Options in Neurology*, *24*(9), 365–381. DOI: 10.1007/s11940-022-00727-2

Saeed, S. (2024). Improved hybrid K-nearest neighbors' techniques in segmentation of low-grade tumor and cerebrospinal fluid.

Saeed, S., & Abdullah, A. (2022). Hybrid graph cut hidden Markov model of K-mean cluster technique. CMC-Computers, Materials & Continua, 1-15.

Saeed, S., Ghani, R., Shahid, Z., Naseeb, U., & Khan, U. A. (2024). Nervous Discrepancy of Spinal Cord Schwannoma Causing Posterior Neck Swelling: Spinal Cord Schwannoma Causing Posterior Neck Swelling. *Pakistan Journal of Health Sciences*, 229-232.

Saeed, S., Jhanjhi, N. Z., Naqvi, M., Humayun, M., & Ponnusamy, V. (2021). Quantitative analysis of COVID-19 patients: A preliminary statistical result of deep learning artificial intelligence framework. In *ICT solutions for improving smart communities in Asia* (pp. 218-242). DOI: 10.4018/978-1-7998-7114-9.ch011

Saeed, S. (2018). Impact of data mining techniques to analyze health care data. *Journal of Medical Sciences and Health.*

Saeed, S. (2021). Implementation of donor recognition and selection for bioinformatics blood bank application. In *Advanced AI techniques and applications in bioinformatics* (Vol. 1, pp. 105–138). CRC Press. DOI: 10.1201/9781003126164-5

Saeed, S., & Abdullah, A. (2021). Combination of brain cancer with hybrid K-NN algorithm using statistical analysis of cerebrospinal fluid (CSF) surgery. *International Journal of Computer Science and Network Security*, *21*(2), 120–130.

Saeed, S., & Abdullah, A. (2021). Comparison analysis of medical health care information of graph cutting using multi-dimension segmentation. *Machine Learning Healthcare: Handling and Managing Data*, *1*(1), 1–23.

Saeed, S., & Abdullah, A. (2022). Hybrid graph cut hidden Markov model of K-mean cluster technique. *CMC-Computers. Materials & Continua*, *1*, 1–15.

Saeed, S., & Abdullah, A. (2022). Hybrid graph cut hidden Markov model of K-mean cluster technique. *Computers, Materials & Continua*, *72*(1), 1–15. DOI: 10.32604/cmc.2022.024085

Saeed, S., Abdullah, A., Jhanjhi, N. Z., Naqvi, M., & Ahmed, S. (2020). Effects of cell phone usage on human health and specifically on the brain. In *Machine learning for healthcare* (pp. 53–68). Chapman and Hall/CRC. DOI: 10.1201/9780429330131-5

Saeed, S., Ghani, R., & Shahid, Z. (2024). Prevalence of low back pain and its associated factors in an underdeveloped country: Pakistan. *Journal of Health and Rehabilitation Research*, *4*(3), 1–7.

Saeed, S., Ghani, R., & Shahid, Z. (2024). Prevalence of low back pain and its associated factors in an underdeveloped country: Pakistan: Prevalence of low back pain in Pakistan. *Journal of Health and Rehabilitation Research*, *4*(3), 1–7.

Saeed, S., Ghani, R., & Shahid, Z. (2024). Prevalence of Low Back Pain and Its Associated Factors in an Underdeveloped Country: Pakistan: Prevalence of Low Back Pain in Pakistan. *Journal of Health and Rehabilitation Research*, *4*(3), 1–7.

Saeed, S., & Haron, H. (2021). A systematic mapping study of low-grade tumor of brain cancer and CSF fluid detecting in MRI images. *Approaches and Applications of Deep Learning in Virtual Medical Care*, *1*(1), 1–25.

Saeed, S., & Haron, H. (2021). Improve correlation matrix of discrete Fourier transformation (CM-DFT) technique for finding the missing values of MRI images. *Mathematical Biosciences and Engineering*, •••, 1–22.

Saeed, S., & Qasim, M. B. (2023). Surgical acute epidural hematoma in the temporal perioral region of the brain. *International Journal of Head and Neck Surgery*, *14*(3), 1–8. DOI: 10.5005/jp-journals-10001-1552

Saeed, S., Shaikh, A., Ali, M., Hussain, M., Ahmed, F., & Mehmood, S. (2017). Implementation of failure enterprise systems in the organizational perspective framework. *International Journal of Advanced Computer Science and Applications*, *8*(5), 54–63. DOI: 10.14569/IJACSA.2017.080508

Saeed, S., Shaikh, A., Memon, M. A., & Naqvi, S. M. R. (2018). Impact of data mining techniques to analyze health care data. *Journal of Medical Imaging and Health Informatics*, *8*(4), 682–690. DOI: 10.1166/jmihi.2018.2385

Saeed, S., Shaikh, A., Memon, M. A., Saleem, M. Q., & Naqvi, S. M. R. (2017). Assessment of brain tumor due to the usage of MATLAB performance. *Journal of Medical Imaging and Health Informatics*, *7*(6), 1454–1460. DOI: 10.1166/jmihi.2017.2187

Sage, A., & Badura, P. (2020). Intracranial hemorrhage detection in head CT using double-branch convolutional neural network, support vector machine, and random forest. *Applied Sciences (Basel, Switzerland)*, *10*(21), 7577. DOI: 10.3390/app10217577

Salah, H., Qasem, H., Omer, H., Bradley, D. A., & Sulieman, A. (2025). Optimizing CT Imaging for Patients with Disabilities: A Survey on Radiation Dose Reduction and Protocol Improvements. *Radiation Physics and Chemistry*, •••, 113164. DOI: 10.1016/j.radphyschem.2025.113164

Salar, H., Anns, K. M., Salar, M., Khan, F., Aman, M., Zafar, U., Ahmad, I., Basharat, S., Murad, R., Salar, K., & Anwar, S. S. M. (2025). From Gut to Gray Matter: A Case Report of Posterior Reversible Encephalopathy Syndrome in a Pediatric Patient with Celiac Disease. *Clinical Case Reports*, *13*(3), e70260. DOI: 10.1002/ccr3.70260 PMID: 40114993

Sampath, T., Srinivasan, T. P., Thamizharasan, S., & Krithaksha, V. (2025). 3D Printing in Medicine. In *Compendium of 3D Bioprinting Technology* (pp. 271–285). CRC Press.

Samuel, A. L. (1959). Some Studies in Machine Learning Using the Game of Checkers. *IBM Journal of Research and Development*, *3*(3), 210–229. DOI: 10.1147/rd.33.0210

Saputra, M. F. A., Widiyaningtyas, T., & Wibawa, A. P. (2018). Illiteracy classification using K means-naïve bayes algorithm. *JOIV: International Journal on Informatics Visualization*, *2*(3), 153–158. DOI: 10.30630/joiv.2.3.129

Sarkodie, B. D., Jimah, B. B., Offei, A. K., Botwe, B., Anim, D., Mensah, Y. B., & Brakohiapa, E. K. (2022). Challenges of practicing neuro-endovascular interventions in a resource-limited country; Ghana in focus. *Neurological Sciences*, *43*(9), 5451–5457. DOI: 10.1007/s10072-022-06222-5 PMID: 35729440

Sarvamangala, D. R., & Kulkarni, R. V. (2022). Convolutional neural networks in medical image understanding: A survey. *Evolutionary Intelligence*, *15*(1), 1–22. DOI: 10.1007/s12065-020-00540-3 PMID: 33425040

Schmidt, T. P., Weiss, M., Hoellig, A., Nikoubashman, O., Schulze-Steinen, H., Albanna, W., Clusmann, H., Schubert, G. A., & Veldeman, M. (2022). Revisiting the timeline of delayed cerebral ischemia after aneurysmal subarachnoid hemorrhage: Toward a temporal risk profile. *Neurocritical Care*, *37*(3), 735–743. DOI: 10.1007/s12028-022-01545-9 PMID: 35790670

Schneider, A. L., Law, C. A., Gottesman, R. F., Krauss, G., Huang, J., Kucharska-Newton, A., Jensen, F. E., Gugger, J. J., Diaz-Arrastia, R., & Johnson, E. L. (2024). Posttraumatic epilepsy and dementia risk. *JAMA Neurology*, *81*(4), 346–353. DOI: 10.1001/jamaneurol.2024.0010 PMID: 38407883

Shaban, M. (2023). Deep learning for Parkinson's disease diagnosis: A short survey. *Computers*, *12*(3), 58. DOI: 10.3390/computers12030058

Shah, K. A., White, T. G., Teron, I., Turpin, J., Dehdashti, A. R., Temes, R. E., Black, K., & Woo, H. H. (2024). Quantitative magnetic resonance angiography as an alternative imaging technique in the assessment of cerebral vasospasm after subarachnoid hemorrhage. *Interventional Neuroradiology : Journal of Peritherapeutic Neuroradiology, Surgical Procedures and Related Neurosciences*, *30*(2), 271–279. DOI: 10.1177/15910199221138167 PMID: 36357992

Sharma, N., Mallela, A. N., Khan, T., Canton, S. P., Kass, N. M., Steuer, F., Jardini, J., Biehl, J., & Andrews, E. G. (2024). Evolution of the meta-neurosurgeon: A systematic review of the current technical capabilities, limitations, and applications of augmented reality in neurosurgery. *Surgical Neurology International*, *15*, 146. DOI: 10.25259/SNI_167_2024 PMID: 38742013

Sharma, P. K., Balachandar, S., Vikram, M. A., & Sukumar, P. D. (2025). Rituximab (monoclonal anti-CD20 antibody) induced posterior reversible encephalopathy syndrome (PRES): A case report and literature review. *Radiology Case Reports*, *20*(3), 1538–1547. DOI: 10.1016/j.radcr.2024.11.070 PMID: 39811052

Shiwlani, A., Khan, M., Sherani, A. M. K., & Qayyum, M. U. (2023). Synergies of AI and smart technology: Revolutionizing cancer medicine, vaccine development, and patient care. *International Journal of Social. Humanities and Life Sciences, 1*(1), 10–18.

Shoukat, S., Tabassum, S., & Shahbaz, H. (2024). Frequency of Cerebral Aneurysm in patients with subarachnoid hemorrhage on CT Cerebral Angiography. *Pakistan Journal of Medical Sciences, 40*(9), 1975. PMID: 39416605

Siddique, S., Shultana, S., & Frizell, S. (2023, September). An enhanced strategy of detecting neurological disorders from magnetic resonance images using deep learning. In *2023 IEEE Sixth International Conference on Artificial Intelligence and Knowledge Engineering (AIKE)* (pp. 99-104). IEEE. DOI: 10.1109/AIKE59827.2023.00024

Singh, K. R., & Dash, S. (2023). Early detection of neurological diseases using machine learning and deep learning techniques: A review. *Artificial Intelligence for Neurological Disorders, 1*, 1–24. DOI: 10.1016/B978-0-323-90277-9.00001-8

Singh, R., Wang, K., Qureshi, M. B., Rangel, I. C., Brown, N. J., Shahrestani, S., Gottfried, O. N., Patel, N. P., & Bydon, M. (2022). Robotics in neurosurgery: Current prevalence and future directions. *Surgical Neurology International, 13*, 373. DOI: 10.25259/SNI_522_2022 PMID: 36128120

Smyrna, G. (2017, January 19). *Briviact (Brivaracetam) prescribing information*. UCB, Inc. Retrieved from https://www.ucb.com/stories-media/Press-Releases/article/UCB-files-BRIVIACT-brivaracetam-CV-in-the-U-S-as-monotherapy-treatment-for-adult-epilepsy-patients-with-partial-onset-seizures

Sommer, F., Goldberg, J. L., McGrath, L.Jr, Kirnaz, S., Medary, B., & Härtl, R. (2021). Image guidance in spinal surgery: A critical appraisal and future directions. *The International Journal of Spine Surgery, 15*(s2), S74–S86. DOI: 10.14444/8142 PMID: 34675032

Soun, J. E., Chow, D. S., Nagamine, M., Takhtawala, R. S., Filippi, C. G., Yu, W., & Chang, P. D. (2021). Artificial intelligence and acute stroke imaging. *AJNR. American Journal of Neuroradiology, 42*(1), 2–11. DOI: 10.3174/ajnr.A6883 PMID: 33243898

Specht, S., Zhukova, I., Westhoff, J. H., Erb, L., Ziegler, A., Kölker, S., Hoffmann, G. F., Hagmann, S., & Syrbe, S. (2024). Fat embolism syndrome in Duchenne muscular dystrophy: Report on a novel case and systematic literature review. *European Journal of Paediatric Neurology, 48*, 91–100. DOI: 10.1016/j.ejpn.2023.11.012 PMID: 38096597

Srichawla, B. S., Fang, T., Kipkorir, V., & Garcia-Dominguez, M. A. (2024). Reversible cerebral vasoconstriction syndrome and posterior reversible encephalopathy syndrome following vaccination: Analysis of the VAERS database and systematic review. *Annals of Medicine and Surgery (London), 86*(3), 1251–1260. DOI: 10.1097/MS9.0000000000001407 PMID: 38463101

Srinivasa Rao, N., Kumar, R., Kavitha, N., T, R., Pydi, H. P., Shankhyan, A., Subbiah, R., & Mann, V. S. (2025). Analyse the mechanical property optimization for FDM/3D-printed polycarbonate using Taguchi and TOPSIS techniques. *Journal of Metals. Materials and Minerals, 35*(1), e2196–e2196. DOI: 10.55713/jmmm.v35i1.2196

Stadsholt, S., Strauss, A., Kintzel, J., Schob, S., Elolf, E., Rutenkröger, M., & Scheer, M. (2024). Posterior reversible enzephalopathie syndrome (PRES) following vestibular schwannoma surgery–Case Report and Review of the current theories on pathophysiology of PRES. *Brain & Spine*, 104167. PMID: 39898006

Stark, M., Mynbaev, O., Malvasi, A., & Tinelli, A. (2024). Revolutionizing patient care: The harmonious blend of artificial intelligence and surgical tradition. *International Journal of Clinical and Experimental Pathology, 17*(2), 47–50. DOI: 10.62347/FRIC2771 PMID: 38455508

Stirrat, T., Martin, R., Baek, G., Thiru, S., Lakhani, D., Umair, M., & Sayah, A. (2024). Pixels to precision: Neuroradiology's leap into 3D printing for personalized medicine. *Journal of Clinical Imaging Science, 14*, 49. DOI: 10.25259/JCIS_119_2024 PMID: 39777212

Strein, M., Holton-Burke, J. P., Stilianoudakis, S., Moses, C., Almohaish, S., & Brophy, G. M. (2023). Levetiracetam-associated behavioral adverse events in neurocritical care patients. *Pharmacotherapy, 43*(2), 122–128. DOI: 10.1002/phar.2760 PMID: 36606737

Streubel, S. O., Luedtke, M. A., Garcia, M. I. O., & Alfi, D. (2023). of the Personalized Approach. *Fundamentals of Craniofacial Malformations: Vol. 2, Treatment Principles*, 321.

Stumpo, V., Staartjes, V. E., Esposito, G., Serra, C., Regli, L., Olivi, A., & Sturiale, C. L. (2021). Machine learning and intracranial aneurysms: from detection to outcome prediction. In *Machine Learning in Clinical Neuroscience: Foundations and Applications* (pp. 319–331). Springer International Publishing.

Suhag, D., Kaushik, S., & Taxak, V. B. (2024). 3D Printing in Biomedicine. In *Handbook of Biomaterials for Medical Applications, Volume 1: Fundamentals* (pp. 185-212). Singapore: Springer Nature Singapore.

Sui, S., Sun, J., Chen, X., & Fan, F. (2023). Risk of epilepsy following traumatic brain injury: A systematic review and meta-analysis. *The Journal of Head Trauma Rehabilitation*, *38*(4), 289–298. DOI: 10.1097/HTR.0000000000000818 PMID: 36730820

Support Vector Machine (SVM) Algorithm - Javatpoint. (n.d.). https://www.javatpoint.com/machine-learning-support-vector-machine-algorithm

Tekerek, U., Nazan, O. D., & Yener, N. A. (2023). Posttraumatic epilepsy in critically ill children with traumatic brain injury. *Child's Nervous System*, 1–8. PMID: 37480521

Tétinou, F., Kanmounye, U. S., Sadler, S., Nitcheu, I., Oriaku, A. J., Ndajiwo, A. B., & Bankole, N. D. A. (2021). Cerebral aneurysms in Africa: A scoping review. *Interdisciplinary Neurosurgery : Advanced Techniques and Case Management*, *26*, 101291. DOI: 10.1016/j.inat.2021.101291

Tharek, A., Muda, A. S., Baseri Hudi, A., & Baseri Hudin, A. (2022). Intracranial hemorrhage detection in CT scan using deep learning. *Asian Journal of Medical Technology*, *2*(1), 1–18. DOI: 10.32896/ajmedtech.v2n1.1-18

Tirupal, T., Mohan, B. C., & Kumar, S. S. (2021). Multimodal medical image fusion techniques–a review. *Current Signal Transduction Therapy*, *16*(2), 142–163. DOI: 10.2174/1574362415666200226103116

Tjoumakaris, S. I., Hanel, R., Mocco, J., Ali-Aziz Sultan, M., Froehler, M., Lieber, B. B., Coon, A., Tateshima, S., Altschul, D. J., Narayanan, S., El Naamani, K., Taussky, P., Hoh, B. L., Meyers, P., Gounis, M. J., Liebeskind, D. S., Volovici, V., Toth, G., Arthur, A., & Wakhloo, A. K. (2024). ARISE I consensus review on the management of intracranial aneurysms. *Stroke*, *55*(5), 1428–1437. DOI: 10.1161/STROKEAHA.123.046208 PMID: 38648283

Tonk, M., Gupta, V., Dhwaj, A., & Sachdeva, M. (2025). Current developments and advancements of 3-dimensional printing in personalized medication and drug screening. *Drug Metabolism and Personalized Therapy*, *39*(4), 167–182. DOI: 10.1515/dmpt-2024-0024 PMID: 39331538

Trakolis, L., & Petridis, A. K. (2024). Clinical management of a ruptured intracranial aneurysm. *Frontiers in Stroke*, *3*, 1450650. DOI: 10.3389/fstro.2024.1450650

Ueda, D., Yamamoto, A., Nishimori, M., Shimono, T., Doishita, S., Shimazaki, A., Katayama, Y., Fukumoto, S., Choppin, A., Shimahara, Y., & Miki, Y. (2019). Deep learning for MR angiography: Automated detection of cerebral aneurysms. *Radiology*, *290*(1), 187–194. DOI: 10.1148/radiol.2018180901 PMID: 30351253

Václavík, D., Volný, O., Cimflová, P., Švub, K., Dvorníková, K., & Bar, M. (2022). The importance of CT perfusion for diagnosis and treatment of ischemic stroke in anterior circulation. *Journal of Integrative Neuroscience*, *21*(3), 92. DOI: 10.31083/j.jin2103092 PMID: 35633173

Vadhavekar, N. H., Sabzvari, T., Laguardia, S., Sheik, T., Prakash, V., Gupta, A., & Patiño, B. B. R.Sr. (2024). Advancements in imaging and neurosurgical techniques for brain tumor resection: A comprehensive review. *Cureus*, *16*(10). Advance online publication. DOI: 10.7759/cureus.72745 PMID: 39618625

Vakharia, V. N. (2020). *Computer-Assisted Planning and Robotics in Epilepsy Surgery* (Doctoral dissertation, UCL (University College London)).

vbookshelf. (2019). vbookshelf/Intracranial-Hemorrhage-Analyzer: Ai powered web app that automatically detects and segments intracranial hemorrhages on brain CT images - Tensorflow.js. https://github.com/vbookshelf/Intracranial-Hemorrhage-Analyzer

Vlachou, M., Siamidi, A., & Protopapa, C. (2025). 3D-printing technologies for pharmaceutical applications. *Fundamentals and future trends of 3D printing in drug delivery*, 29-46.

Vyas, T., Yadav, R., Solanki, C., Darji, R., Desai, S., & Tanwar, S. (2022). Deep learning-based scheme to diagnose Parkinson's disease. *Expert Systems: International Journal of Knowledge Engineering and Neural Networks*, *39*(3), e12739. DOI: 10.1111/exsy.12739

Wallace, N., Schaffer, N. E., Aleem, I. S., & Patel, R. (2020). 3D-printed patient-specific spine implants: A systematic review. *Clinical Spine Surgery*, *33*(10), 400–407. DOI: 10.1097/BSD.0000000000001026 PMID: 32554986

Wang, A. C., & Heros, R. C. (2016). Subarachnoid hemorrhage grading scales. *Journal of Neurosurgery*, *124*(2), 296–298. DOI: 10.3171/2015.3.JNS15336 PMID: 26381258

Wang, B., Liao, X., Ni, Y., Zhang, L., Liang, J., Wang, J., Liu, Y., Sun, X., Ou, Y., Wu, Q., Shi, L., Yang, Z., & Lan, L. (2022). High-resolution medical image reconstruction based on residual neural network for diagnosis of cerebral aneurysm. *Frontiers in Cardiovascular Medicine*, *9*, 1013031. DOI: 10.3389/fcvm.2022.1013031 PMID: 36337881

Wang, D. M., Li, J., Liu, J. R., & Hu, H. Y. (2012). Diffusion tensor imaging predicts long-term motor functional outcome in patients with acute supratentorial intracranial hemorrhage. *Cerebrovascular Diseases (Basel, Switzerland), 34*(3), 199–205. DOI: 10.1159/000341857 PMID: 23006600

Wang, G. X.. (2021). Advanced neuroimaging in surgical planning for cerebral aneurysms. *Neurosurgical Review, 44*, 1997–2010.

Wang, J., Wang, Y., Wang, R., Wang, Q., Wen, M., Wang, J., Sheng, L., Zheng, Y., & Xi, T. (2025). A Review on 3D Printing Processes in Pharmaceutical Engineering and Tissue Engineering: Applications, Trends and Challenges. *Advanced Materials Technologies, 10*(2), 2400620. DOI: 10.1002/admt.202400620

Wang, X., & Huang, X. (2024). Risk factors and predictive indicators of rupture in cerebral aneurysms. *Frontiers in Physiology, 15*, 1454016. DOI: 10.3389/fphys.2024.1454016 PMID: 39301423

Wiles, M. D., Braganza, M., Edwards, H., Krause, E., Jackson, J., & Tait, F. (2023). Management of traumatic brain injury in the non-neurosurgical intensive care unit: A narrative review of current evidence. *Anaesthesia, 78*(4), 510–520. DOI: 10.1111/anae.15898 PMID: 36633447

Woźniak, M., Siłka, J., & Wieczorek, M. (2023). Deep neural network correlation learning mechanism for CT brain tumor detection. *Neural Computing & Applications, 35*(20), 14611–14626. DOI: 10.1007/s00521-021-05841-x

Wu, R., Hu, F., Liu, C., & Liang, J. (2024). The value of modified hijdra score in patients with aneurysmal subarachnoid hemorrhage. *Heliyon, 10*(7), e28550. DOI: 10.1016/j.heliyon.2024.e28550 PMID: 38590907

Xiao, Z. K., Wang, B., Liu, J. H., Yang, Y. B., Jie, N., Mao, X. Y., Gong, X. Y., Liu, A. H., & Duan, Y. H. (2025). Risk factors for the development of delayed cerebral ischemia after aneurysmal subarachnoid hemorrhage: A systematic review and meta-analysis. *World Neurosurgery, 193*, 427–446. DOI: 10.1016/j.wneu.2024.09.104 PMID: 39343384

Yang, C., & Li, Y. (2022). Review of the prevention and treatment of hydrocephalus after aneurysmal subarachnoid hemorrhage. *World Neurosurgery, 168*, 134–138. DOI: 10.1016/j.wneu.2022.08.089 PMID: 36041720

Yang, C., Zhao, Z., Yang, B., Wang, K., Zhu, G., & Miao, H. (2024). Sex differences in outcome of aneurysmal subarachnoid hemorrhage and its relation to postoperative cerebral ischemia. *Neurocritical Care, 41*(3), 985–996. DOI: 10.1007/s12028-024-02028-9 PMID: 38954369

Yu, N., Nguyen, T., Cho, Y. D., Kavanagh, N. M., Ghassib, I., & Giannobile, W. V. (2019). Personalized scaffolding technologies for alveolar bone regenerative medicine. *Orthodontics & Craniofacial Research, 22*(S1), 69–75. DOI: 10.1111/ocr.12275 PMID: 31074155

Zacharia, B. E., Hickman, Z. L., Grobelny, B. T., DeRosa, P., Kotchetkov, I., Ducruet, A. F., & Connolly, E. S. (2010). Epidemiology of aneurysmal subarachnoid hemorrhage. *Neurosurgery Clinics, 21*(2), 221–233. PMID: 20380965

Zahid, M. J., Mavani, P., Awuah, W. A., Alabdulrahman, M., Punukollu, R., Kundu, A., Mago, A., Maher, K., Adebusoye, F. T., & Khan, T. N. (2024). Sculpting the future: A narrative review of 3D printing in plastic surgery and prosthetic devices. *Health Science Reports, 7*(6), e2205. DOI: 10.1002/hsr2.2205 PMID: 38915353

Zeb, S., Nizamullah, F. N. U., Abbasi, N., & Fahad, M. (2024). AI in healthcare: Revolutionizing diagnosis and therapy. *International Journal of Multidisciplinary Sciences and Arts, 3*(3), 118–128. DOI: 10.47709/ijmdsa.v3i3.4546

Zhang, D., Sheng, Y., Wang, C., Chen, W., & Shi, X. (2024). Global traumatic brain injury intracranial pressure: From monitoring to surgical decision. *Frontiers in Neurology, 15*, 1423329. DOI: 10.3389/fneur.2024.1423329 PMID: 39355091

Zhao, Z., Poyhonen, J., & Cai, C. X., Sophie Woodley Hooper, F., Ma, Y., Hu, Y., ... & Tsz Ho Tse, Z. (2021). Augmented reality technology in image-guided therapy: State-of-the-art review. *Proceedings of the Institution of Mechanical Engineers, Part H: Journal of Engineering in Medicine, 235*(12), 1386-1398.

Zhao, D., Li, Y., & Cui, J. (2024). The factors associated with the modified Fisher grade in patients with aneurysmal subarachnoid hemorrhage. *Frontiers in Physiology, 15*, 1373925. DOI: 10.3389/fphys.2024.1373925 PMID: 39086933

Zhou, S. K., Greenspan, H., Davatzikos, C., Duncan, J. S., Van Ginneken, B., Madabhushi, A., Prince, J. L., Rueckert, D., & Summers, R. M. (2021). A review of deep learning in medical imaging: Imaging traits, technology trends, case studies with progress highlights, and future promises. Proceedings of the IEEE. Institute of Electrical and Electronics Engineers, 109(5), 820. DOI: 10.1109/JPROC.2021.3054390

Zhou, C., Zheng, L., Huang, W., Cheng, X., & Zhang, L. (2024). CT Angiography Image Postprocessing and Data Analysis. In *Whole Body Computed Tomography Angiography* (pp. 43–65). Springer Nature Singapore. DOI: 10.1007/978-981-97-1733-0_2

Zhu, Y., Guo, S., Ravichandran, D., Ramanathan, A., Sobczak, M. T., Sacco, A. F., Patil, D., Thummalapalli, S. V., Pulido, T. V., Lancaster, J. N., Yi, J., Cornella, J. L., Lott, D. G., Chen, X., Mei, X., Zhang, Y. S., Wang, L., Wang, X., Zhao, Y., & Song, K. (2025). 3D-Printed Polymeric Biomaterials for Health Applications. *Advanced Healthcare Materials*, *14*(1), 2402571. DOI: 10.1002/adhm.202402571 PMID: 39498750

Ziebart, A., Dremel, J., Hetjens, S., Nieuwkamp, D. J., Linn, F. H., Etminan, N., & Rinkel, G. J. (2024). Case fatality and functional outcome after spontaneous subarachnoid haemorrhage: A systematic review and meta-analysis of time trends and regional variations in population-based studies. *European Stroke Journal*, *9*(3), 555–565. DOI: 10.1177/23969873241232823 PMID: 38353205

Zimmermann, L. L., Martin, R. M., & Girgis, F. (2017, December). Treatment options for posttraumatic epilepsy. *Current Opinion in Neurology*, *30*(6), 580–586. DOI: 10.1097/WCO.0000000000000505 PMID: 29049053

Zivkovic, Z. (2004). Improved adaptive Gaussian mixture model for background subtraction. Proceedings - International Conference on Pattern Recognition, 2, 28–31. DOI: 10.1109/ICPR.2004.1333992

Zoabi, A., Redenski, I., Oren, D., Kasem, A., Zigron, A., Daoud, S., Moskovich, L., Kablan, F., & Srouji, S. (2022). 3D printing and virtual surgical planning in oral and maxillofacial surgery. *Journal of Clinical Medicine*, *11*(9), 2385. DOI: 10.3390/jcm11092385 PMID: 35566511

About the Contributors

Soobia Saeed is working as a lecturer, at Taylors University, Malaysia. Previously, she was a Director of ORIC at Sohail University formerly Jinnah Medical and Dental College (JMDC) and Assistant professor in Sohail university as well. she was leading an ethical review committee in JMDC and led many other industrial projects and pharmaceutical projects. She has an experience in pharmaceutical collaboration as well. She did Ph. D in computing engineering from Universiti Teknologi Malaysia (UTM), Malaysia. Her PhD thesis is relevant to Artificial intelligence in Healthcare. Her research interest in neurosurgery, oncology, neurosciences, and artificial intelligence encapsulating 90 impactful articles that contribute to the frontiers of knowledge in machine learning, artificial intelligence, computational neuroscience, bioinformatics and computing, and ubiquitous computing. This comprehensive body of work reflects her commitment to advancing the understanding and application of cutting-edge technologies to address contemporary challenges. The bulk of her contributions lies in machine learning, computational neurosciences, and artificial intelligence, where she has explored innovative approaches to address complex problems. These articles, published in journals indexed in the Emerging Sources Citation Index (ESCI), Science Citation Index (SCI), highlighting the clinical relevance and impact of my research in the medical domain and Institute for Scientific Information (ISI), underscoring the significance of her work in shaping the future computational neuroscience and other medical diseases solved by artificial intelligence.

Mohsin Qadeer is an Associate Professor at Agha Khan University Hospital and Medicare Cardiac and General Hospital (MGCH). He is one of the best neurosurgeons in Karachi, with a high patient satisfaction rate. He completed his MBBS and FCPS from Karachi, Pakistan. He completed his house job at Liaquat National Hospital as a house officer and resident neurosurgeon. He has an expert specialization in neurosurgery, which involves surgical treatment of neurological conditions such as peripheral nerve injury, spinal arthritis, cerebrospinal fluid leakage, brain tumors, etc. He has many publications, including national and international publications. Dr. Mohsin Qadeer has authored over 21 impactful articles. Dr. Mohsin Qadeer is associated with renowned hospitals, including Medicare Cardiac and General Hospital (MGCH), the National Medical Complex (NMC), Agha Khan Hospital University, and Ziauddin Hospital. He continued serving in different neurosurgery departments for years, treating all kinds of neurological conditions. A neurosurgeon also specializes in providing pre- and post-surgical care to patients. While working in neurosurgery, he focuses on the treatment of neurological conditions by using surgical methods. His exposure throughout the years of professional practice resulted in the enrichment of treatment skills across the vast field of neurosurgery. He has also been working on risk assessment of neurological conditions as well as their prevention and management. Based on existing conditions, he provides customized treatment plans for patients of all age groups. His expertise in advanced neurosurgery makes him one of the top certified neurosurgeons in Karachi. Currently he supervises many neurosurgeon residents in MGCH and Agha Khan University Hospital, where he contributes to research work in the neurosurgery field.

Index

Symbols

A

B

C

D

G

I

M

N

P

S

V

www.ingramcontent.com/pod-product-compliance
Lightning Source LLC
LaVergne TN
LVHW080901300926
849162LV00003B/505

* 9 7 9 8 3 3 7 3 2 8 0 7 2 *